ECG STAMPEDE

Workbook

Null Publishing
Houston, TX
ISBN 978-1-949510-30-0

Authors

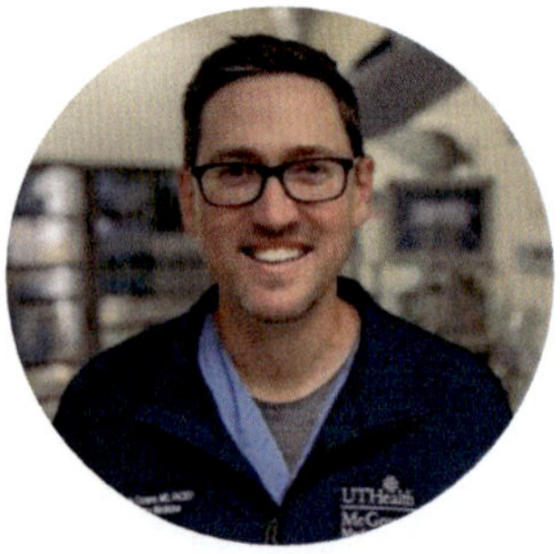

Benjamin L. Cooper, MD, MEd, FACEP

Dr. Cooper is a board-certified emergency medicine physician and associate professor at McGovern Medical School at UTHealth Houston. He serves as the assistant medical director of emergency services at Memorial Hermann Hospital in the Texas Medical Center.

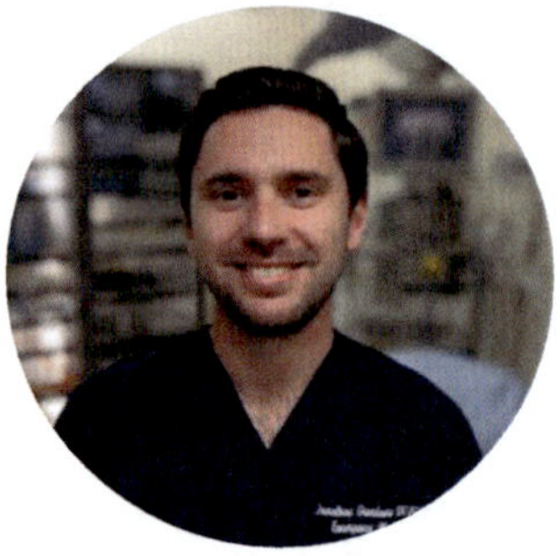

Jonathan A. Giordano, DO, MS, MEd

Dr. Giordano is a board-certified emergency medicine physician and associate professor at Columbia University, where he serves as the director of education, innovation, and research, and the medical education fellowship director.

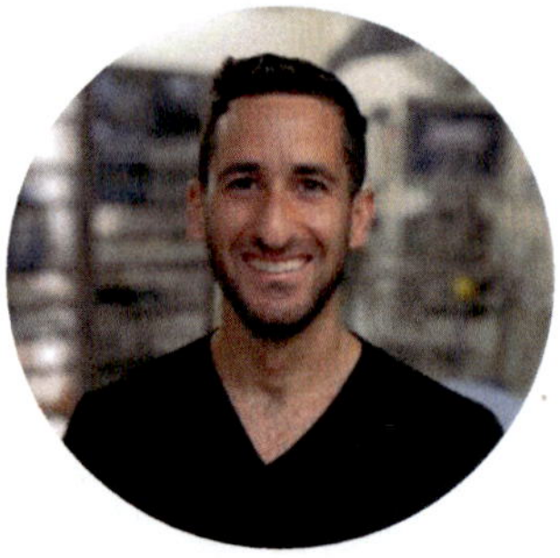

Tom T. Fadial, MD

Dr. Fadial is a board-certified emergency medicine physician in Los Angeles, CA. He is also the creator of ddxof.com, where there's an algorithm for the evaluation and management of just about every chief complaint.

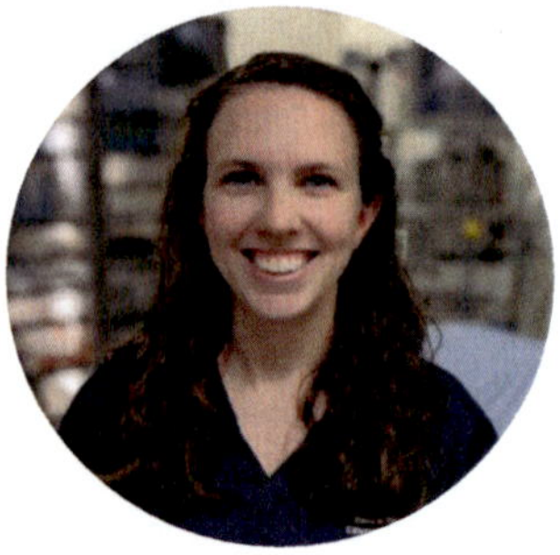

Catherine E. Reynolds, MD

Dr. Reynolds is a board-certified emergency medicine physician and assistant professor at McGovern Medical School at UTHealth Houston. She serves as the chief of service for emergency medicine at Lyndon B. Johnson General Hospital in Houston, TX.

Acknowledgements

We would like to acknowledge those that played a significant role in the development of ECG Stampede: Workbook. Thank you to Drs. Sunny Elagandhala and Brandon O'Keefe Rafaeli for their expert review. Most of all, thank you to the countless UTHealth Houston emergency medicine residents that lent their time and minds to vetting every single case over five years to bring you, the reader, the best electrocardiographic learning experience on the planet.

Dedicated to Ali.

May our hearts beat in synchrony.

Preface

These cases were submitted, vetted, and carefully selected over the course of five years through a weekly emergency medicine conference at UTHealth Houston. The outcomes for every case are known and the diagnoses were all confirmed. Each ECG in this text came from a real patient with a real medical condition deserving attention. It is the greatest honor of my life to have taken care of many of them in their time of need, and to translate meaningful knowledge about their condition so that you, the reader, may be better prepared to care for your next patient.

The workbook is intentionally case-based, and it is divided into two sections – The Cases, and The Explanations. Each case starts with a brief prompt of the patient's age, sex, and presenting complaint, and is followed by five items – rate, rhythm, axis, intervals, signs of ischemia. The five items following each case are there to remind you to use a systematic approach when interpreting each ECG. It is our belief that, if you do so, you will be able to diagnose every critical condition that an electrocardiogram can reveal. Practice is the best way to learn electrocardiography, and errors are essential to learning. May this book serve as a safe place for you to make errors and learn.

I tried my best to cover every critical diagnosis in each ECG; however, it's entirely possible that I missed some. If you discover an explanation that was confusing or a diagnosis that was not covered, please reach out to me. I am committed to making this text authoritative and accurate.

This book is best consumed once you have a foundational knowledge of electrocardiography. Please consider completing the ECG Stampede curriculum prior to using this book. The ECG Stampede curriculum can be purchased in book form on Amazon or can be completed online with video companions and practice guides at **ecgstampede.com**. If you're interested in practicing your skills on the fly, the website has a free, fun, interactive, gamified experience in ECG triage. There's also an ECG Stampede application that can be downloaded in the Apple and Google Play stores.

Thank you for your purchase of this book. Nearly all funds gained from these proceeds go right back into making ECG Stampede your one-stop shop for electrocardiographic education.

Ben
ben@ecgstampede.com

Table of Contents

The Cases

#1 – 63-year-old female presents with weakness

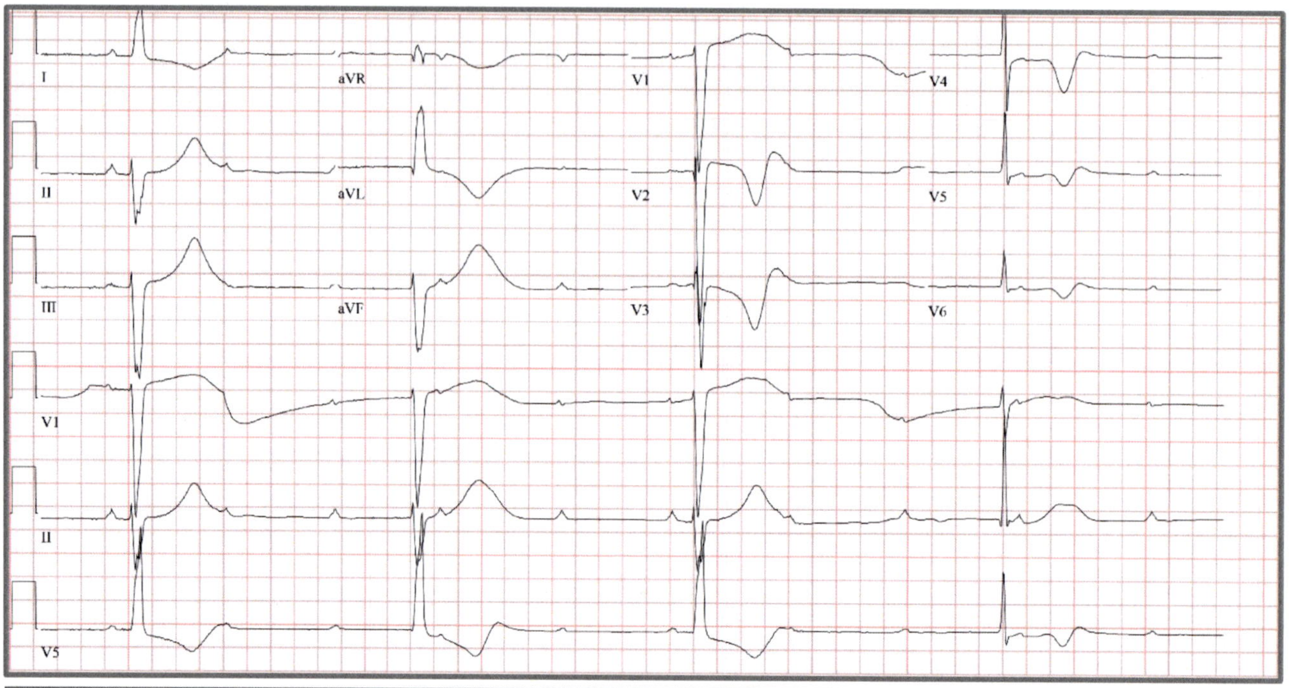

Rate: Rhythm: Axis: Intervals: Ischemia:

#2 – 57-year-old male presents with chest pain

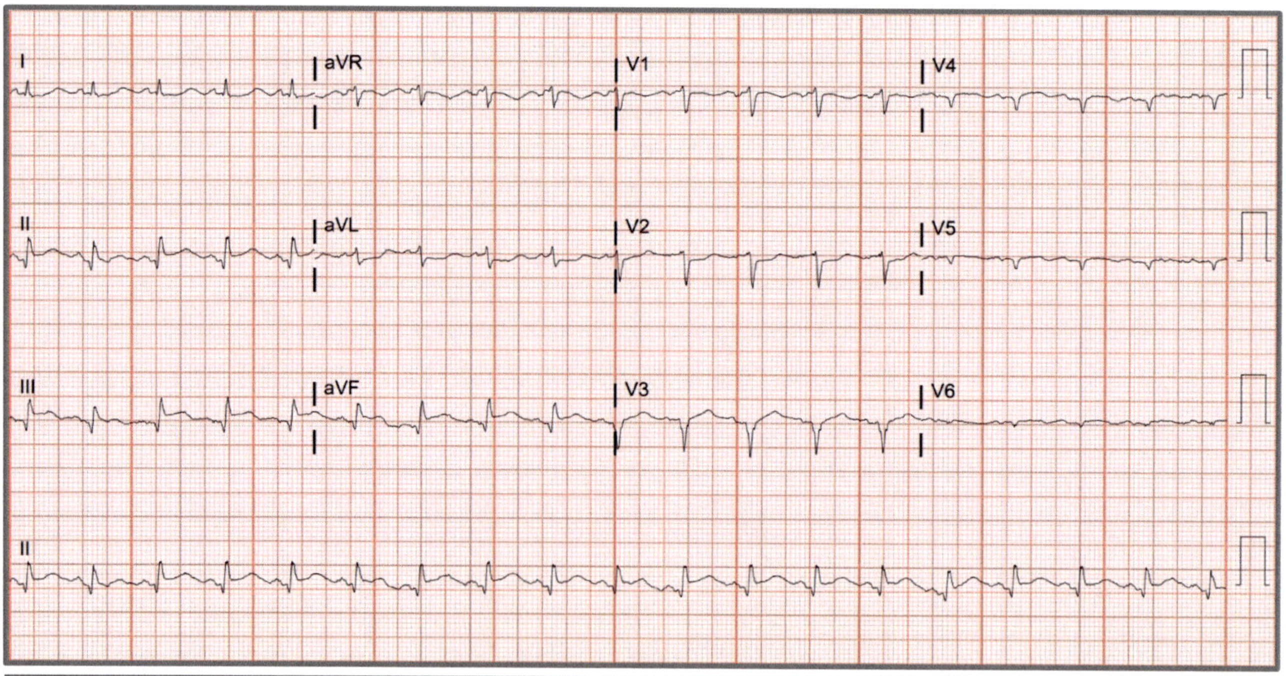

Rate: Rhythm: Axis: Intervals: Ischemia:

#3 – 63-year-old male presents with lower back pain

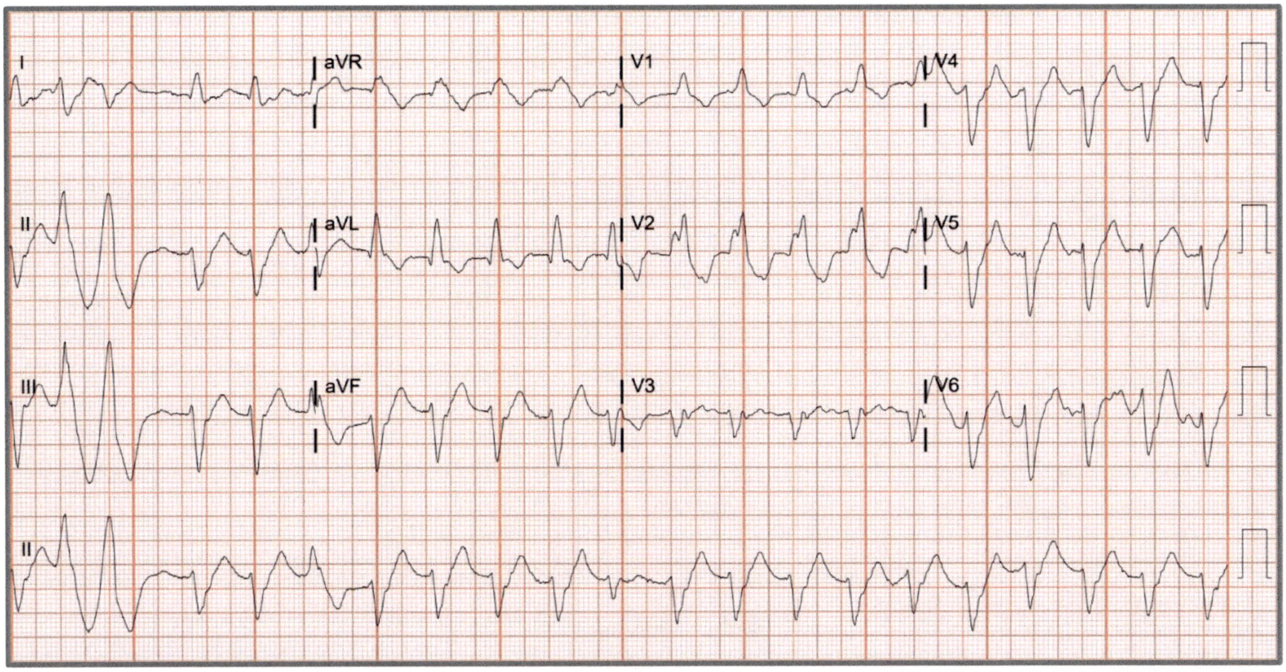

Rate:	Rhythm:	Axis:	Intervals:	Ischemia:

⇩ **Prior ECG** ⇩

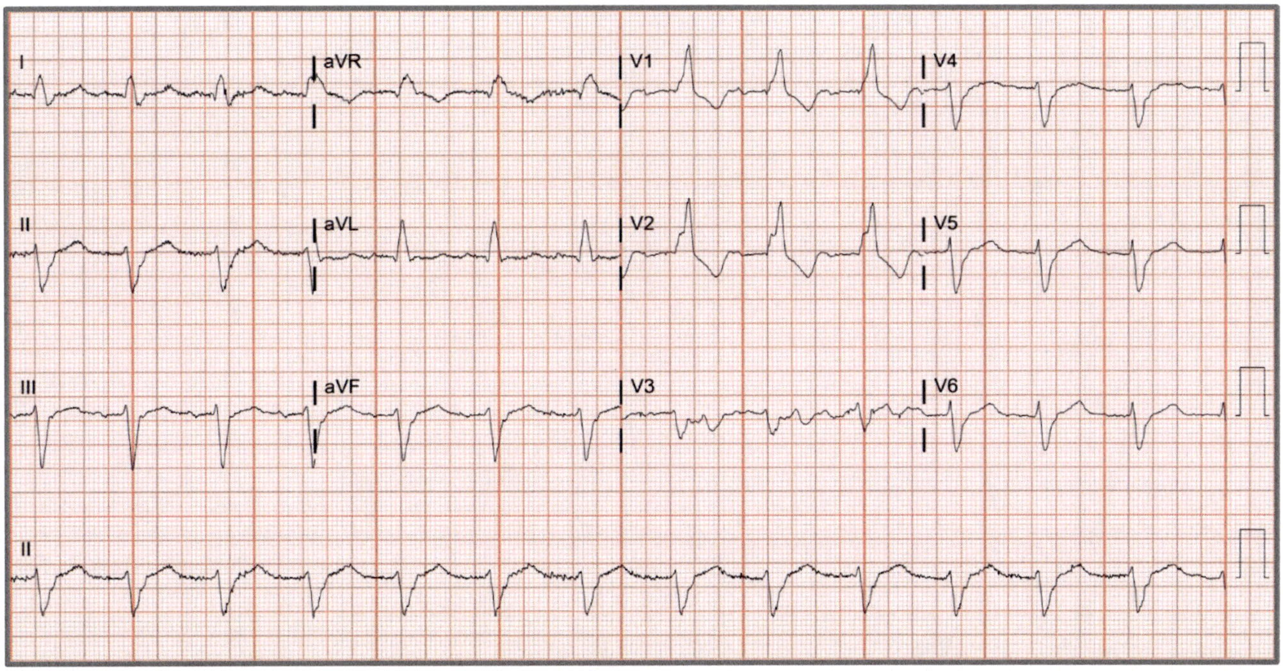

Rate:	Rhythm:	Axis:	Intervals:	Ischemia:

#4 – 94-year-old male presents with dyspnea

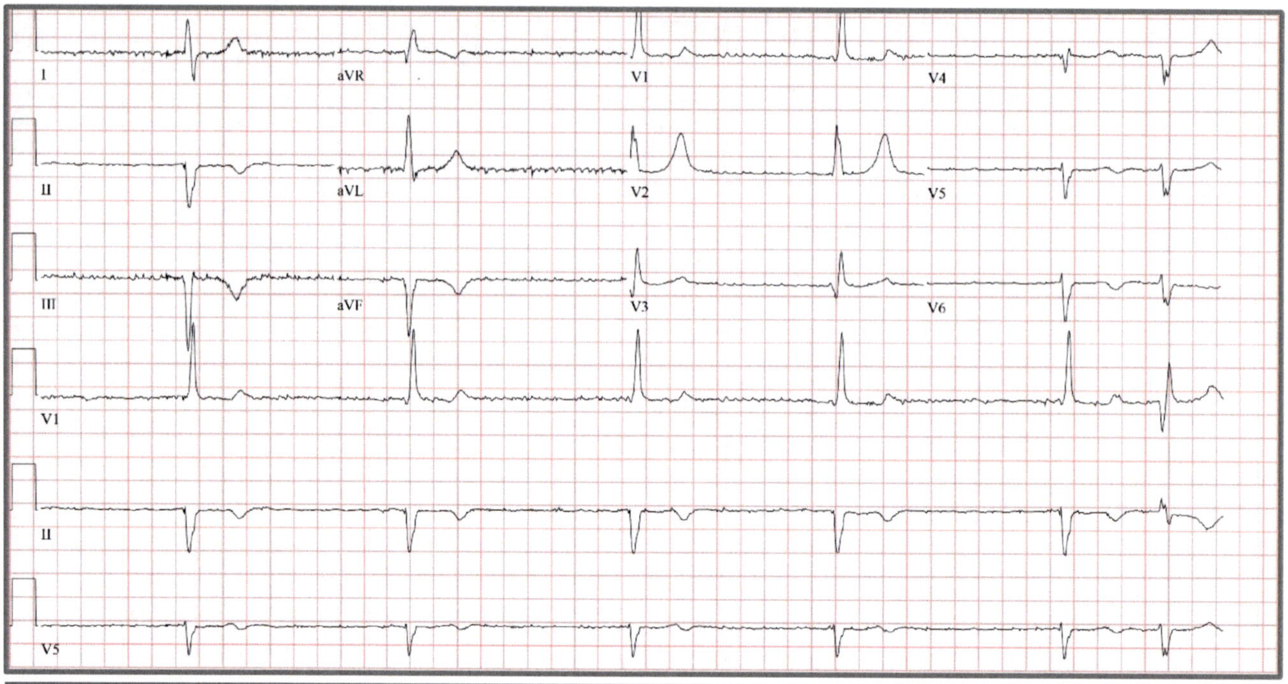

Rate: Rhythm: Axis: Intervals: Ischemia:

#5 – 72-year-old female presents with typical chest pain

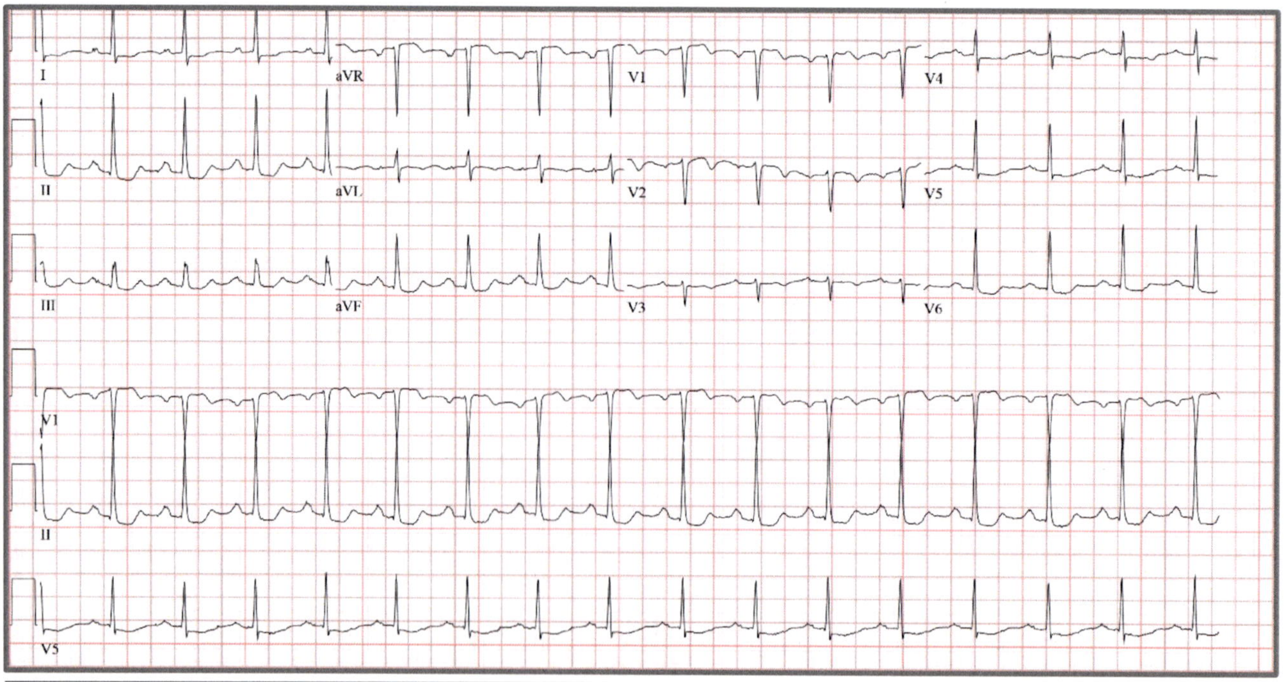

Rate: Rhythm: Axis: Intervals: Ischemia:

#6 – 58-year-old male presents with palpitations for 12 hours

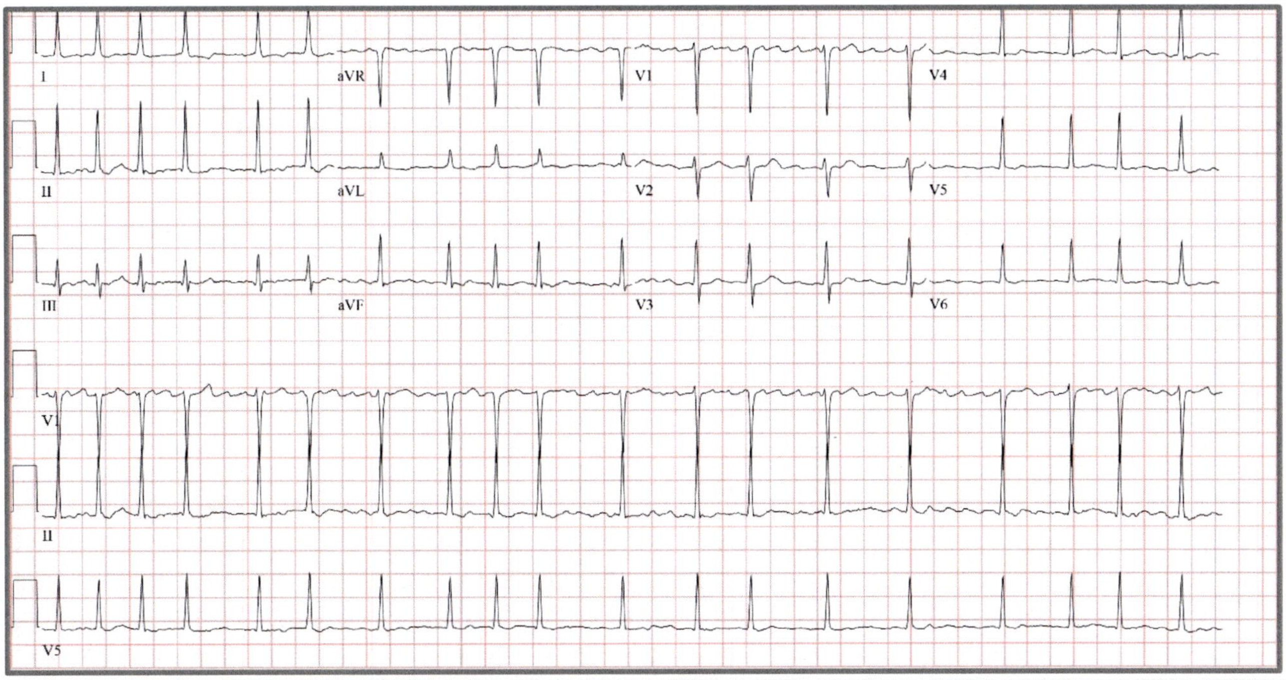

Rate:		Rhythm:		Axis:		Intervals:		Ischemia:	

#7 – 71-year-old male presents with altered mental status

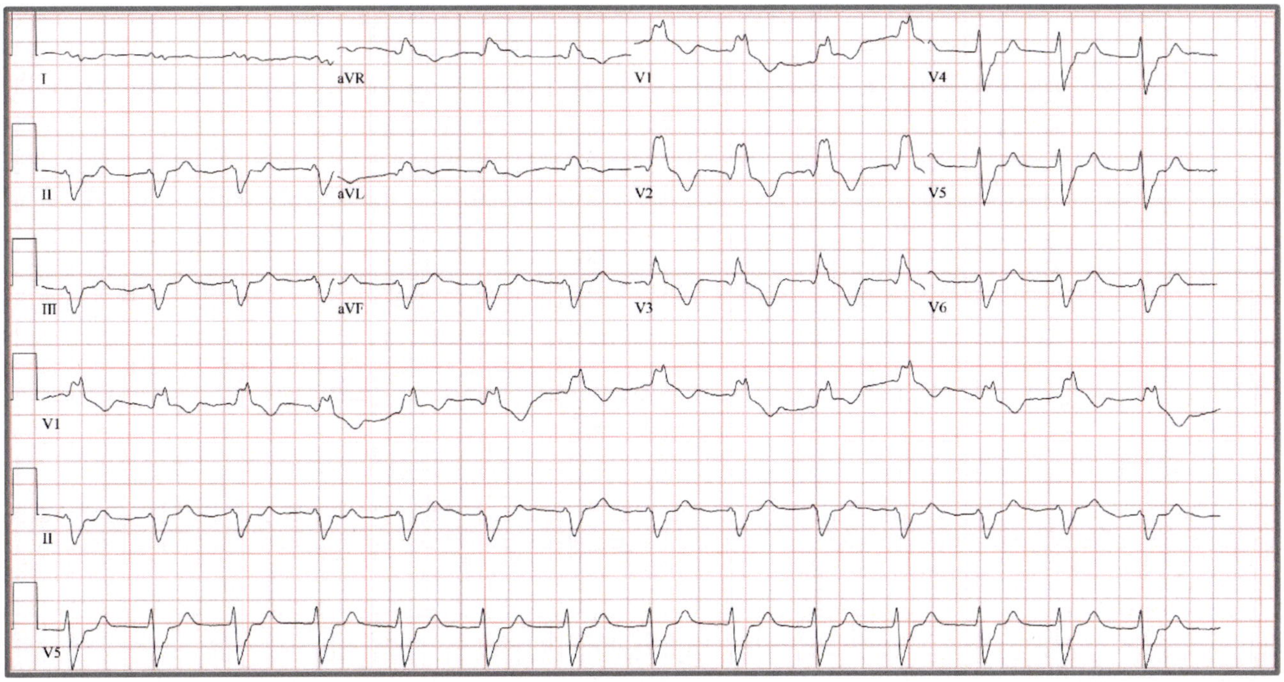

Rate:		Rhythm:		Axis:		Intervals:		Ischemia:	

#8 – 60-year-old male presents with defibrillator firing

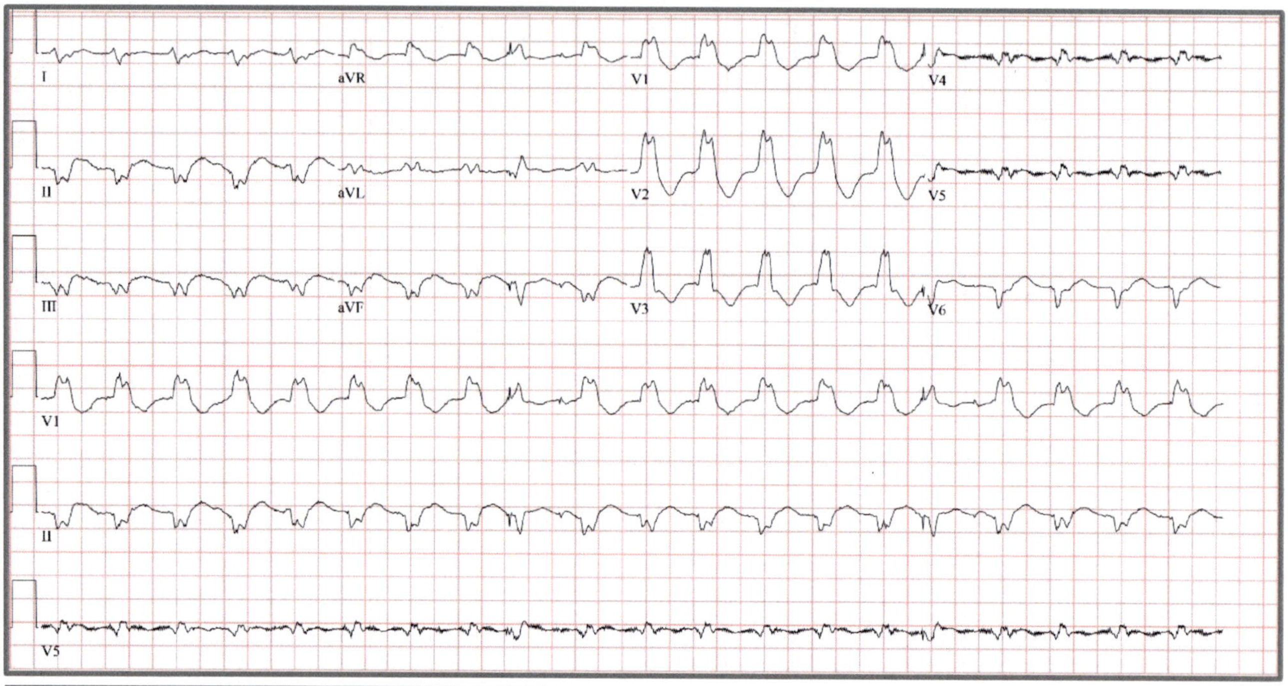

Rate: Rhythm: Axis: Intervals: Ischemia:

#9 – 49-year-old female presents with weakness

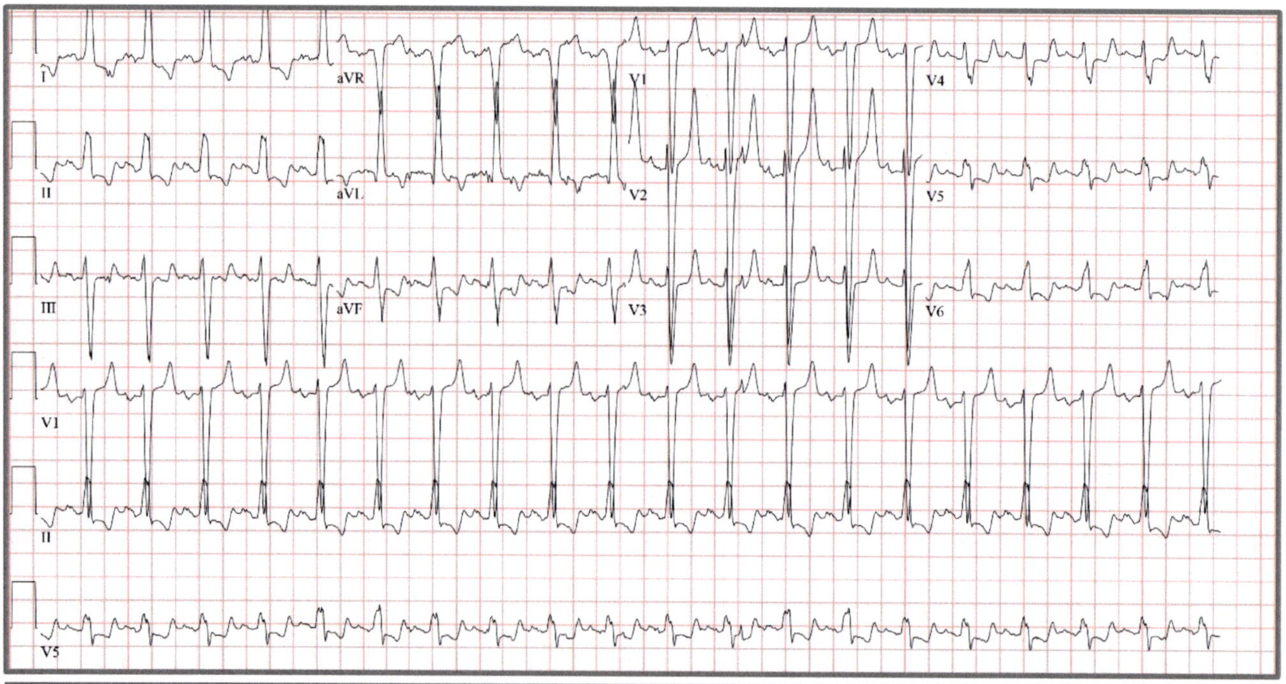

Rate: Rhythm: Axis: Intervals: Ischemia:

#10 – 19-year-old male presents with pleuritic chest pain

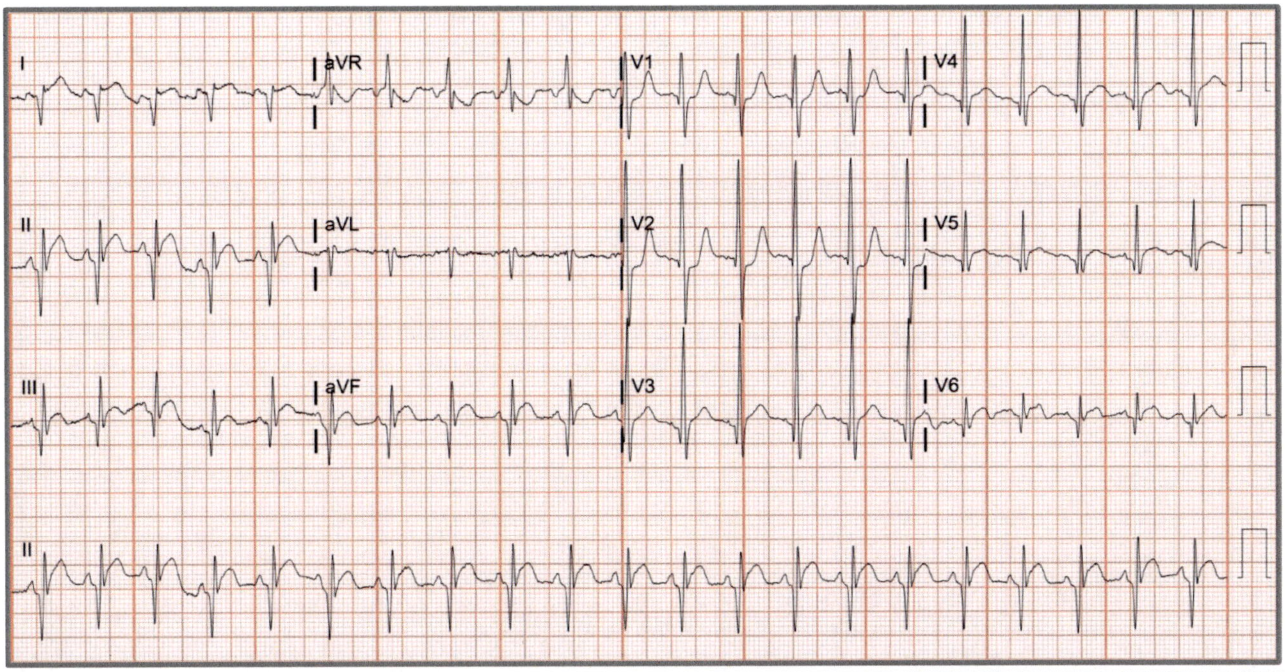

Rate: Rhythm: Axis: Intervals: Ischemia:

#11 – 63-year-old male presents with dizziness

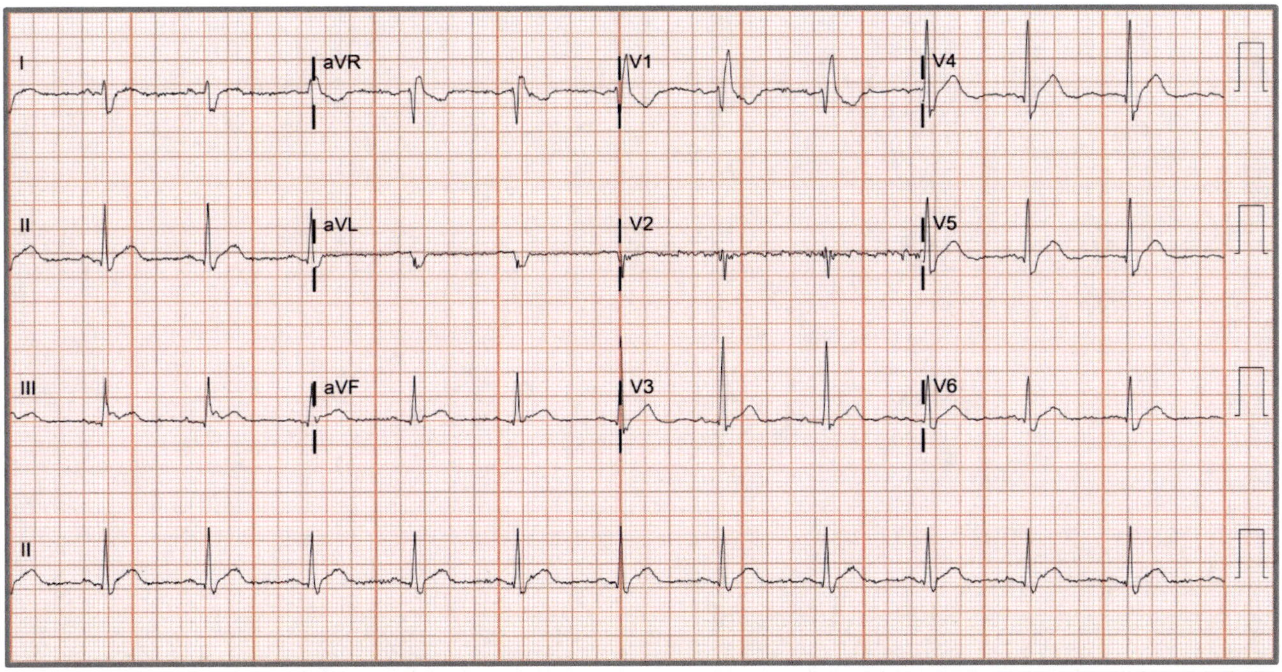

Rate: Rhythm: Axis: Intervals: Ischemia:

#12 – 67-year-old male presents with chest pain

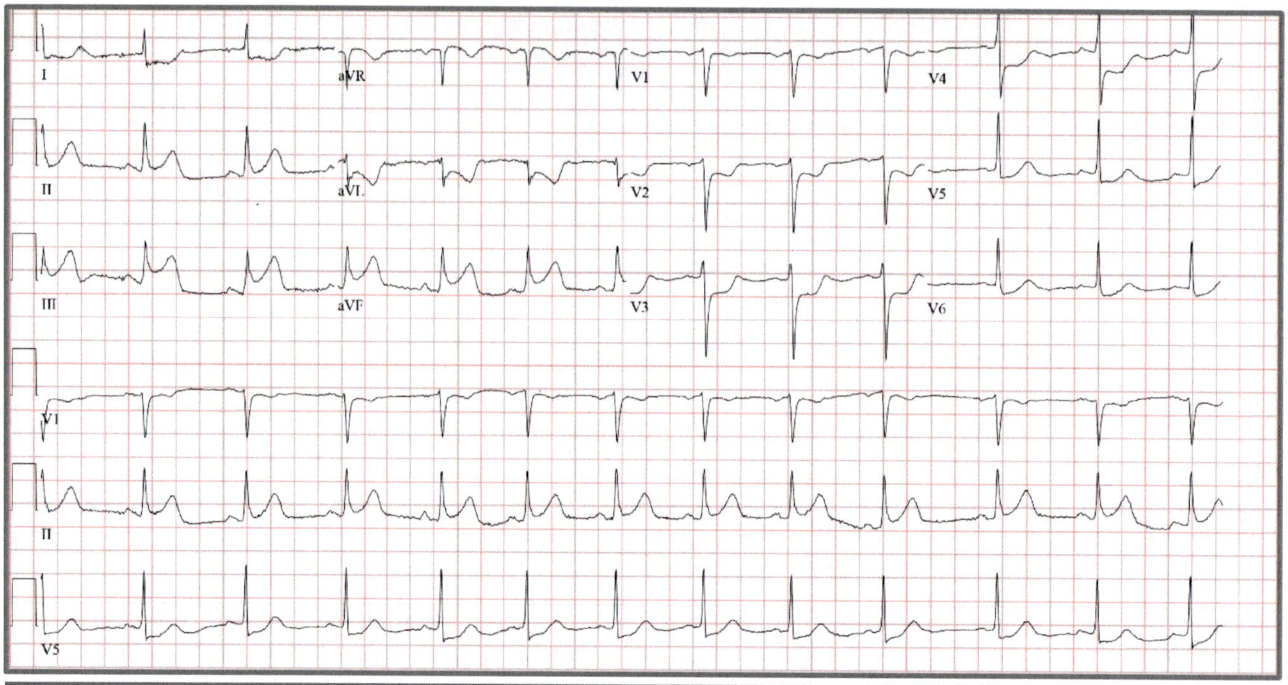

Rate: **Rhythm:** **Axis:** **Intervals:** **Ischemia:**

#13 – 31-year-old male presents with weakness

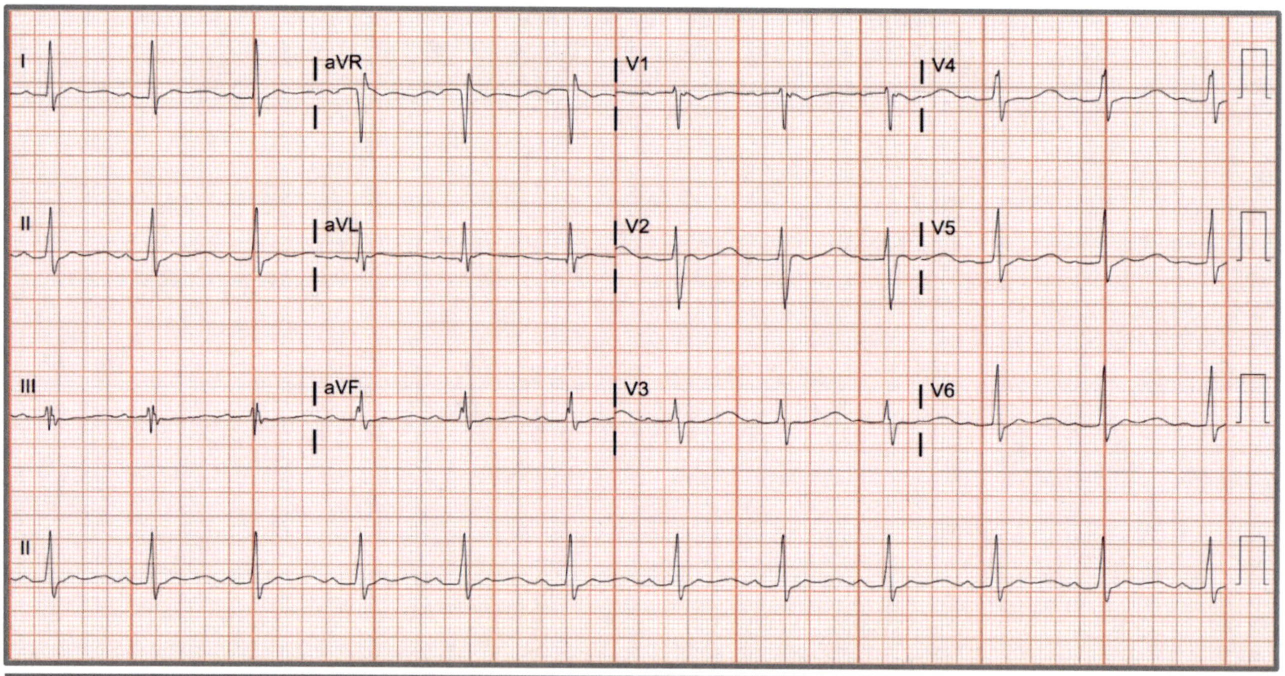

Rate: **Rhythm:** **Axis:** **Intervals:** **Ischemia:**

#14 – 81-year-old female presents with dizziness

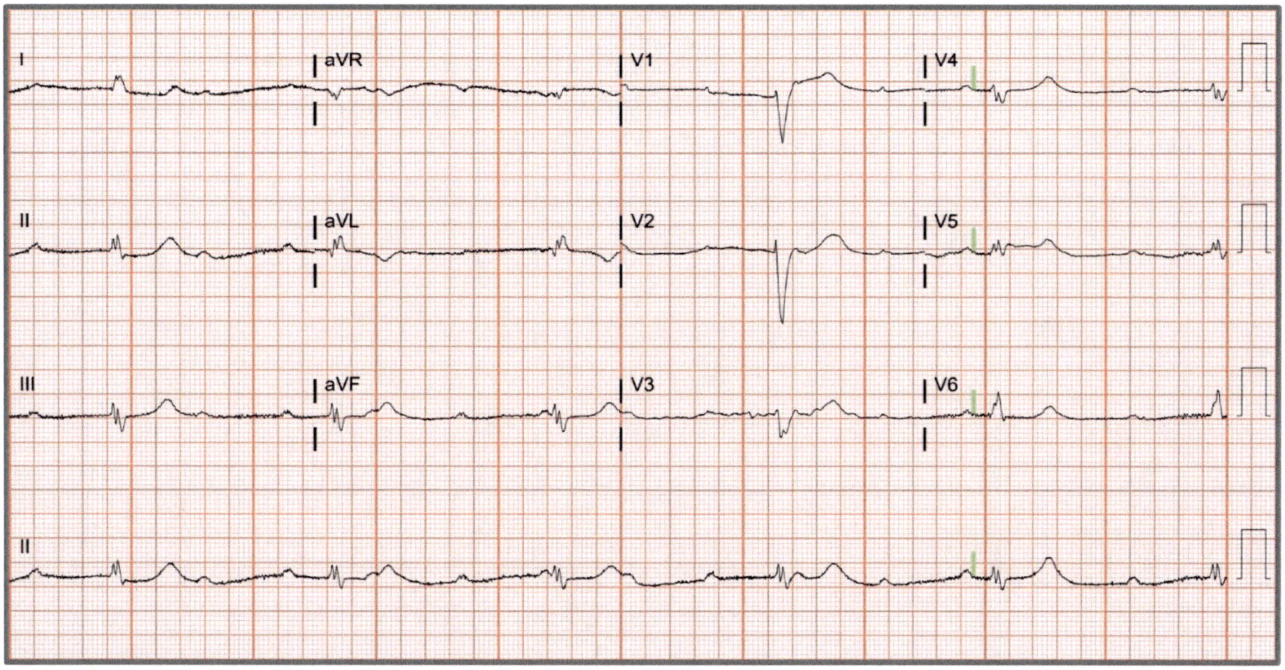

Rate:		Rhythm:		Axis:		Intervals:		Ischemia:	

#15 – 50-year-old male presents with chest pain

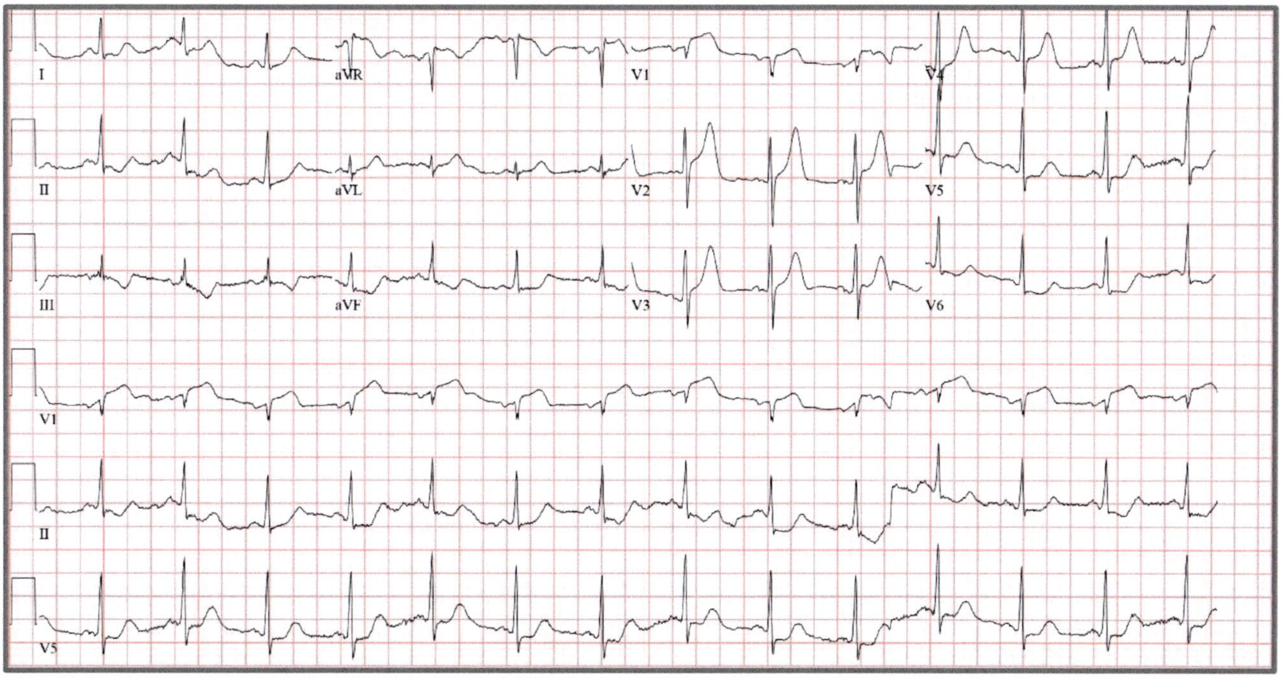

Rate:		Rhythm:		Axis:		Intervals:		Ischemia:	

#16 – 40-year-old female presents with palpitations

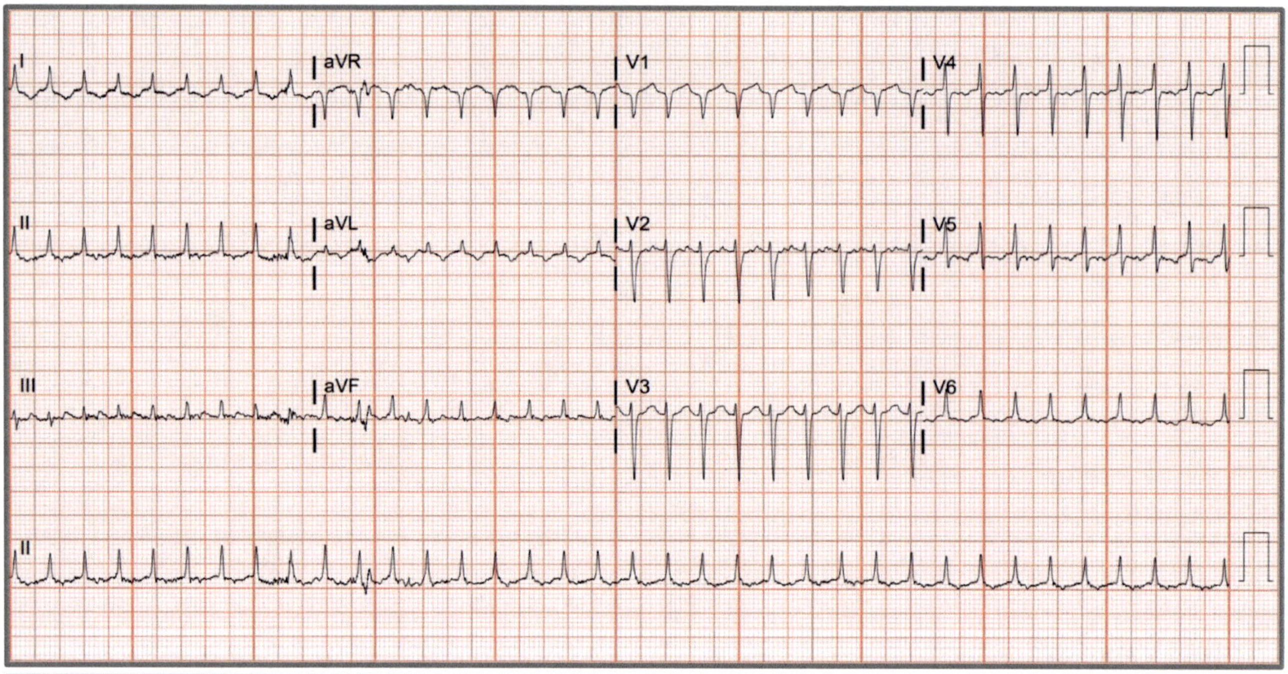

Rate: Rhythm: Axis: Intervals: Ischemia:

⇩ Post-conversion ECG ⇩

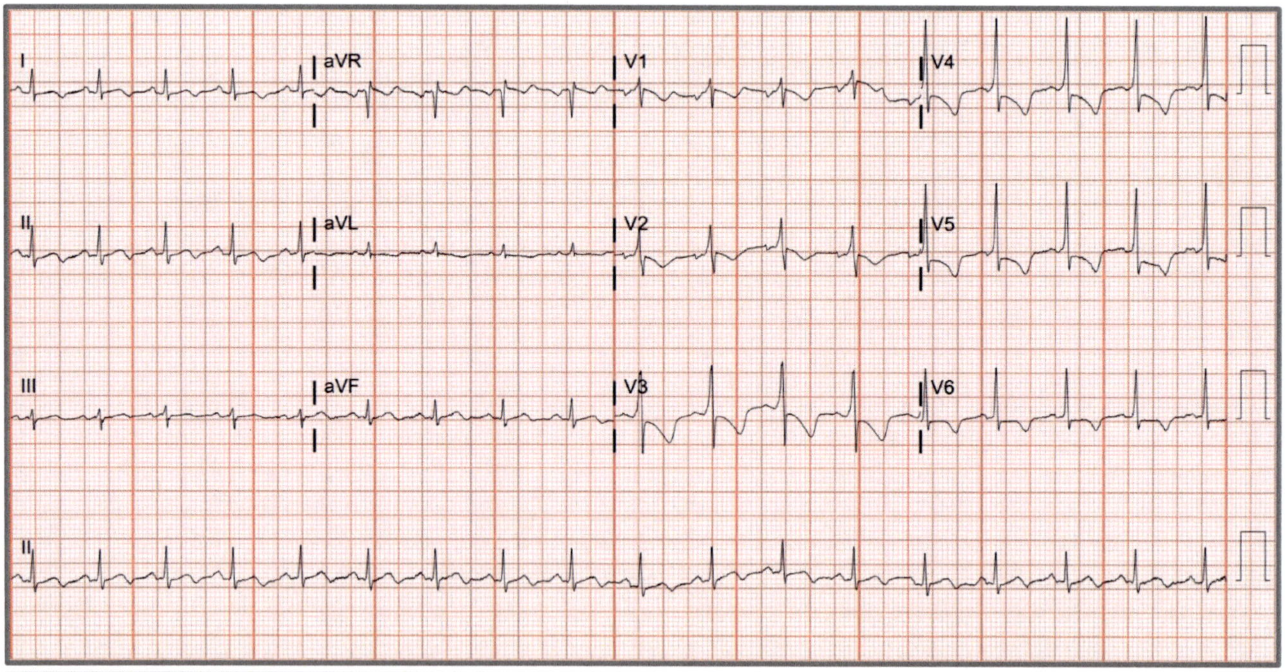

Rate: Rhythm: Axis: Intervals: Ischemia:

#17 – 69-year-old female presents with post-op infection

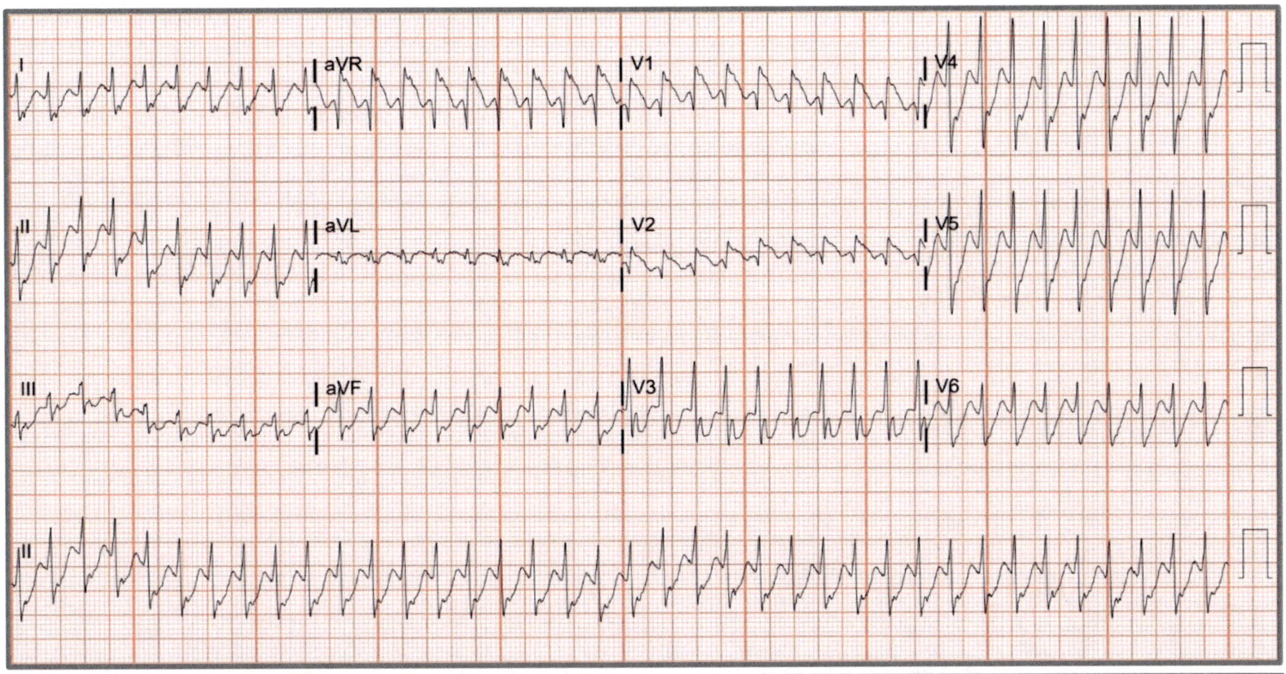

Rate: Rhythm: Axis: Intervals: Ischemia:

#18 – 61-year-old female presents with inactive chest pain

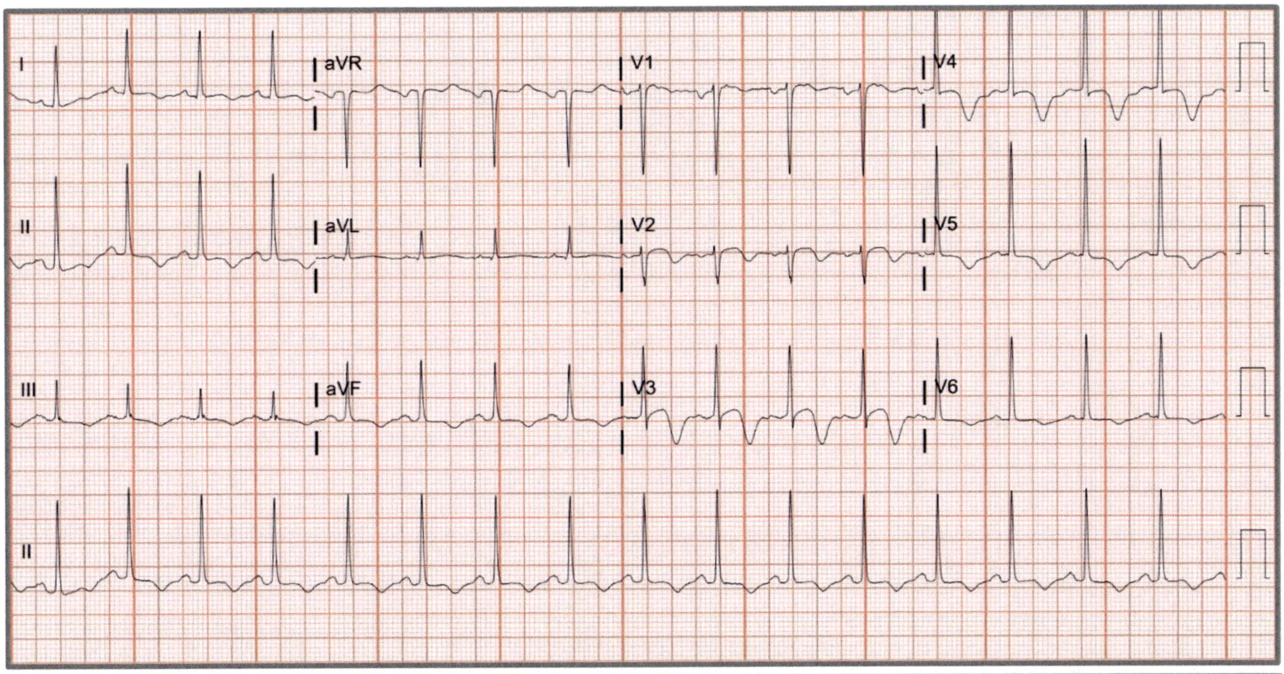

Rate: Rhythm: Axis: Intervals: Ischemia:

#19 – 83-year-old female presents with palpitations

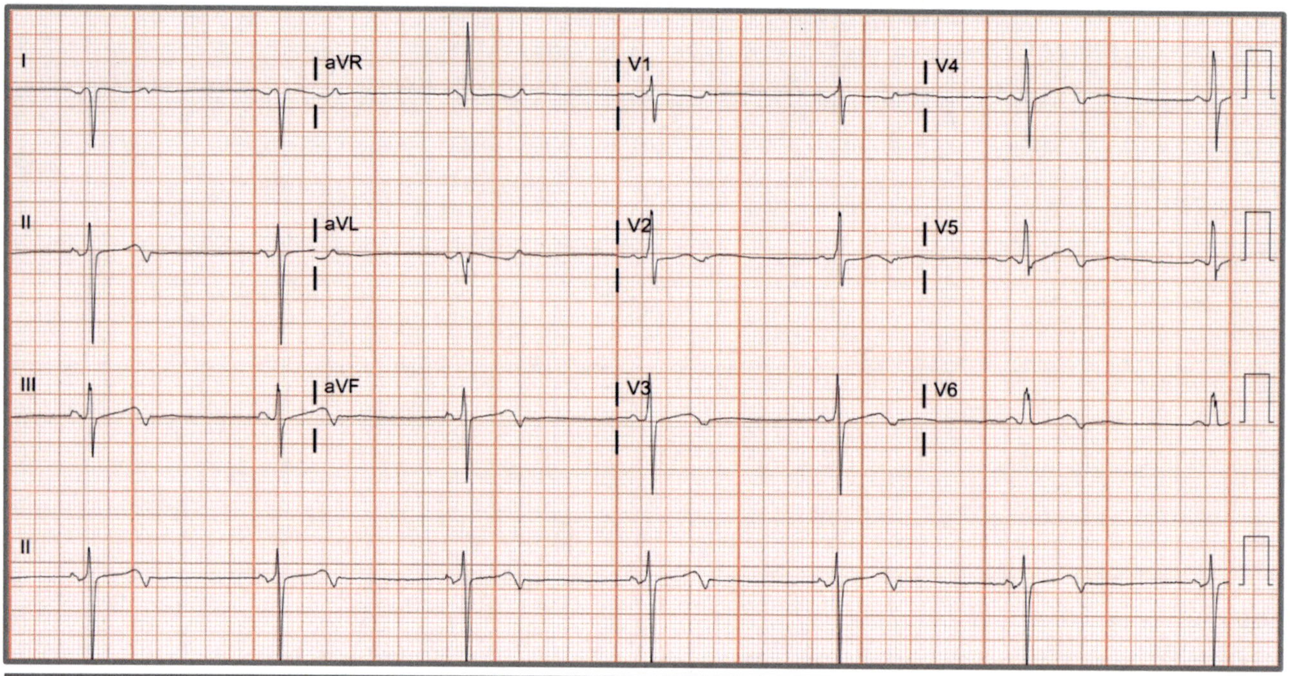

Rate:	Rhythm:	Axis:	Intervals:	Ischemia:

⇩ Repeat ECG ⇩

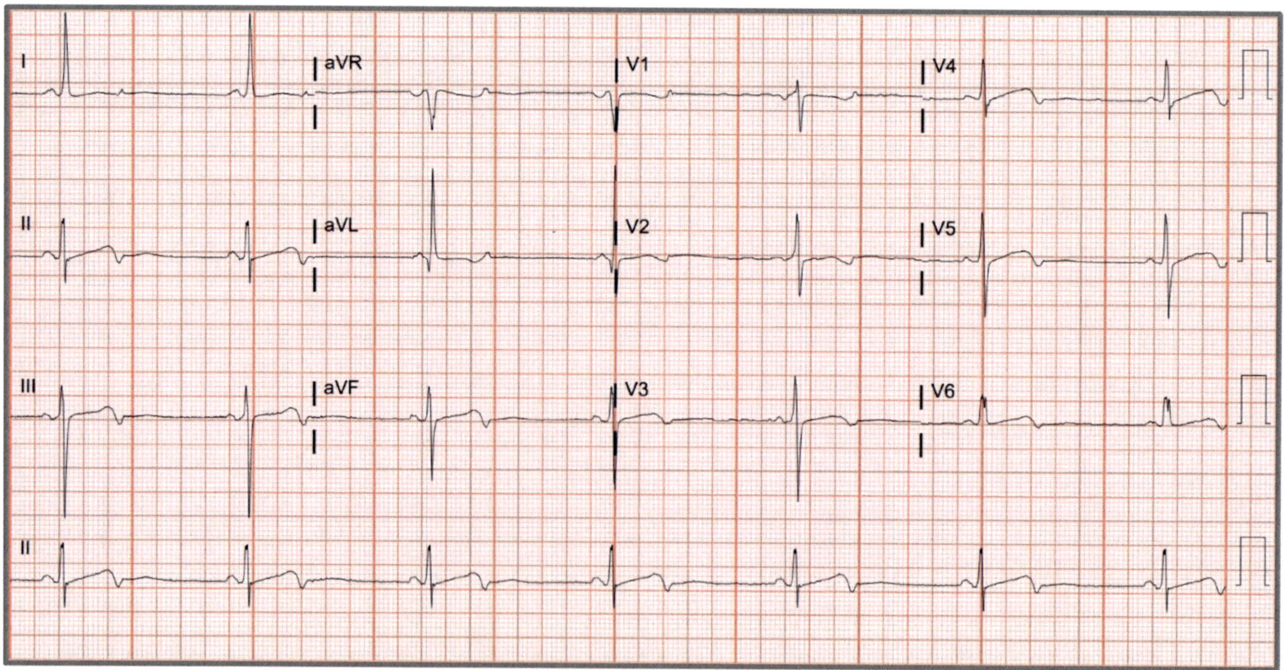

Rate:	Rhythm:	Axis:	Intervals:	Ischemia:

#20 – 67-year-old male presents with syncope

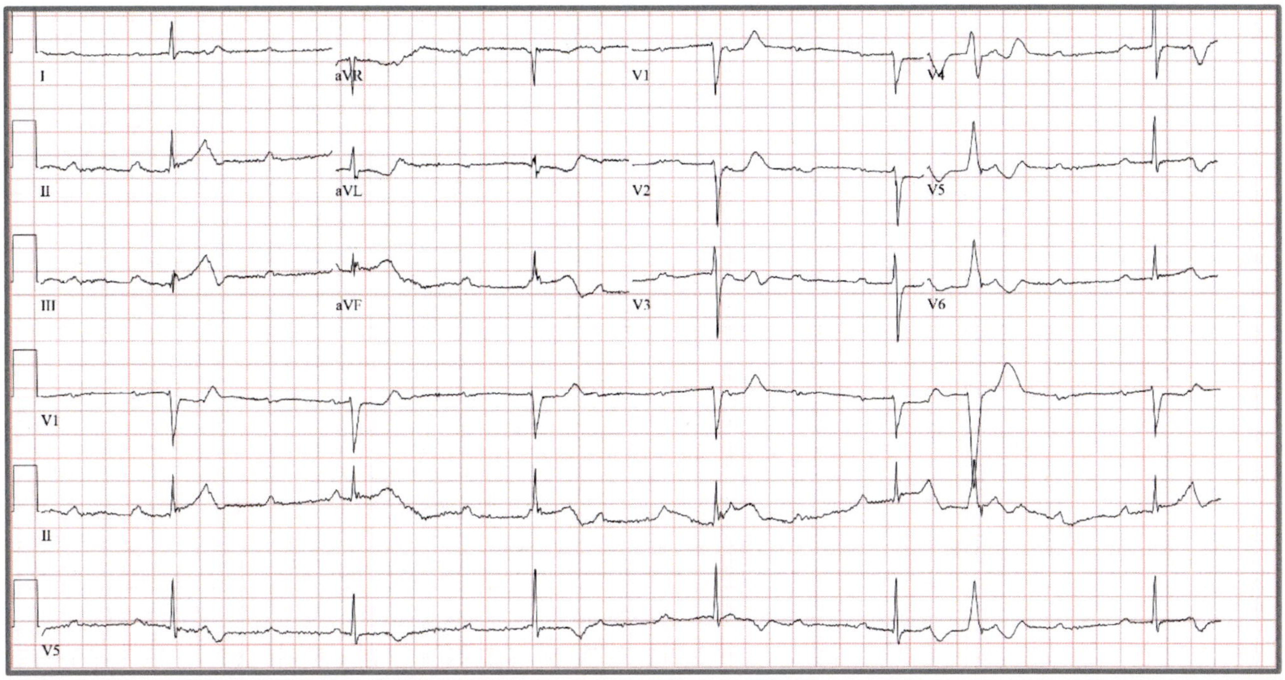

Rate:	Rhythm:	Axis:	Intervals:	Ischemia:

#21 – 62-year-old male presents with dyspnea

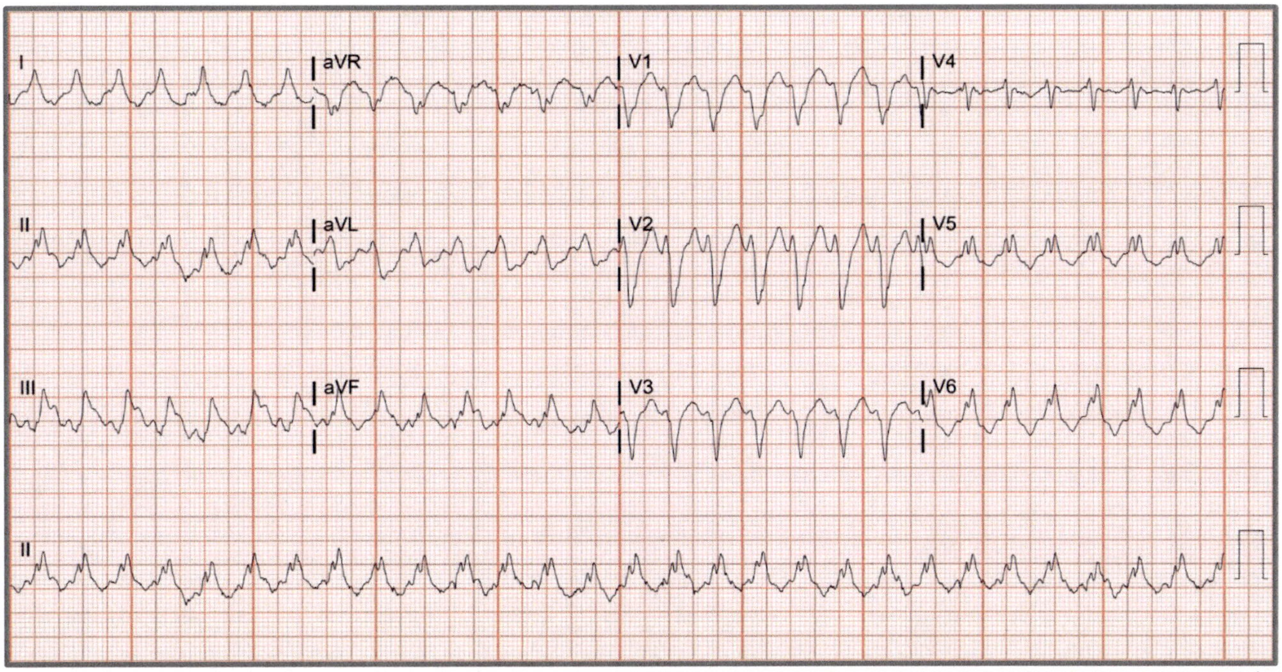

Rate:	Rhythm:	Axis:	Intervals:	Ischemia:

#22 – 73-year-old male presents with palpitations

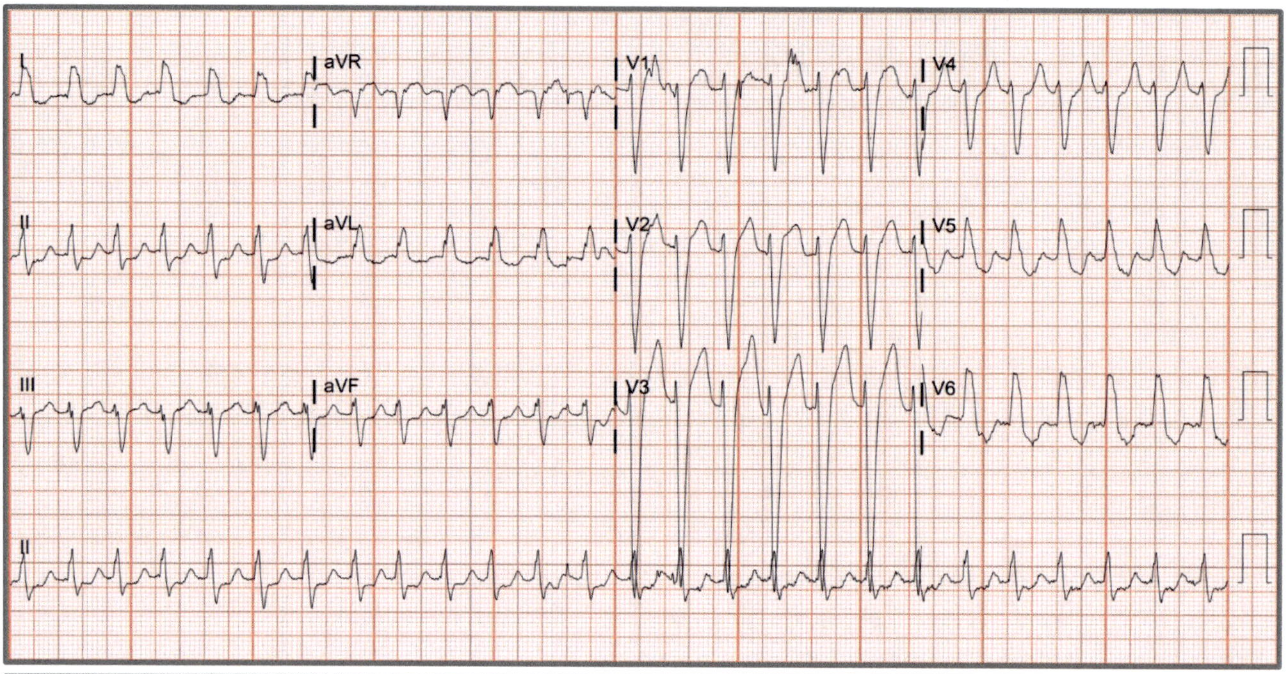

Rate: **Rhythm:** **Axis:** **Intervals:** **Ischemia:**

⇩ Prior ECG ⇩

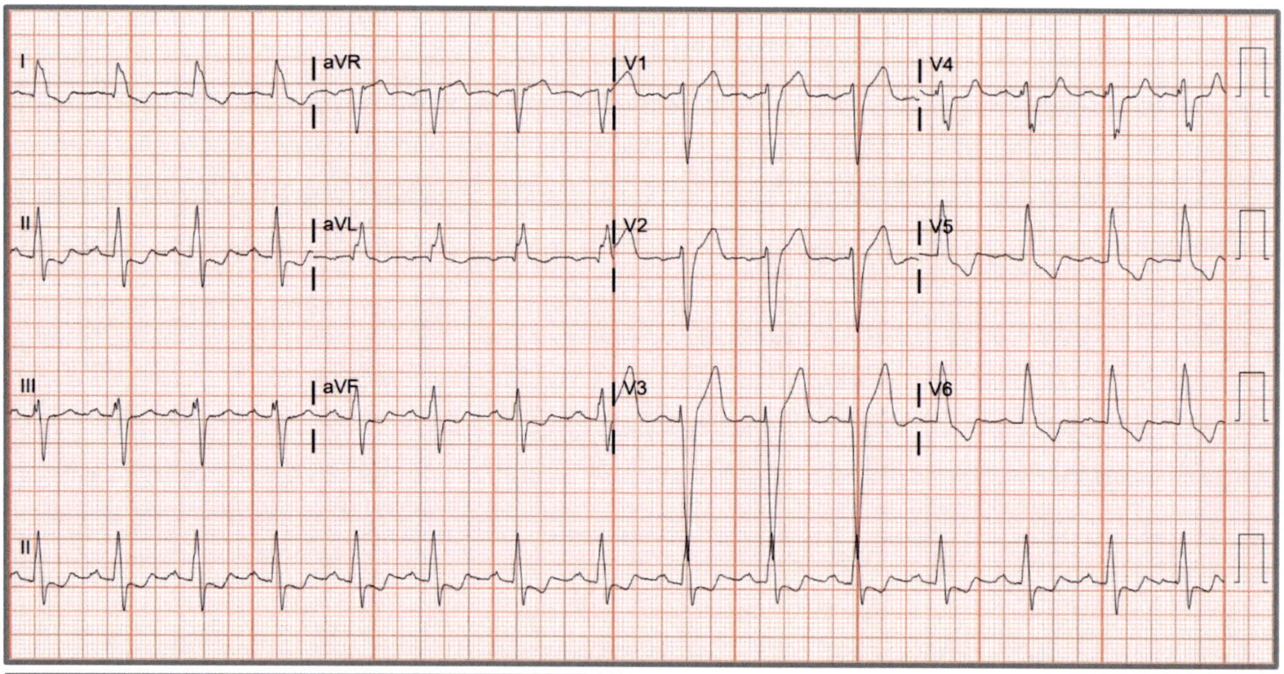

Rate: **Rhythm:** **Axis:** **Intervals:** **Ischemia:**

#23 – 47-year-old male presents with chest pain

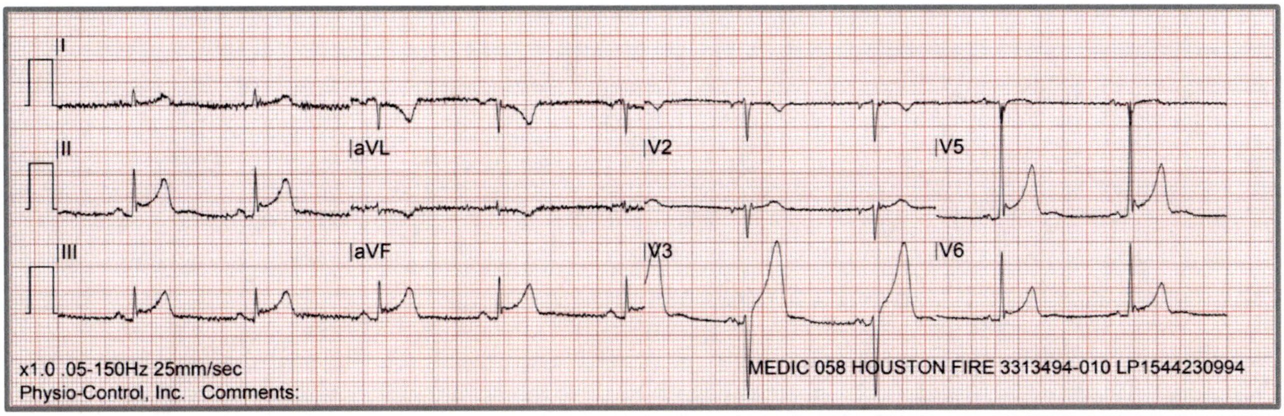

Rate:		Rhythm:		Axis:		Intervals:		Ischemia:	

#24 – 82-year-old female presents with episodic syncope

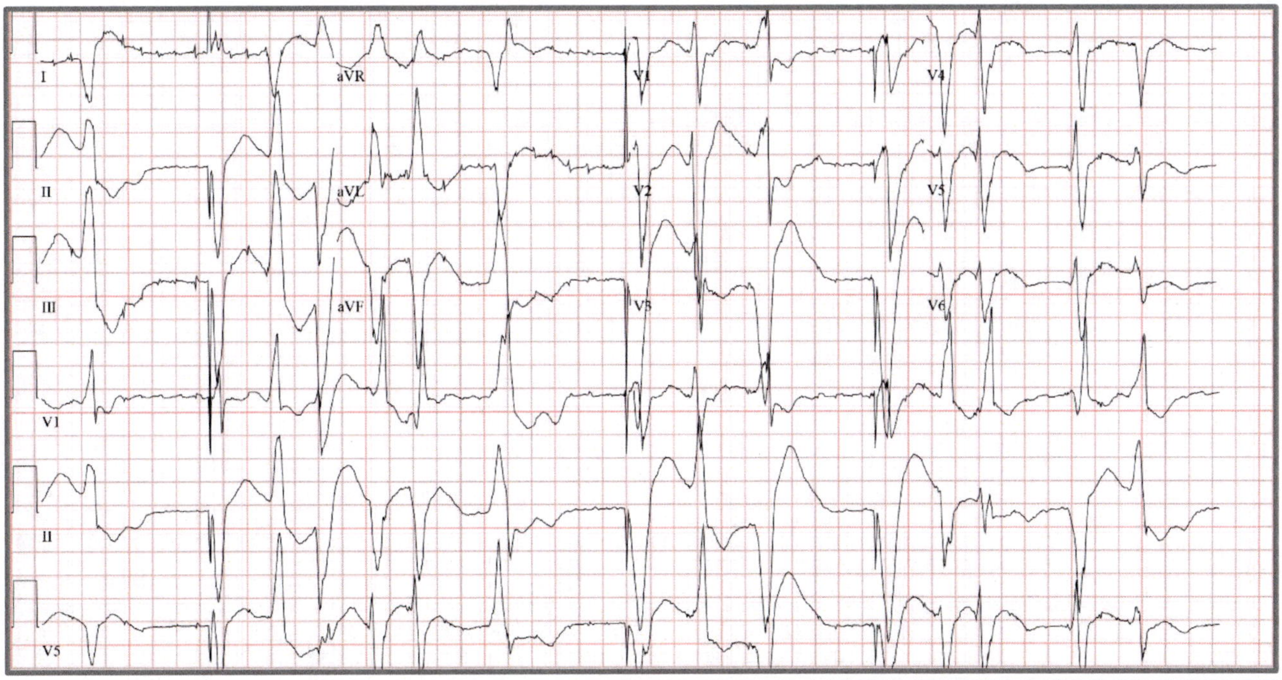

Rate:		Rhythm:		Axis:		Intervals:		Ischemia:	

#25 – 59-year-old male presents status post arrest

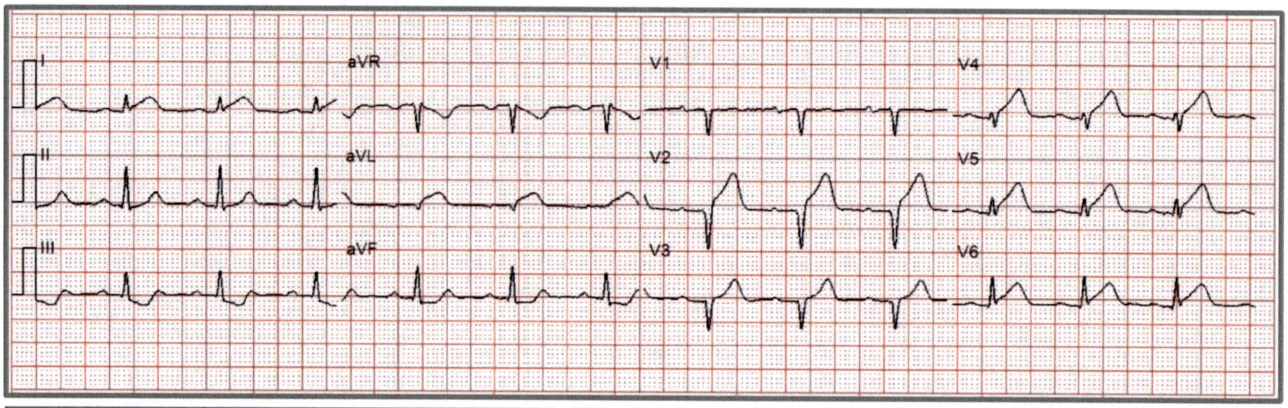

Rate: **Rhythm:** **Axis:** **Intervals:** **Ischemia:**

#26 – 79-year-old female presents with syncope

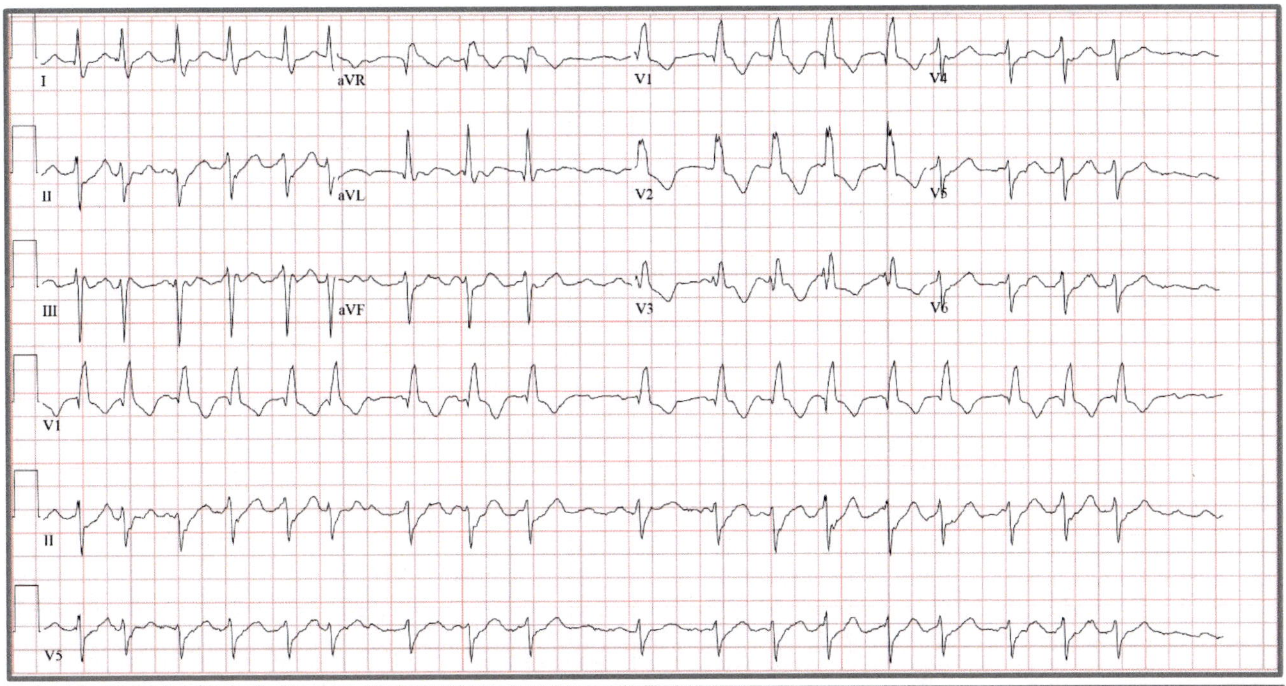

Rate:		Rhythm:		Axis:		Intervals:		Ischemia:	

⇩ Post-conversion ECG ⇩

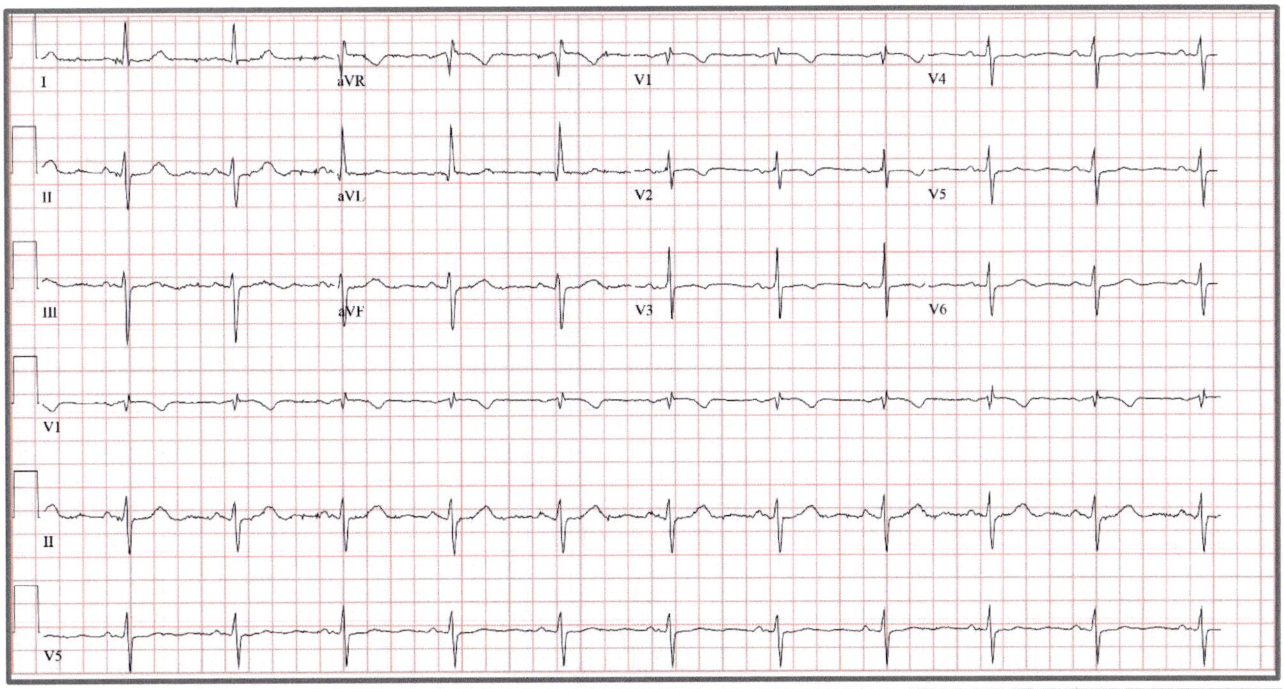

Rate:		Rhythm:		Axis:		Intervals:		Ischemia:	

#27 – 67-year-old female presents with syncope

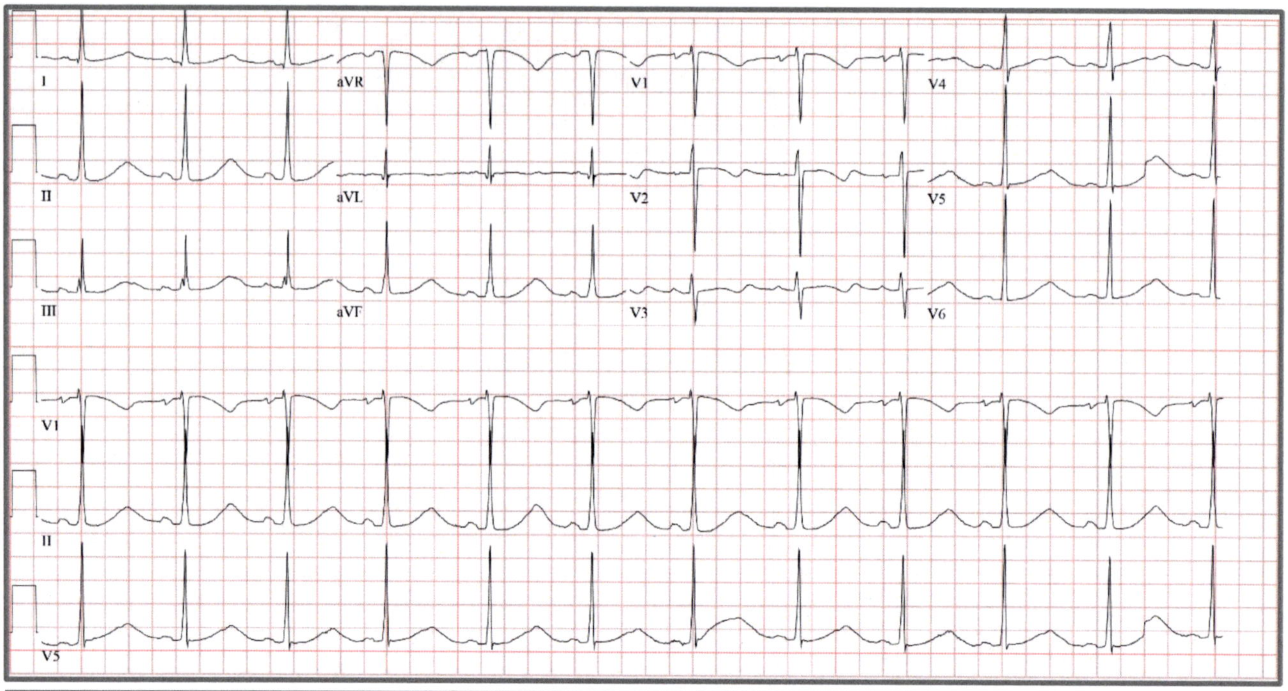

Rate: **Rhythm:** **Axis:** **Intervals:** **Ischemia:**

#28 – 89-year-old male presents with dyspnea

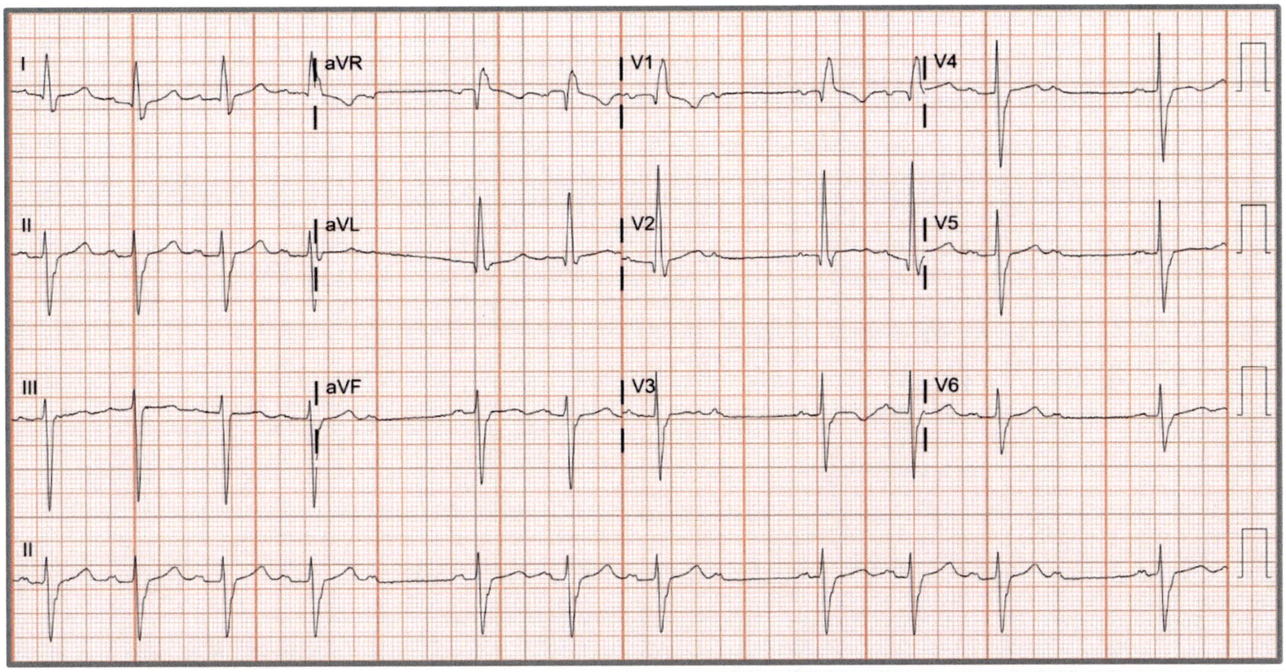

Rate: **Rhythm:** **Axis:** **Intervals:** **Ischemia:**

⇩ Repeat ECG ⇩

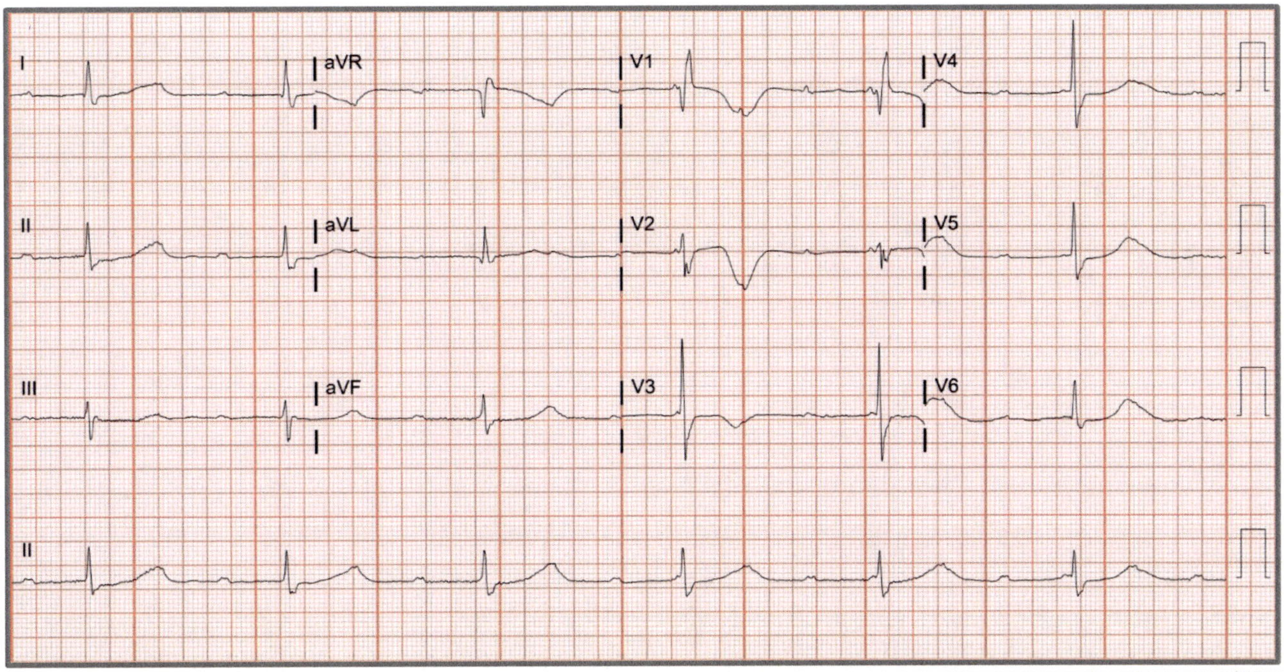

Rate: **Rhythm:** **Axis:** **Intervals:** **Ischemia:**

#29 – 52-year-old male presents with palpitations

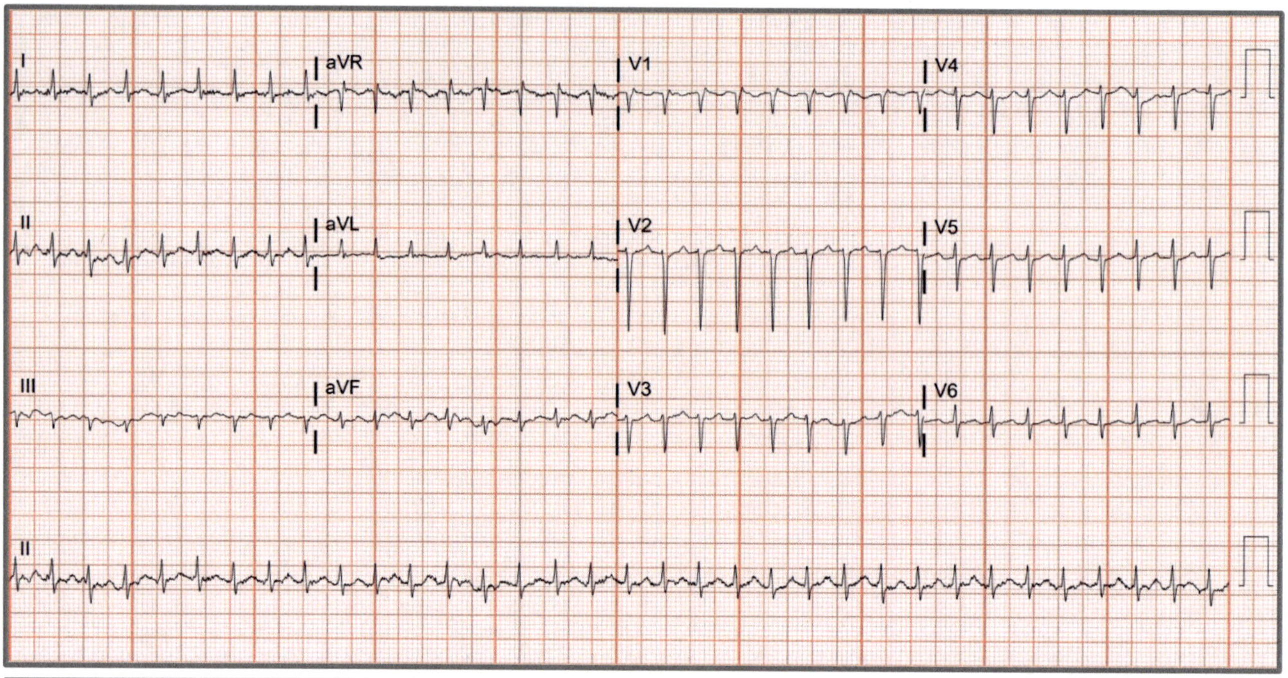

Rate: **Rhythm:** **Axis:** **Intervals:** **Ischemia:**

#30 – 46-year-old male presents with ICD firing

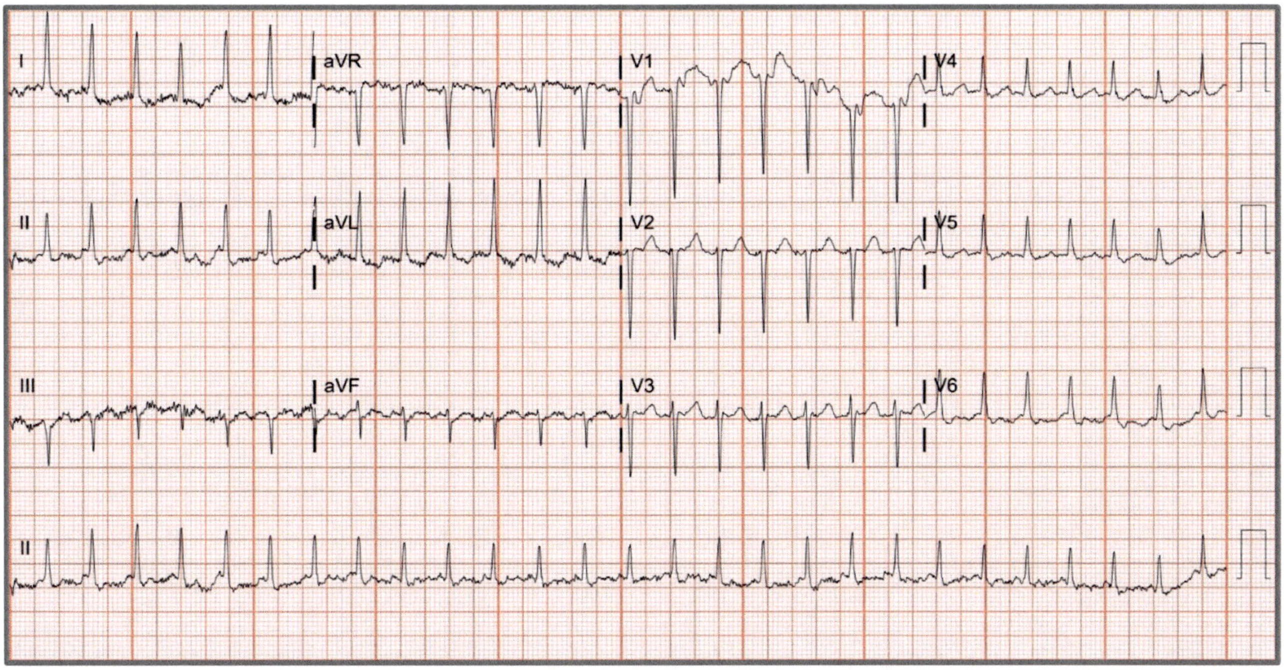

Rate: Rhythm: Axis: Intervals: Ischemia:

⇩ Repeat ECG with Lewis Lead ⇩

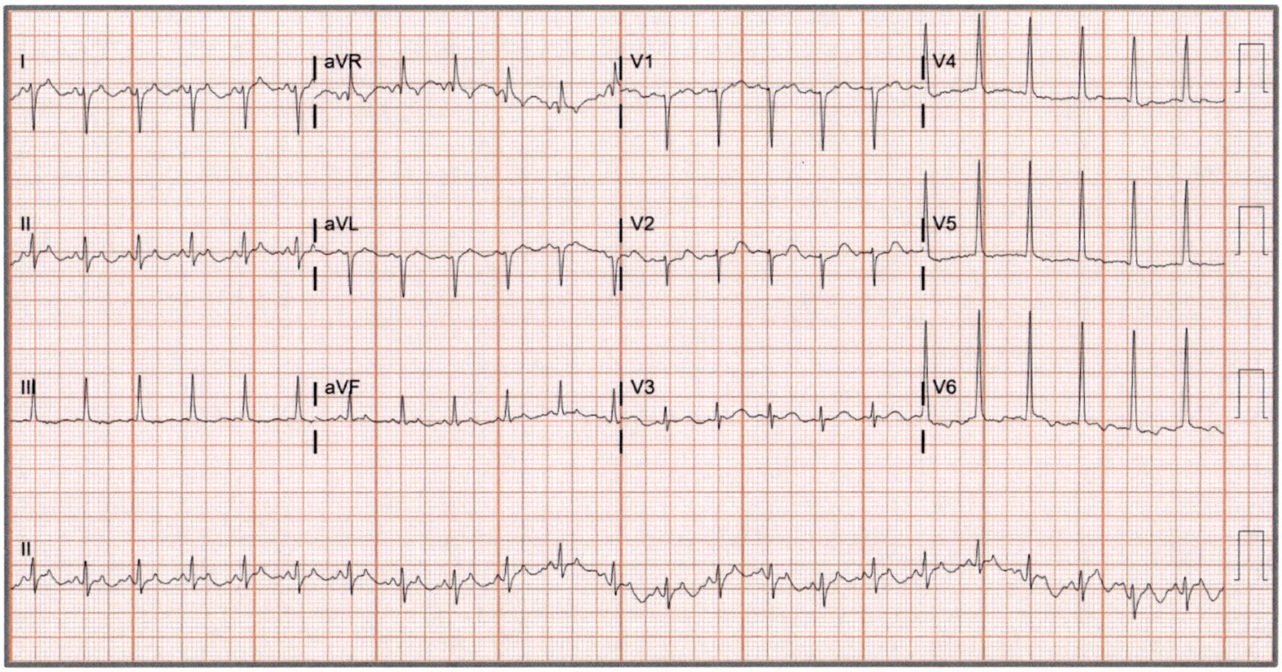

Rate: Rhythm: Axis: Intervals: Ischemia:

#31 – 26-year-old male presents with palpitations

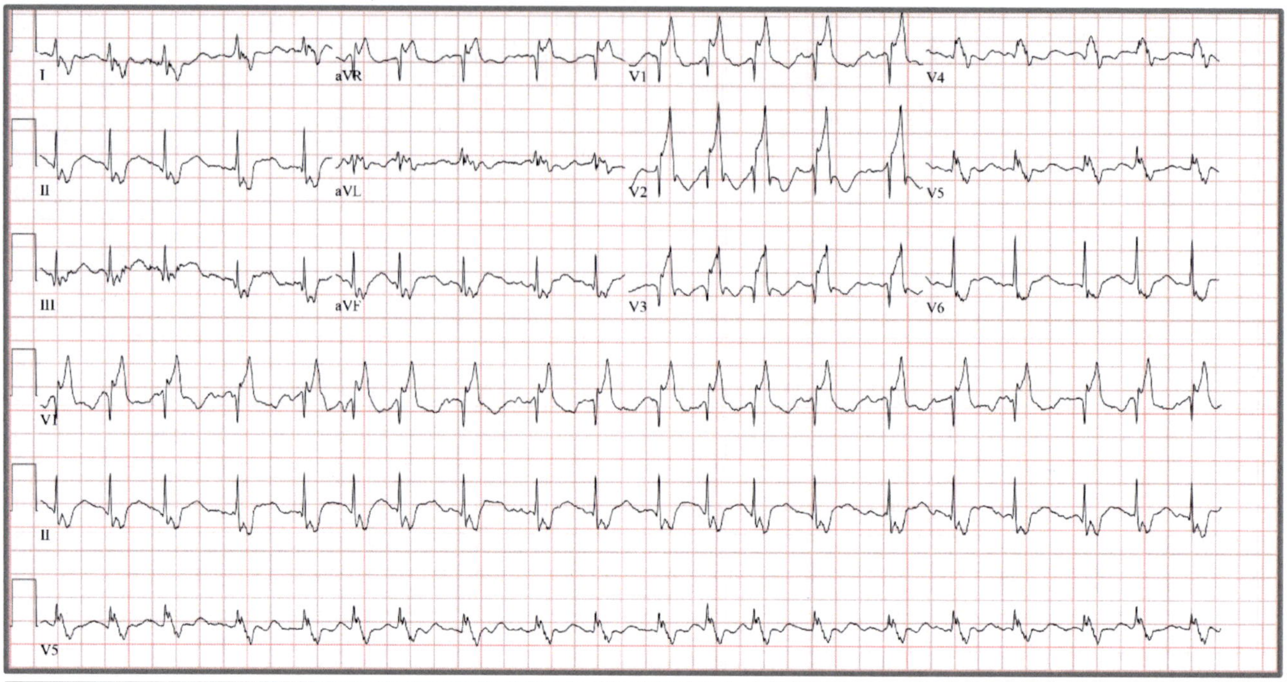

Rate: Rhythm: Axis: Intervals: Ischemia:

#32 – 36-year-old male presents with palpitations

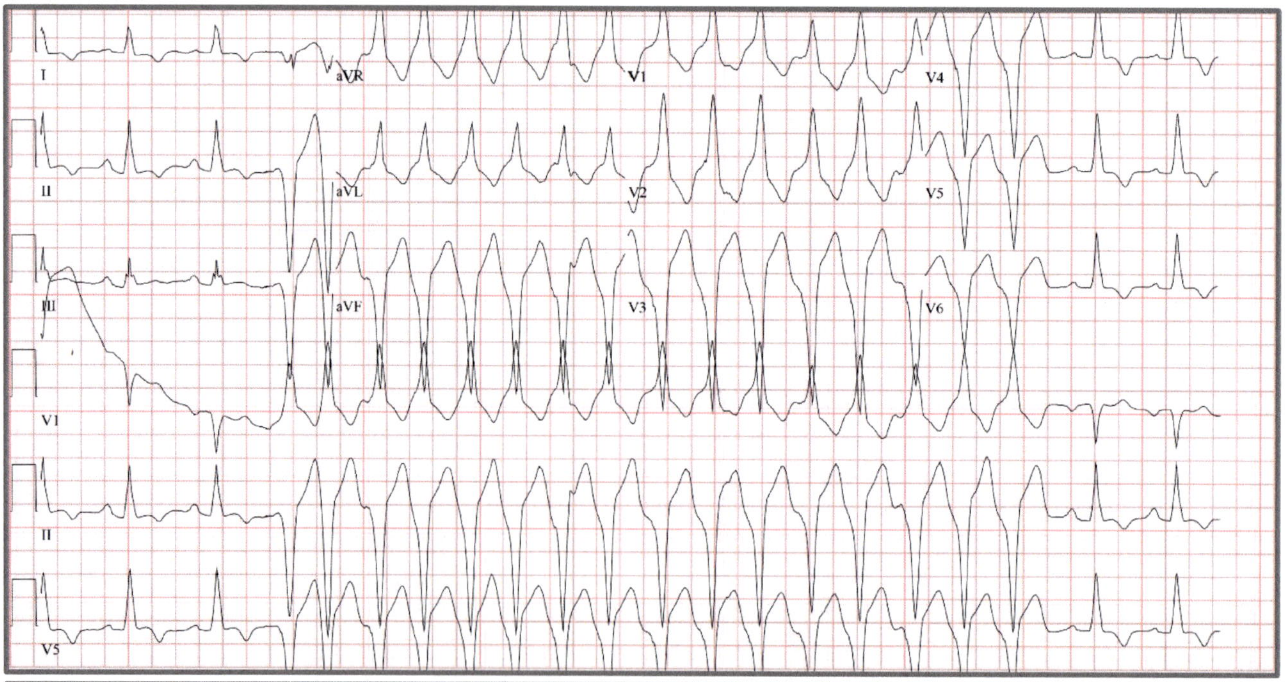

Rate: Rhythm: Axis: Intervals: Ischemia:

#33 – 60-year-old male presents with confusion & chest pain

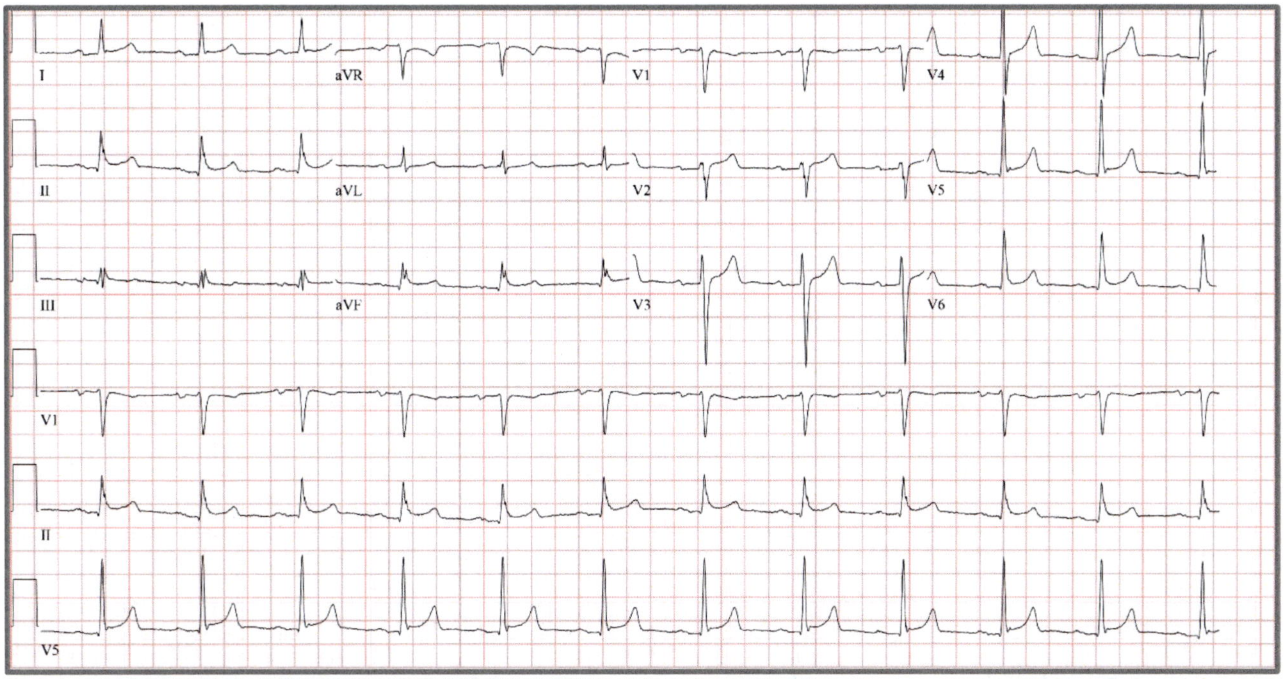

Rate: | **Rhythm:** | **Axis:** | **Intervals:** | **Ischemia:**

#34 – 64-year-old male presents with bradycardia

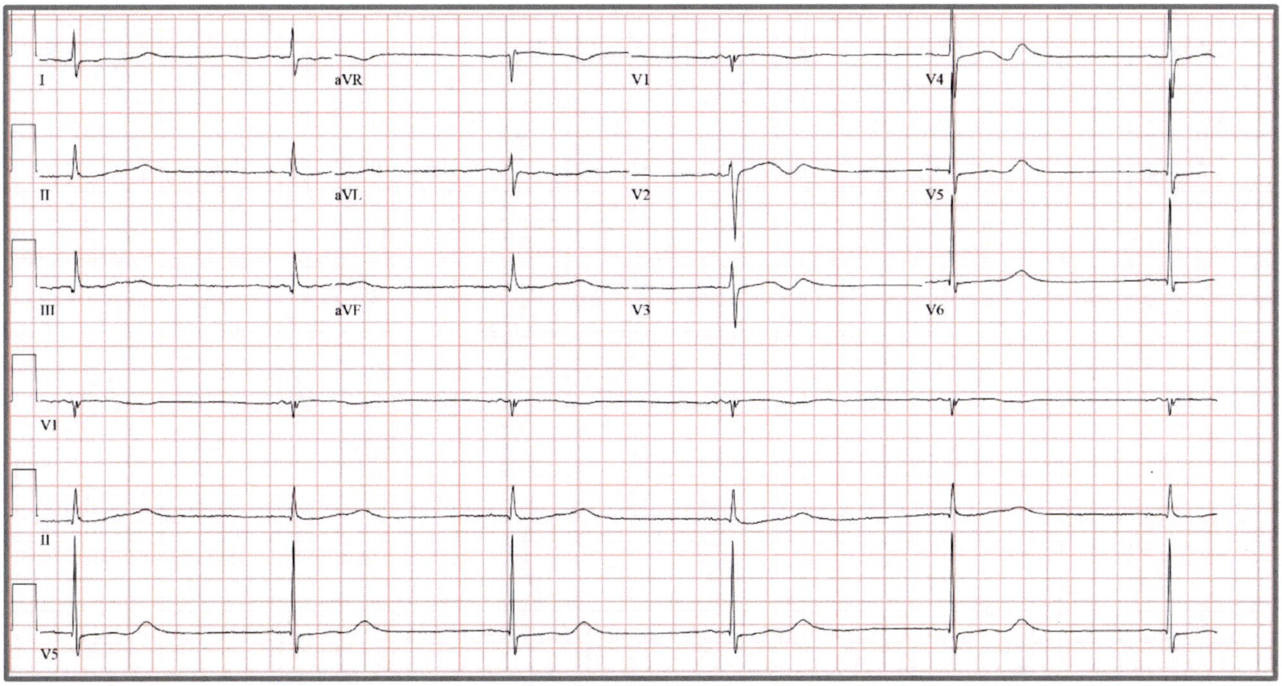

Rate: | **Rhythm:** | **Axis:** | **Intervals:** | **Ischemia:**

#35 – 71-year-old male presents with dyspnea & chest pain

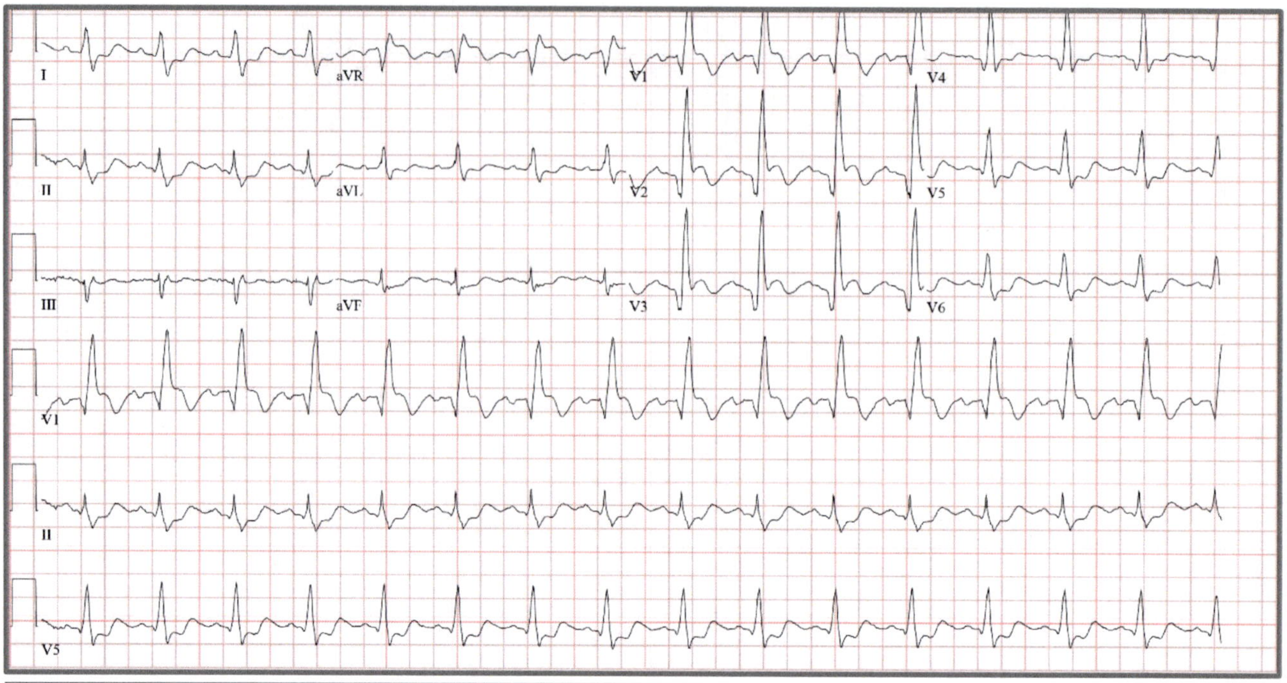

Rate: **Rhythm:** **Axis:** **Intervals:** **Ischemia:**

#36 – 29-year-old male presents with pleuritic chest pain

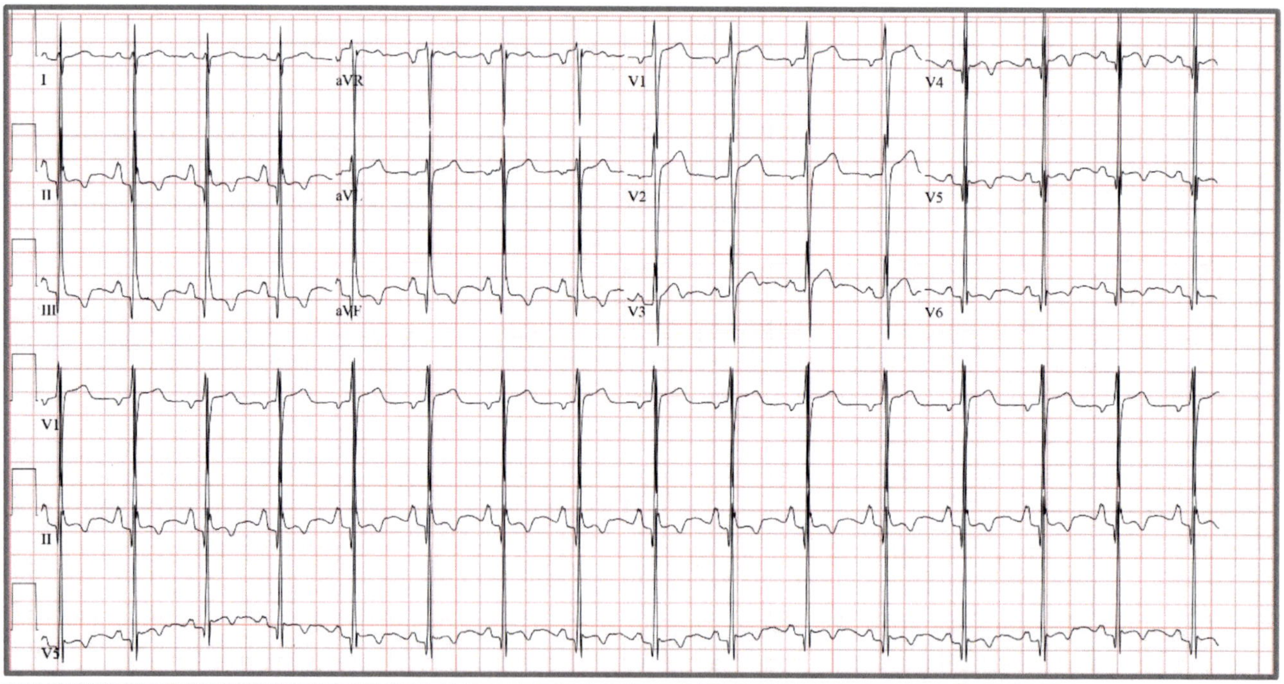

Rate: **Rhythm:** **Axis:** **Intervals:** **Ischemia:**

#37 – 30-year-old male presents status post amitriptyline OD

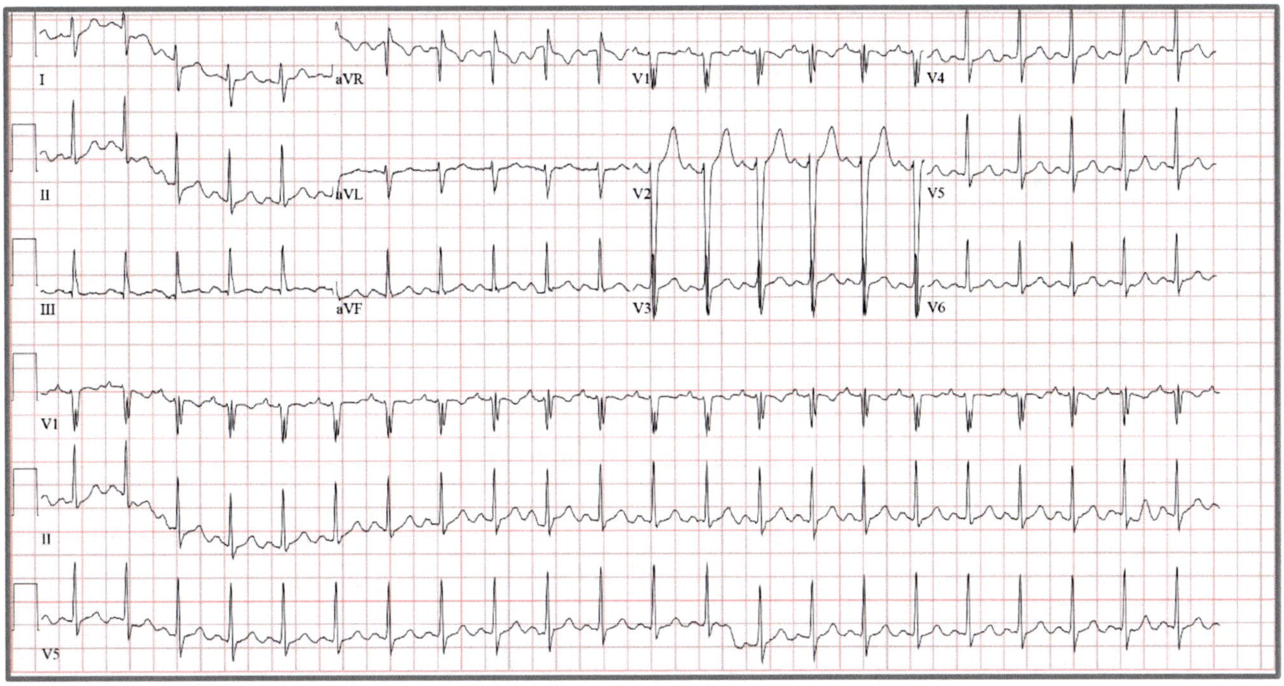

Rate:	Rhythm:	Axis:	Intervals:	Ischemia:

#38 – 38-year-old female presents with upper abdominal pain

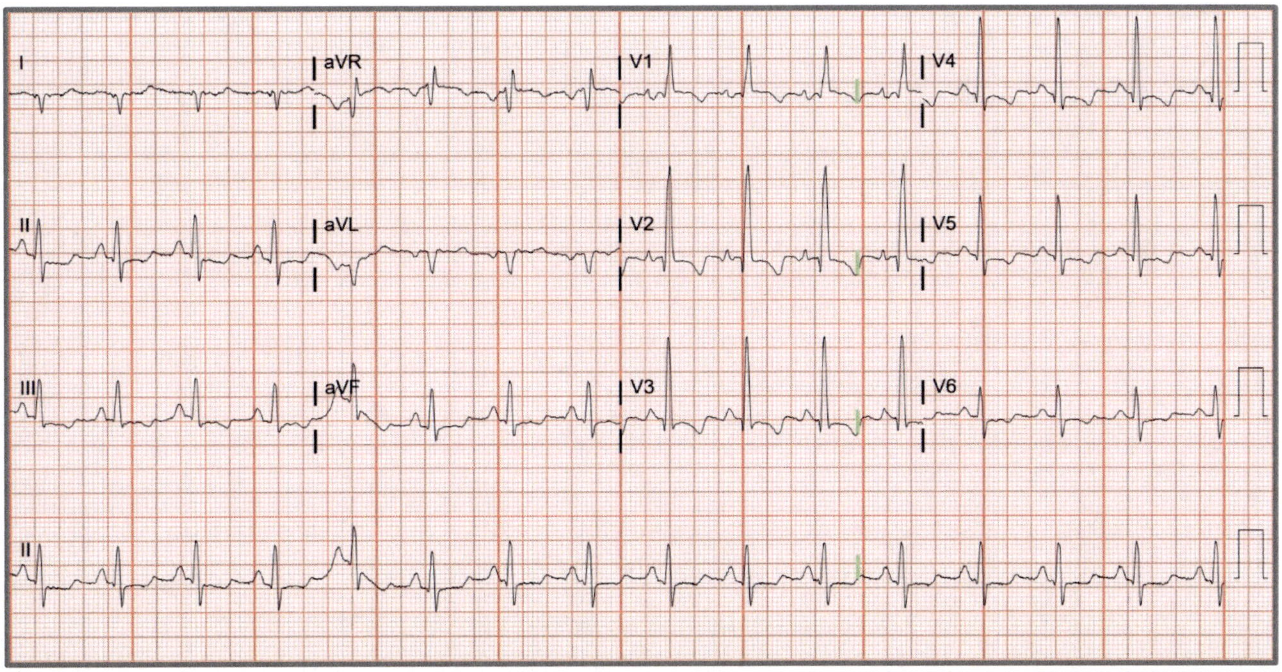

Rate:	Rhythm:	Axis:	Intervals:	Ischemia:

#39 – 96-year-old male presents with palpitations

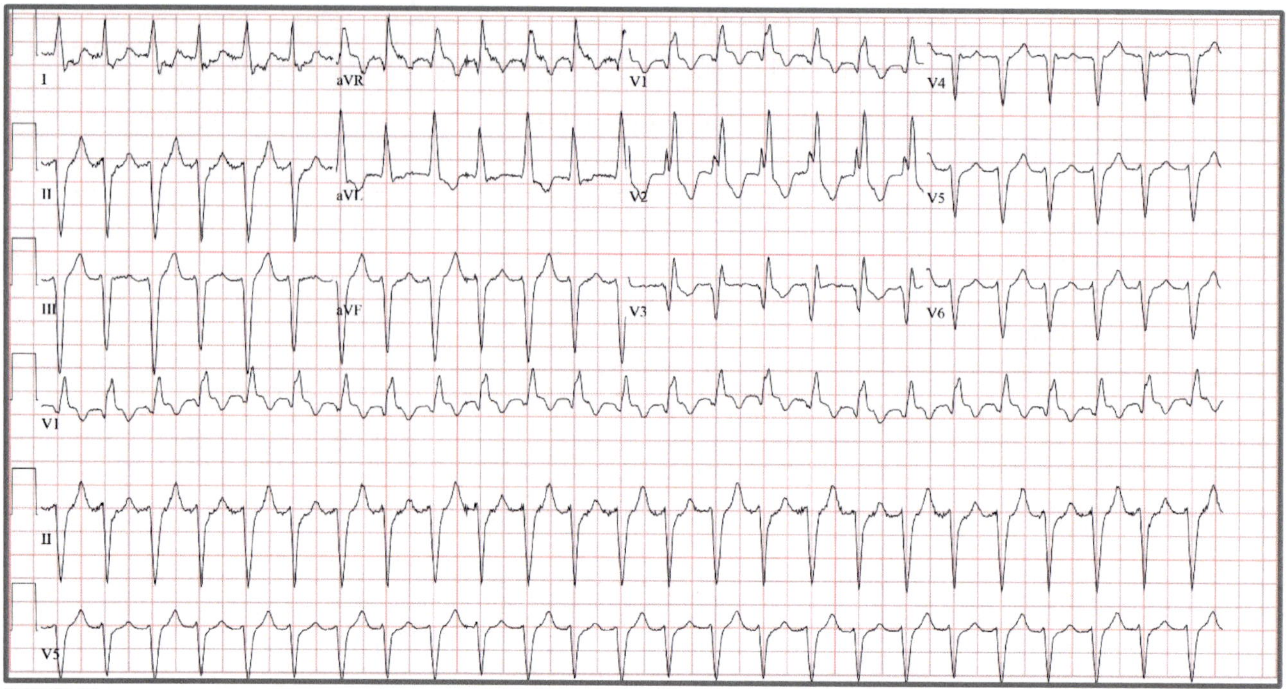

Rate: Rhythm: Axis: Intervals: Ischemia:

#40 – 65-year-old male presents with dyspnea

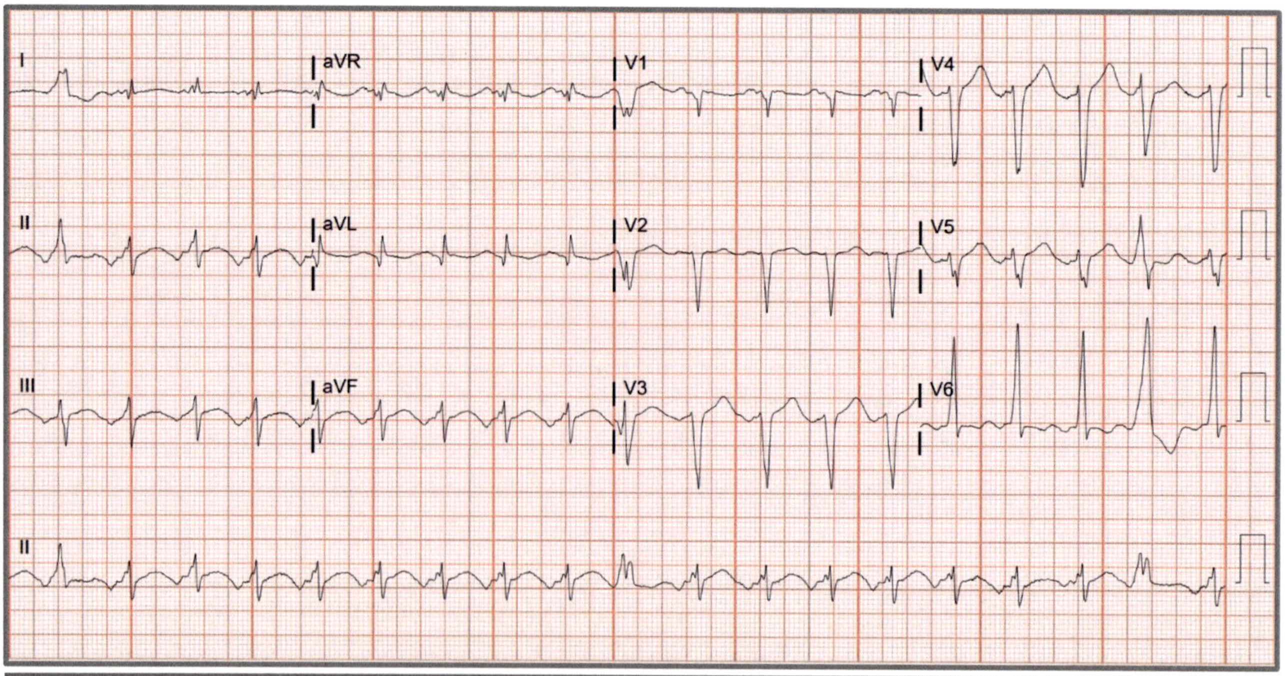

Rate: Rhythm: Axis: Intervals: Ischemia:

#41 – 69-year-old female presents with foot pain

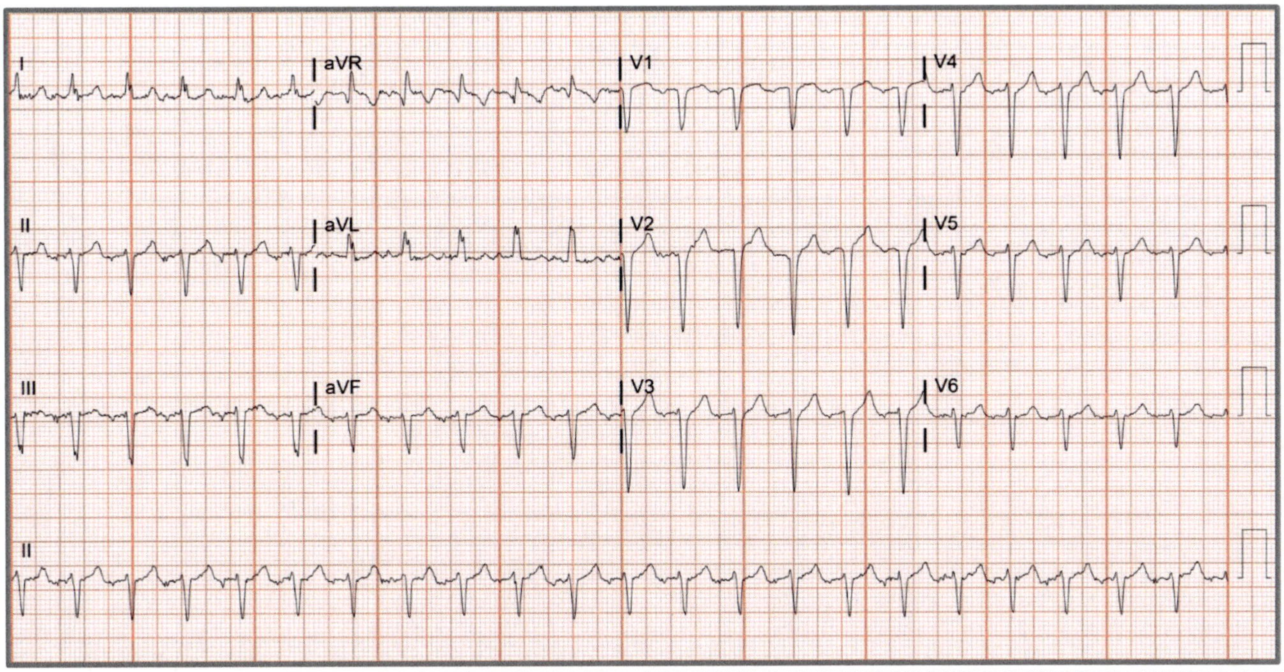

Rate:	Rhythm:	Axis:	Intervals:	Ischemia:

⇩ Post-conversion ECG ⇩

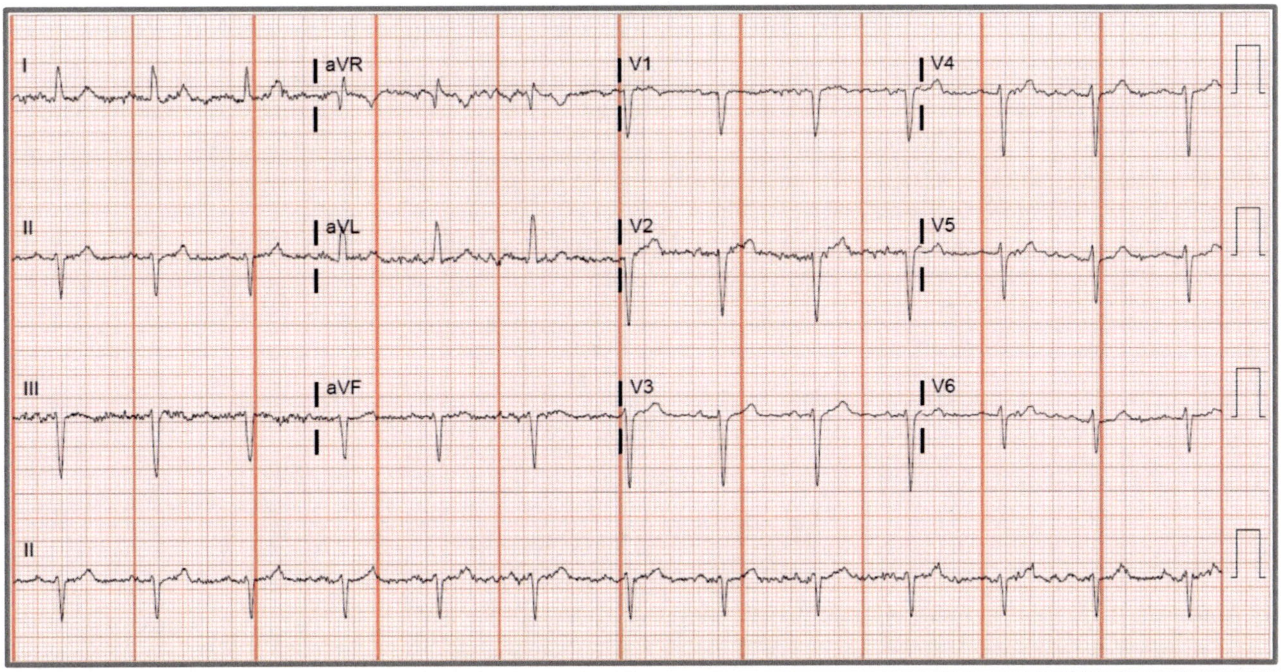

Rate:	Rhythm:	Axis:	Intervals:	Ischemia:

#42 – 31-year-old female presents with arrest

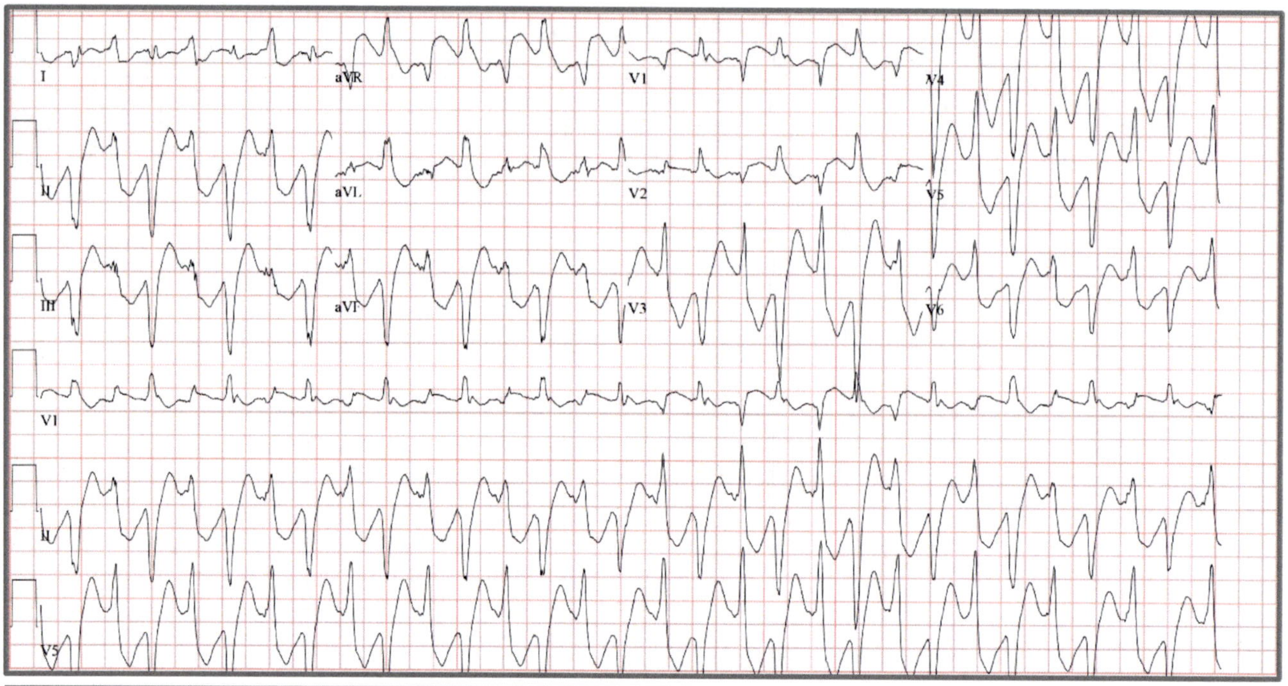

Rate: Rhythm: Axis: Intervals: Ischemia:

#43 – 44-year-old male presents with syncope

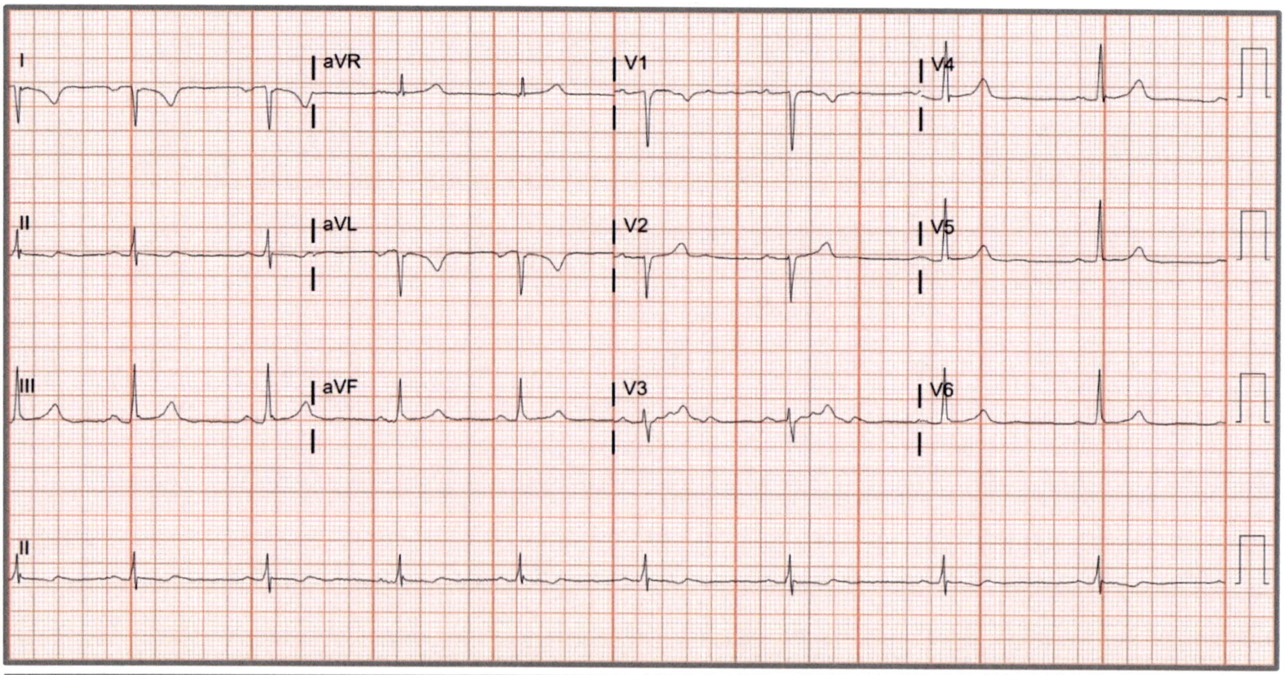

Rate: Rhythm: Axis: Intervals: Ischemia:

#44 – 53-year-old female presents with chest pain

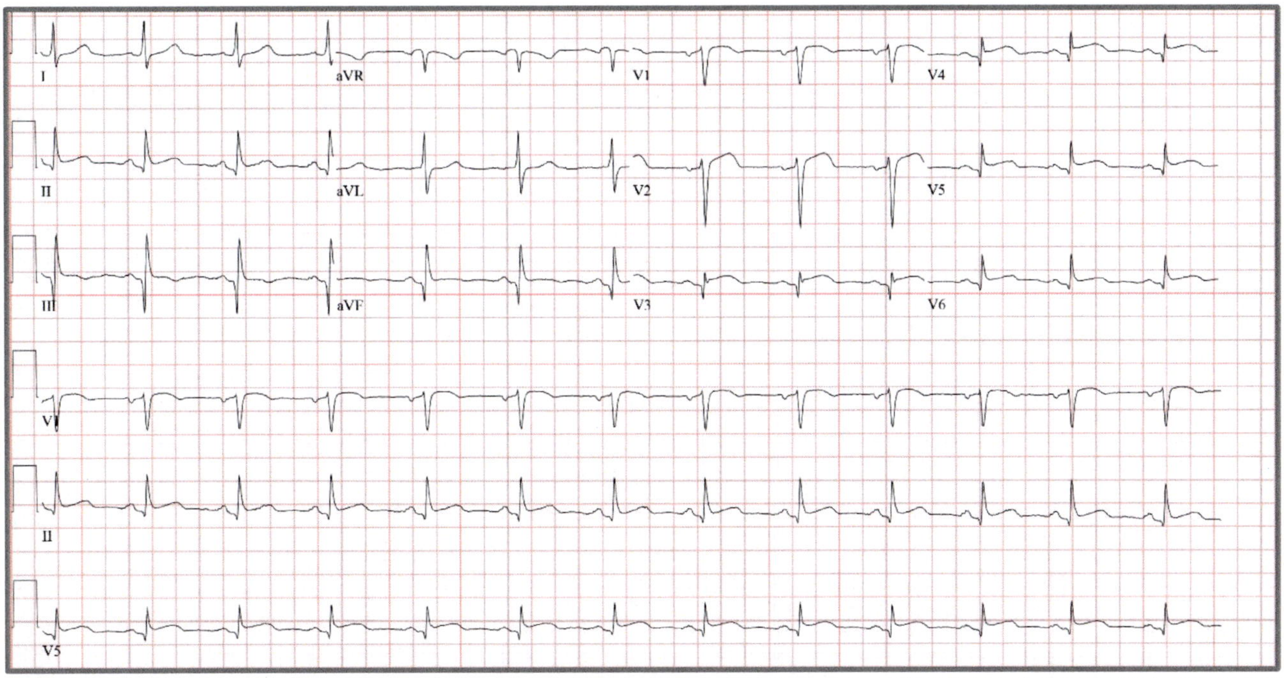

Rate: Rhythm: Axis: Intervals: Ischemia:

#45 – 76-year-old male presents with right leg edema

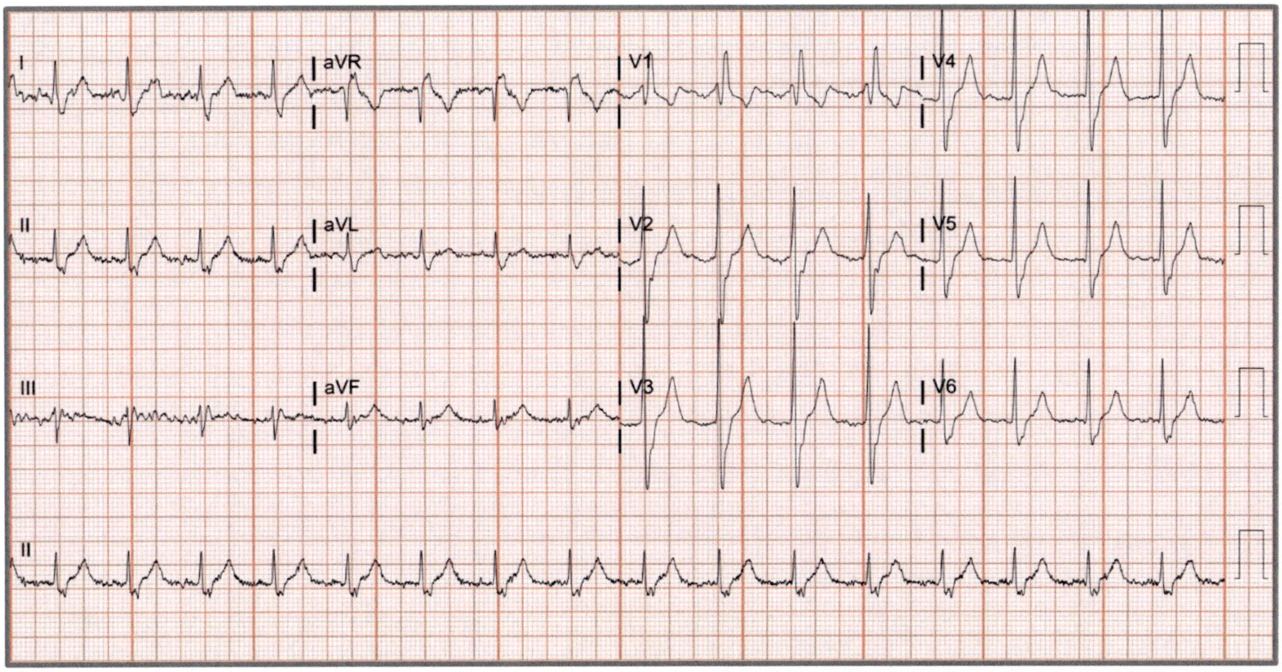

Rate: Rhythm: Axis: Intervals: Ischemia:

#46 – 51-year-old male presents as callback for abnormal labs

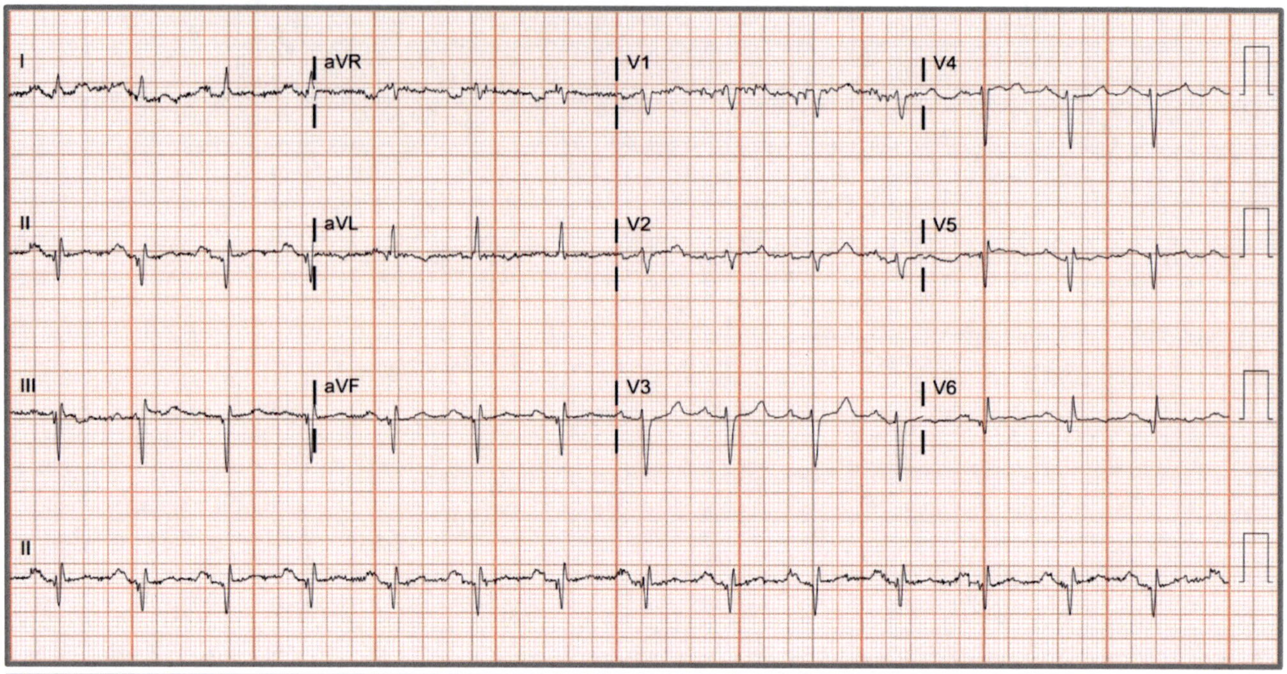

Rate: **Rhythm:** **Axis:** **Intervals:** **Ischemia:**

#47 – 36-year-old male presents with chest pain

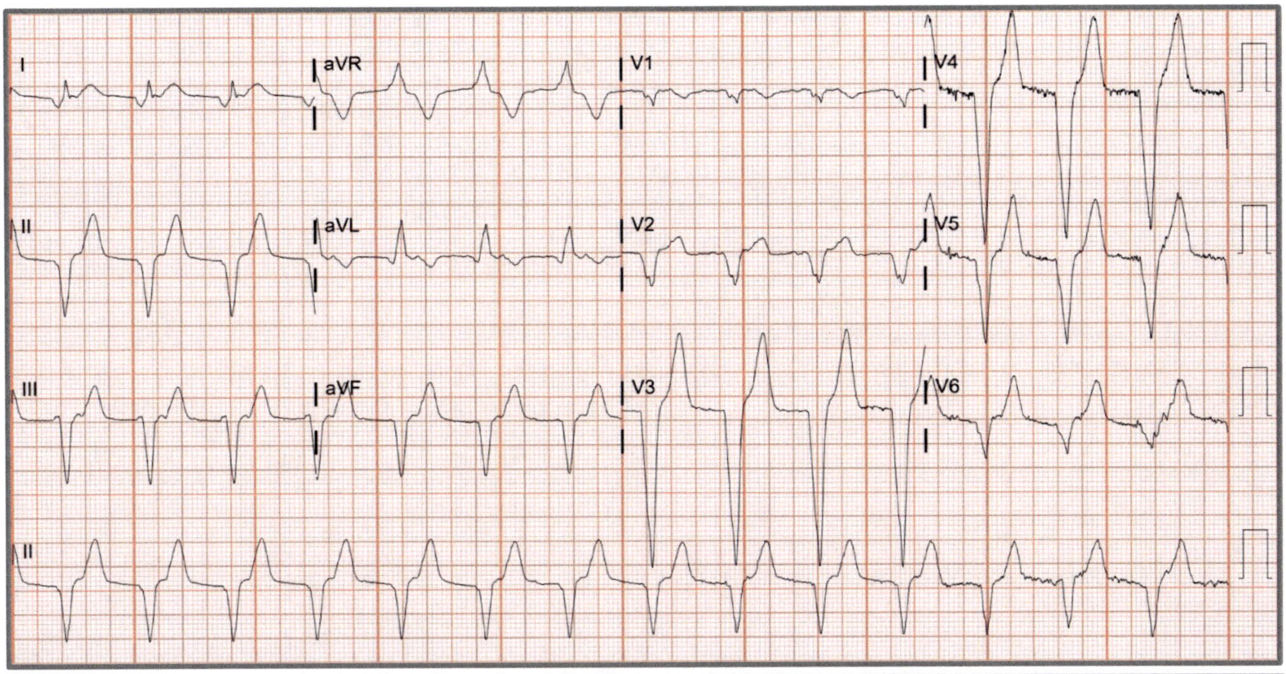

Rate: Rhythm: Axis: Intervals: Ischemia:

⇩ Prior ECG ⇩

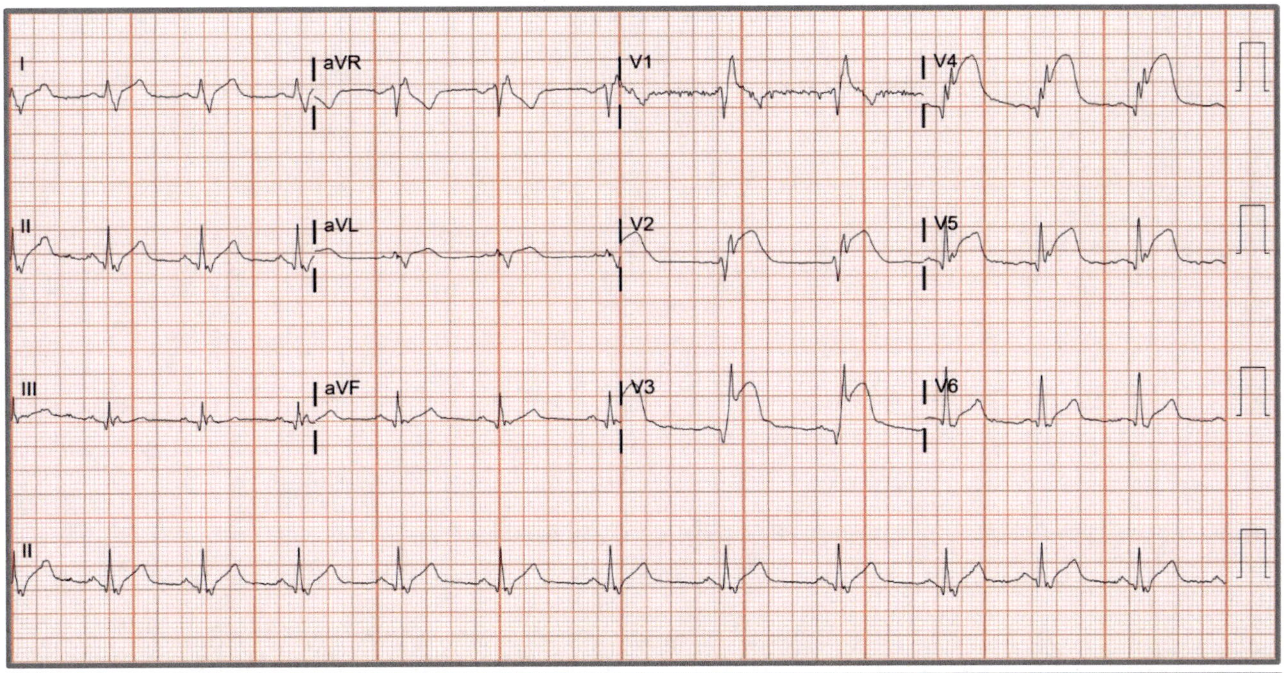

Rate: Rhythm: Axis: Intervals: Ischemia:

#48 – 61-year-old female presents with stuttering chest pain

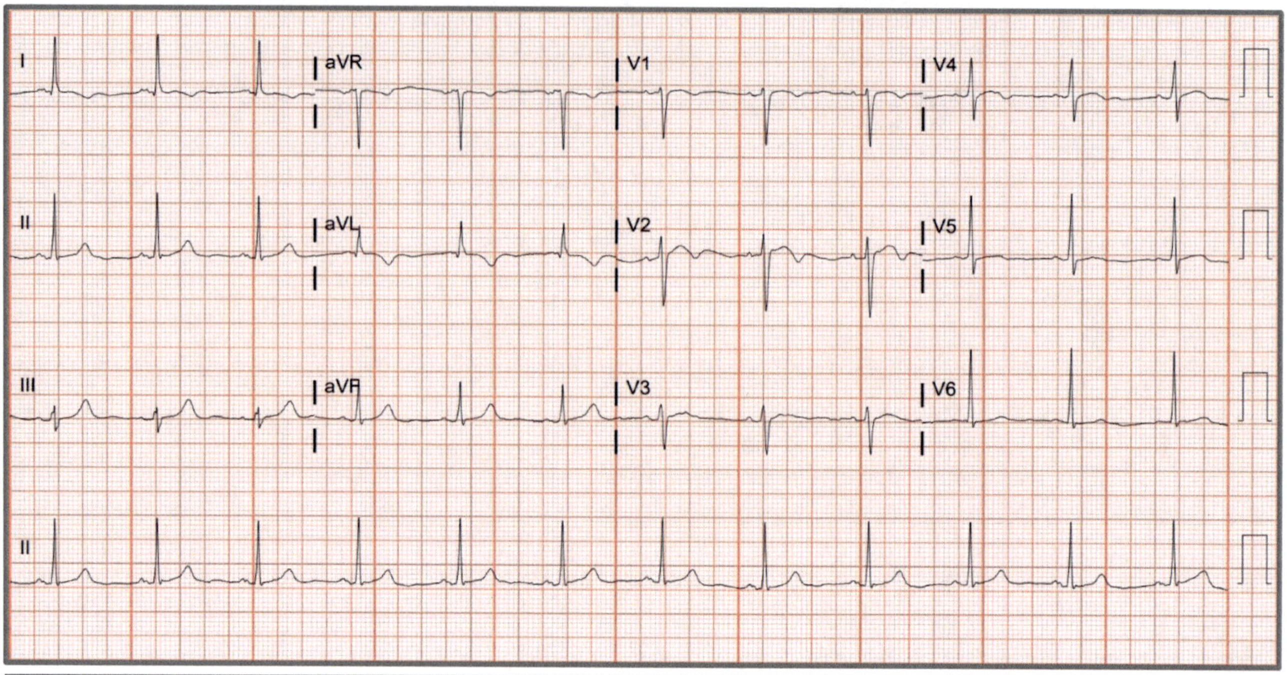

Rate:	Rhythm:	Axis:	Intervals:	Ischemia:

#49 – 70-year-old female presents with chest pain

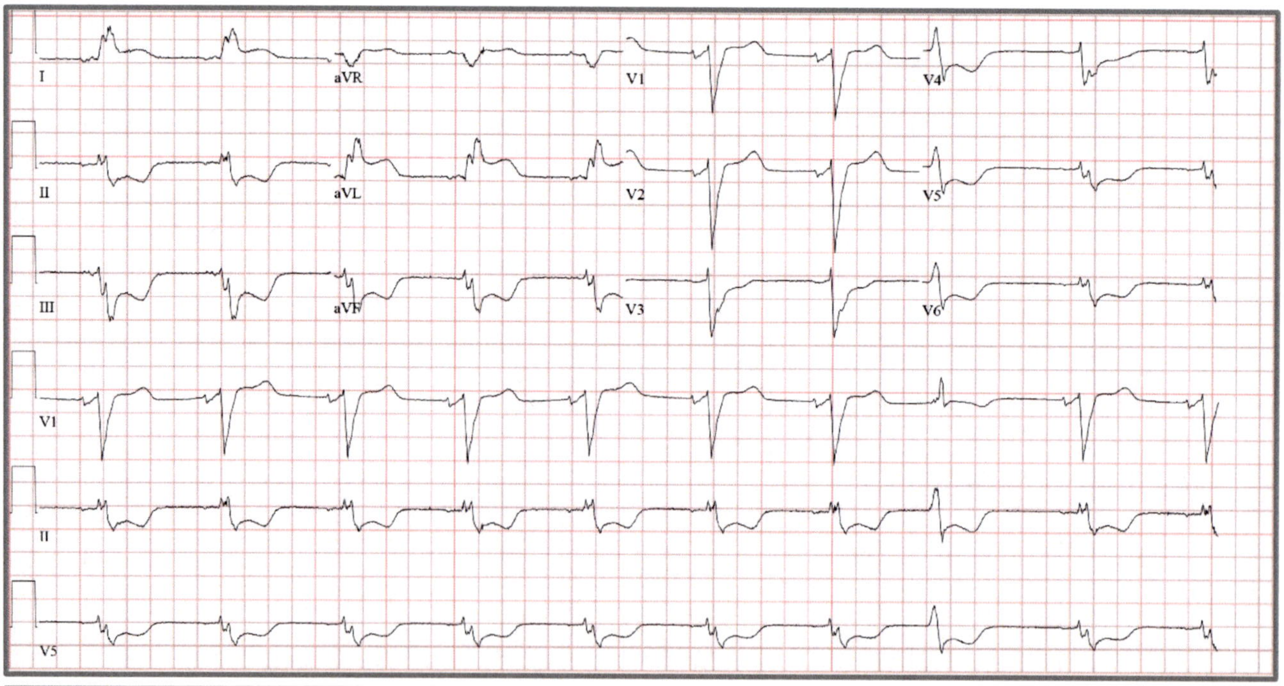

Rate:	Rhythm:	Axis:	Intervals:	Ischemia:

#50 – 51-year-old female presents with chest wall spasms

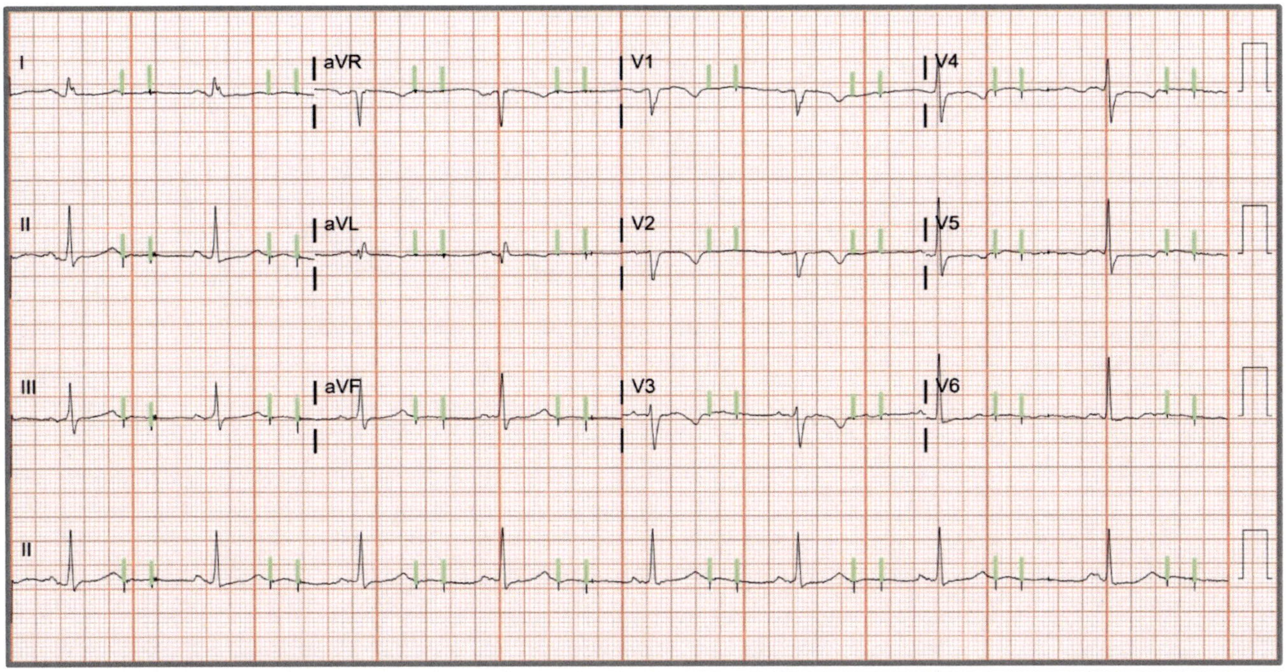

Rate:		Rhythm:		Axis:		Intervals:		Ischemia:	

#51 – 72-year-old male presents with dizziness

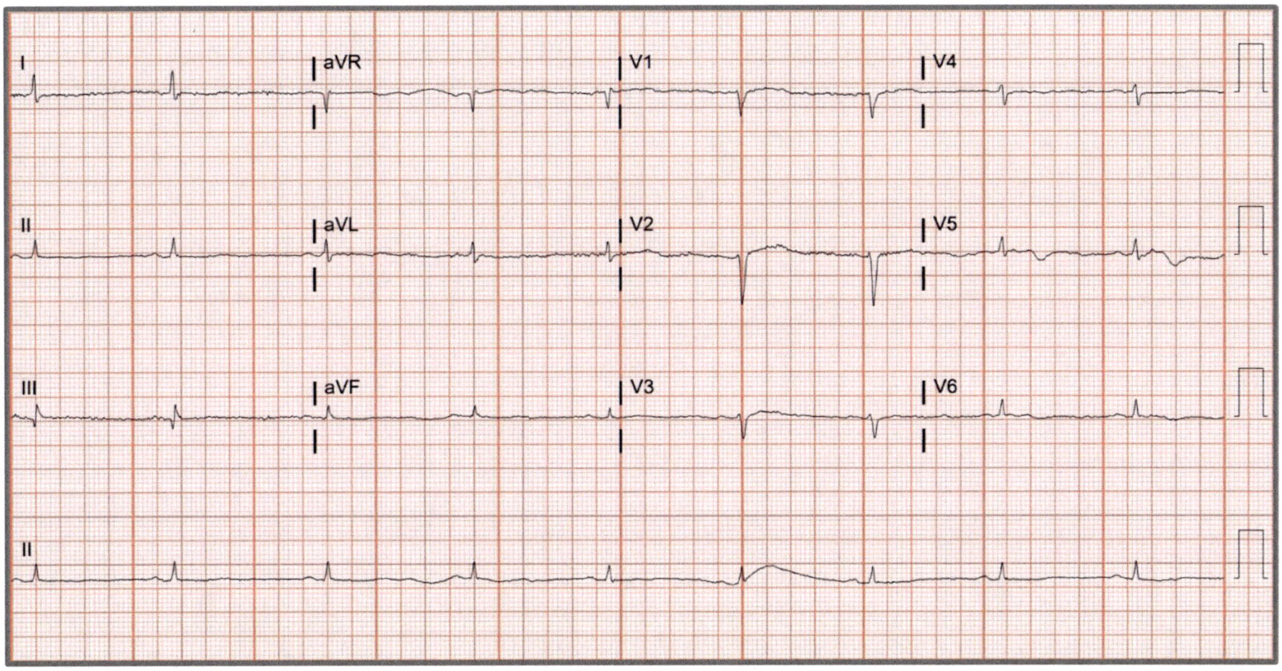

Rate:		Rhythm:		Axis:		Intervals:		Ischemia:	

#52 – 58-year-old female presents with chest pain

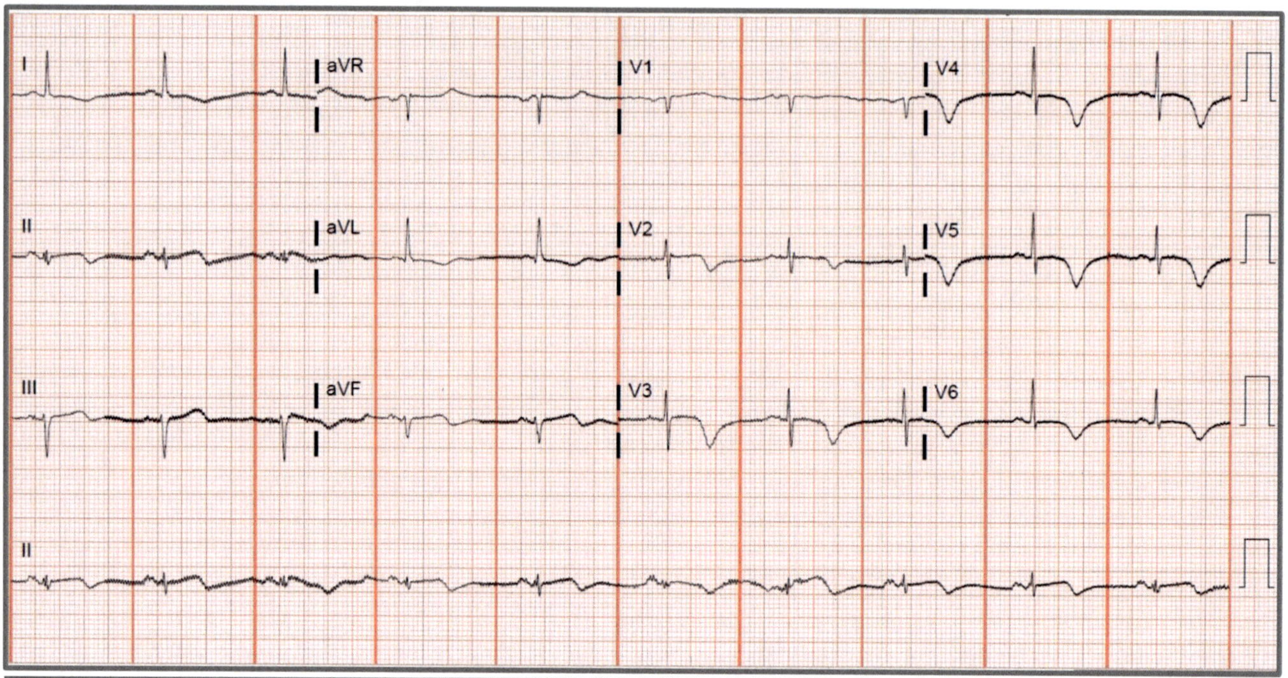

Rate: **Rhythm:** **Axis:** **Intervals:** **Ischemia:**

#53 – 81-year-old male presents with chest pain

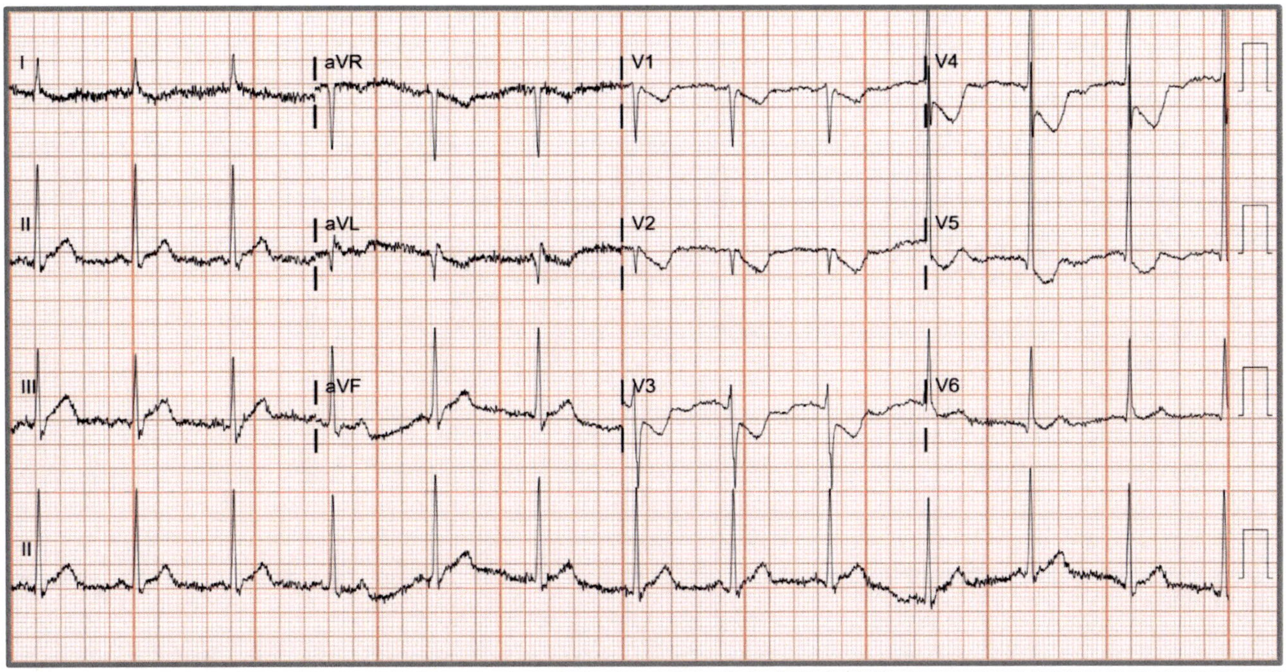

Rate: **Rhythm:** **Axis:** **Intervals:** **Ischemia:**

⇩ Repeat ECG with Posterior Leads ⇩

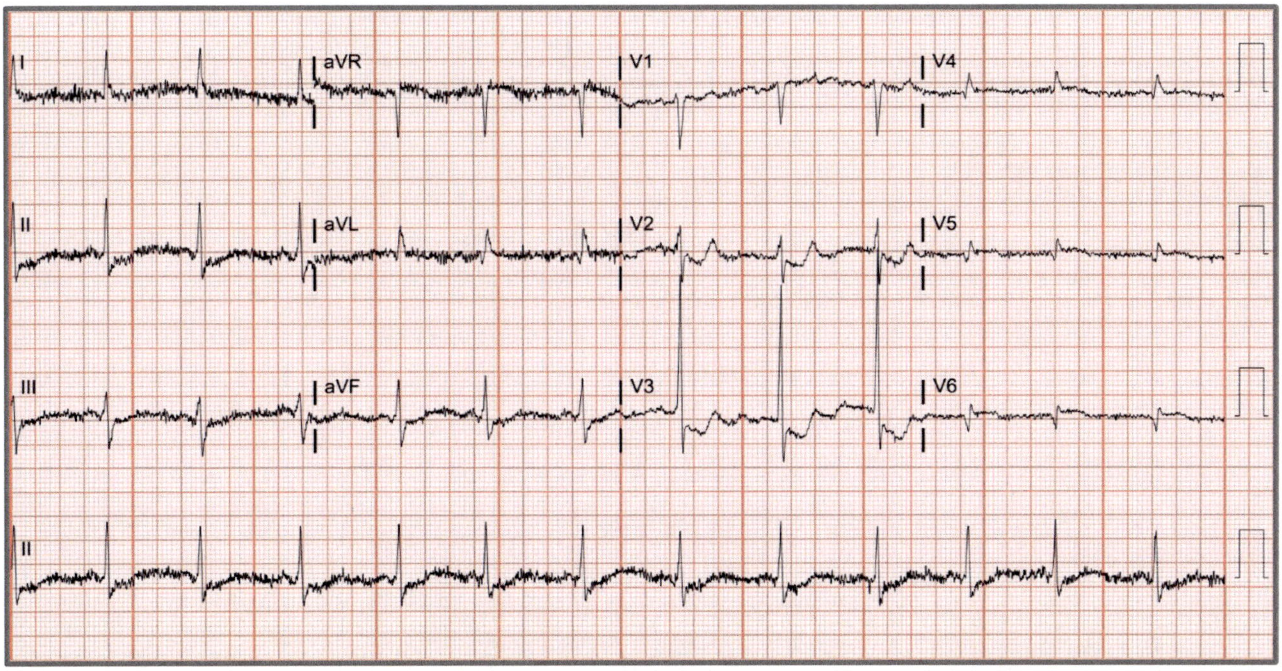

Rate: **Rhythm:** **Axis:** **Intervals:** **Ischemia:**

#54 – 81-year-old male presents with chest pain

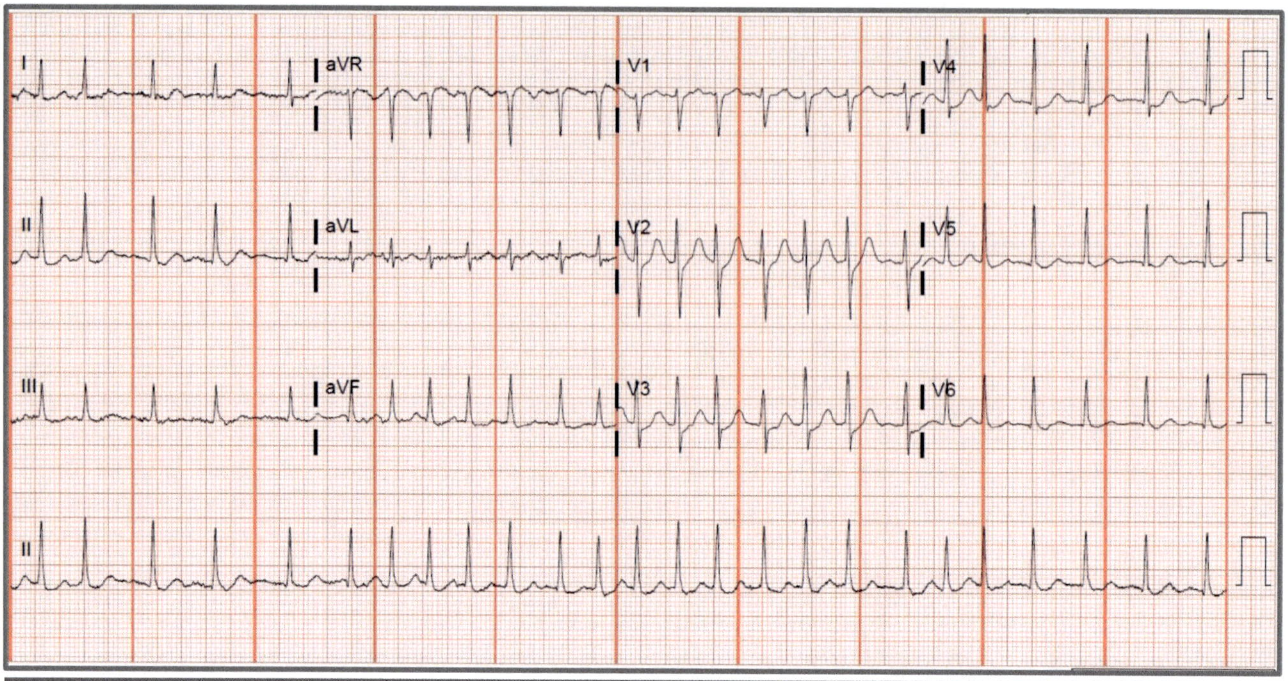

Rate: Rhythm: Axis: Intervals: Ischemia:

#55 – 71-year-old male presents with palpitations

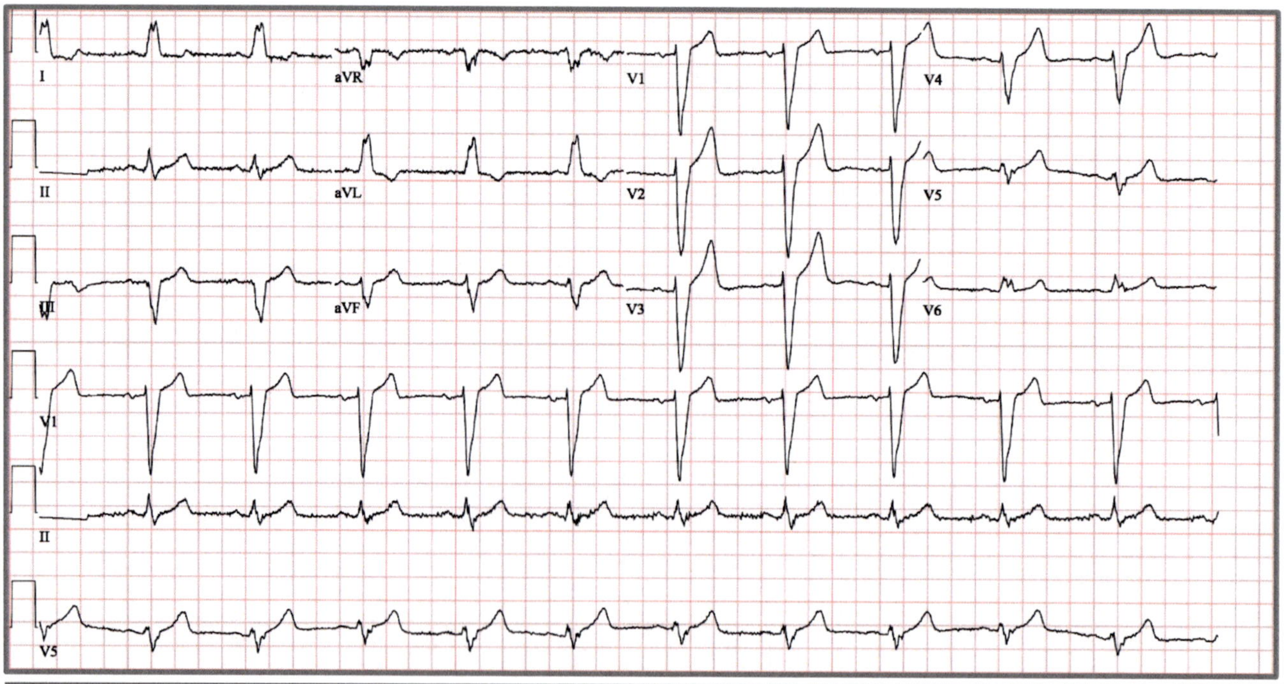

Rate: Rhythm: Axis: Intervals: Ischemia:

#56 – 67-year-old male presents with dyspnea

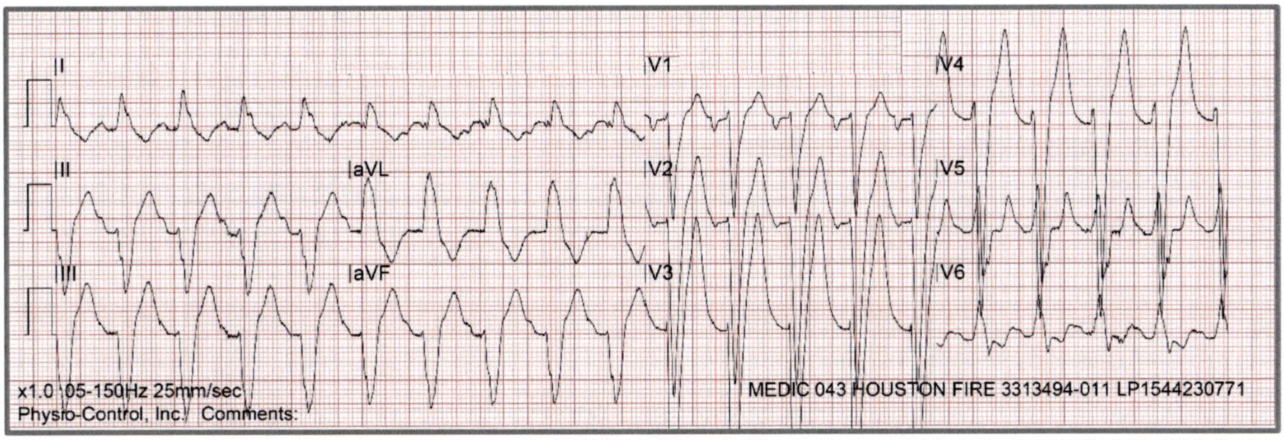

Rate: | **Rhythm:** | **Axis:** | **Intervals:** | **Ischemia:**

#57 – 61-year-old female presents with palpitations

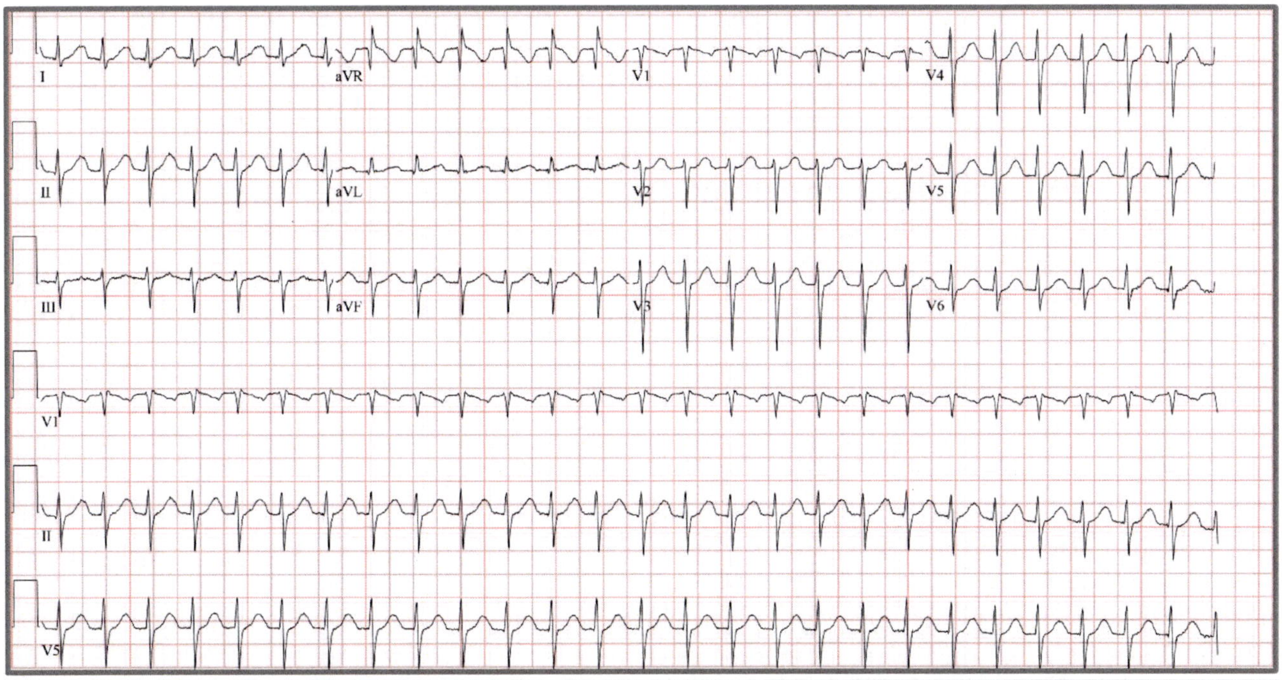

Rate: | **Rhythm:** | **Axis:** | **Intervals:** | **Ischemia:**

#58 – 61-year-old female presents with palpitations

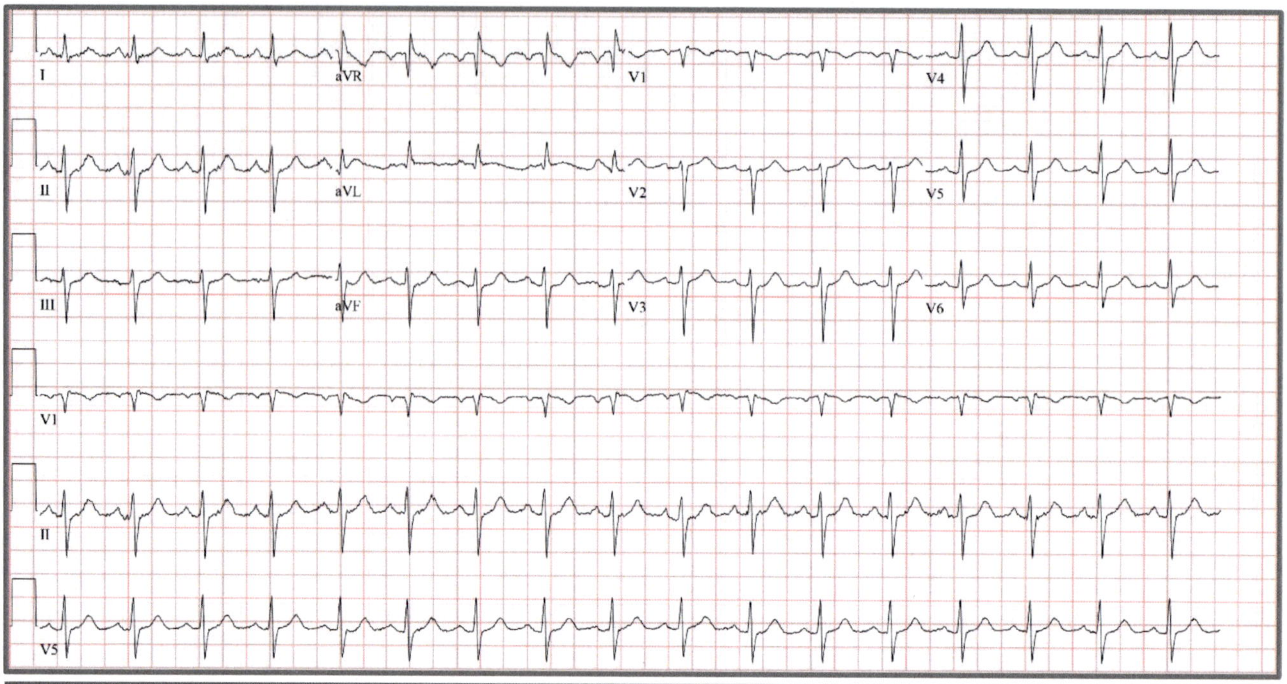

Rate: Rhythm: Axis: Intervals: Ischemia:

#59 – 39-year-old female presents with syncope

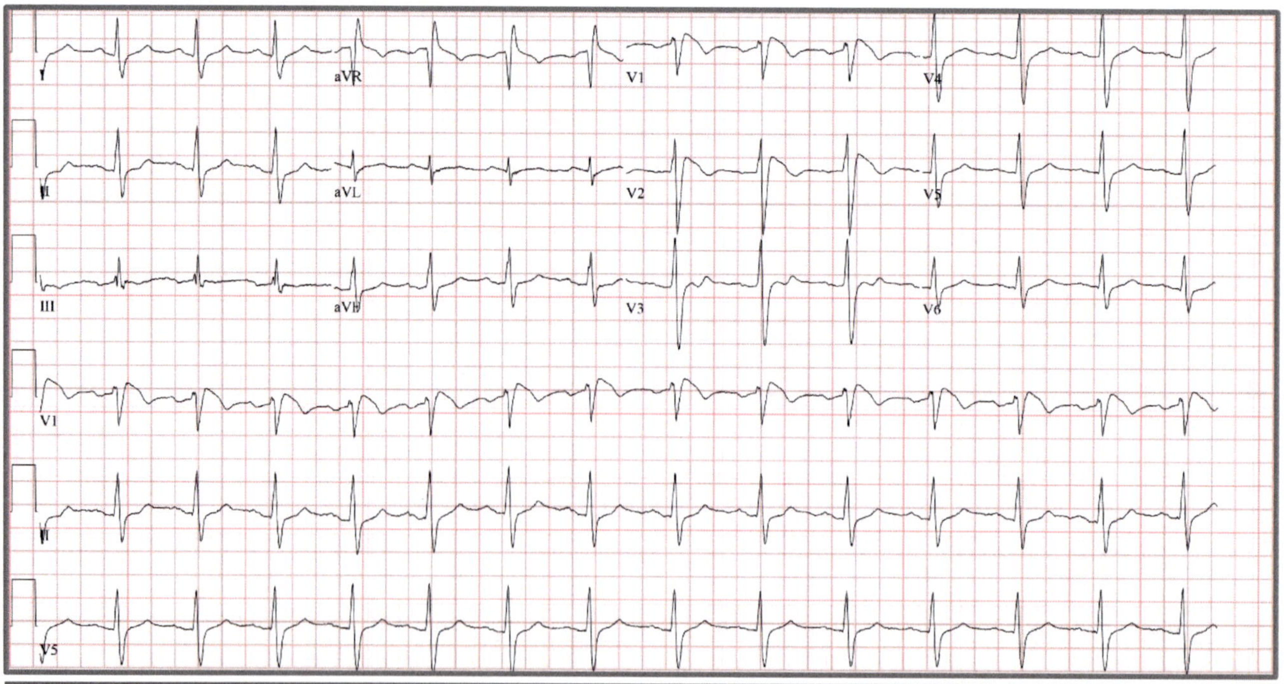

Rate: Rhythm: Axis: Intervals: Ischemia:

#60 – 40-year-old male found down

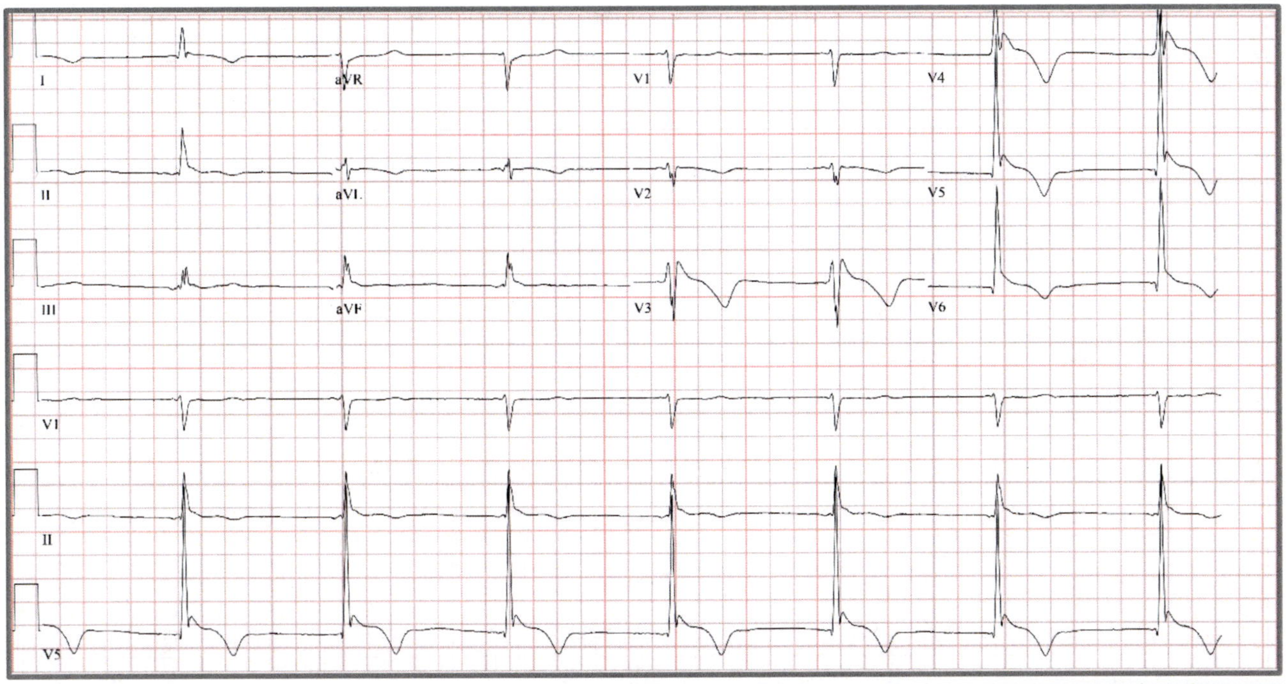

Rate:	Rhythm:	Axis:	Intervals:	Ischemia:

#61 – 53-year-old female found down

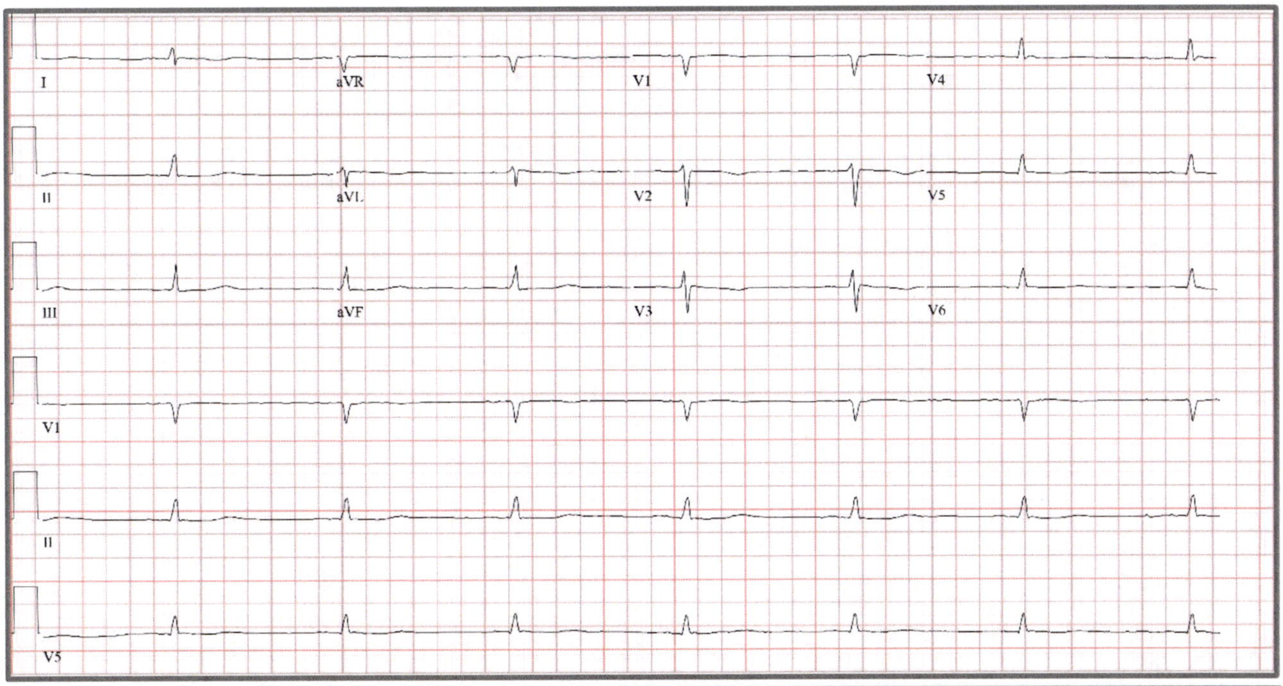

Rate:	Rhythm:	Axis:	Intervals:	Ischemia:

#62 – 62-year-old female presents with chest pain

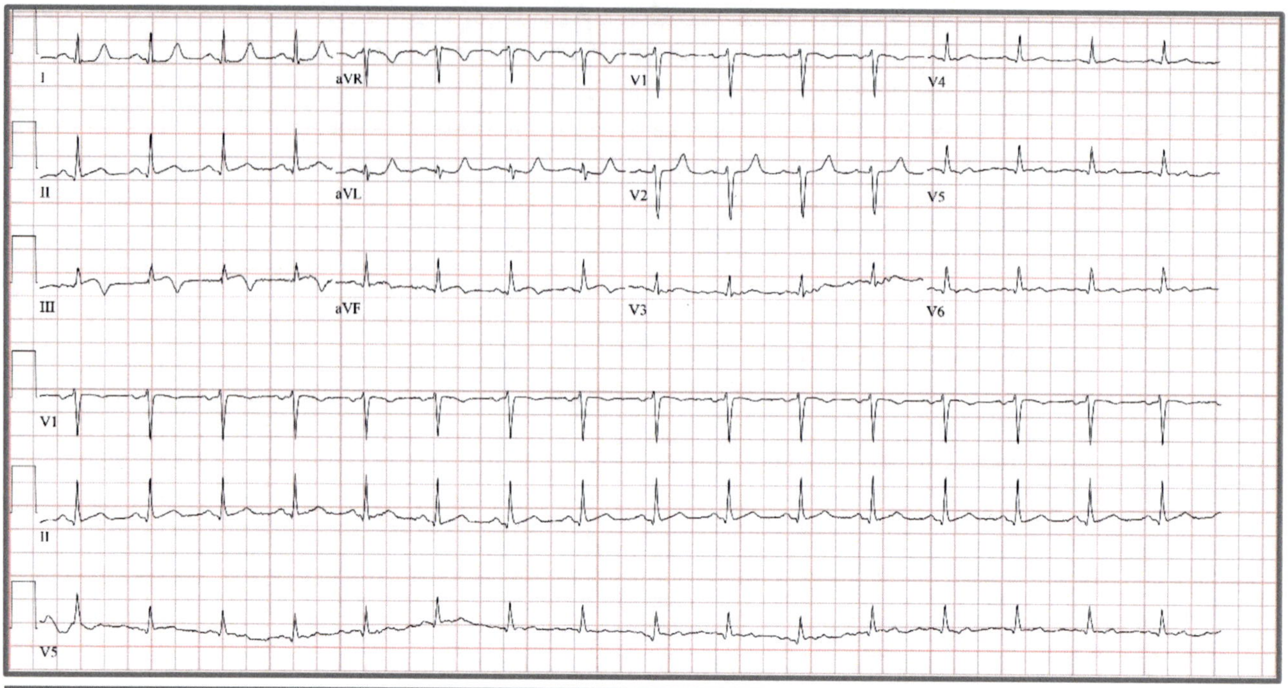

Rate:	Rhythm:	Axis:	Intervals:	Ischemia:

#63 – 70-year-old female presents with altered mentation

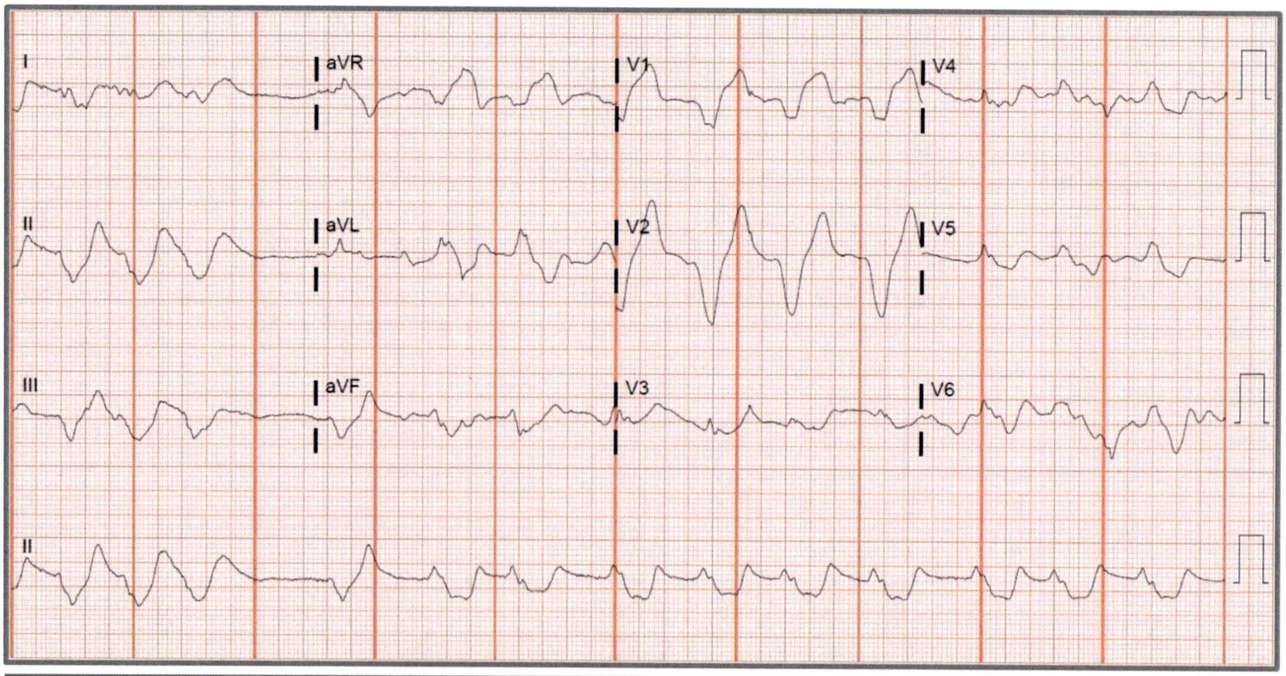

Rate:	Rhythm:	Axis:	Intervals:	Ischemia:

#64 – 50-year-old female presents with vomiting

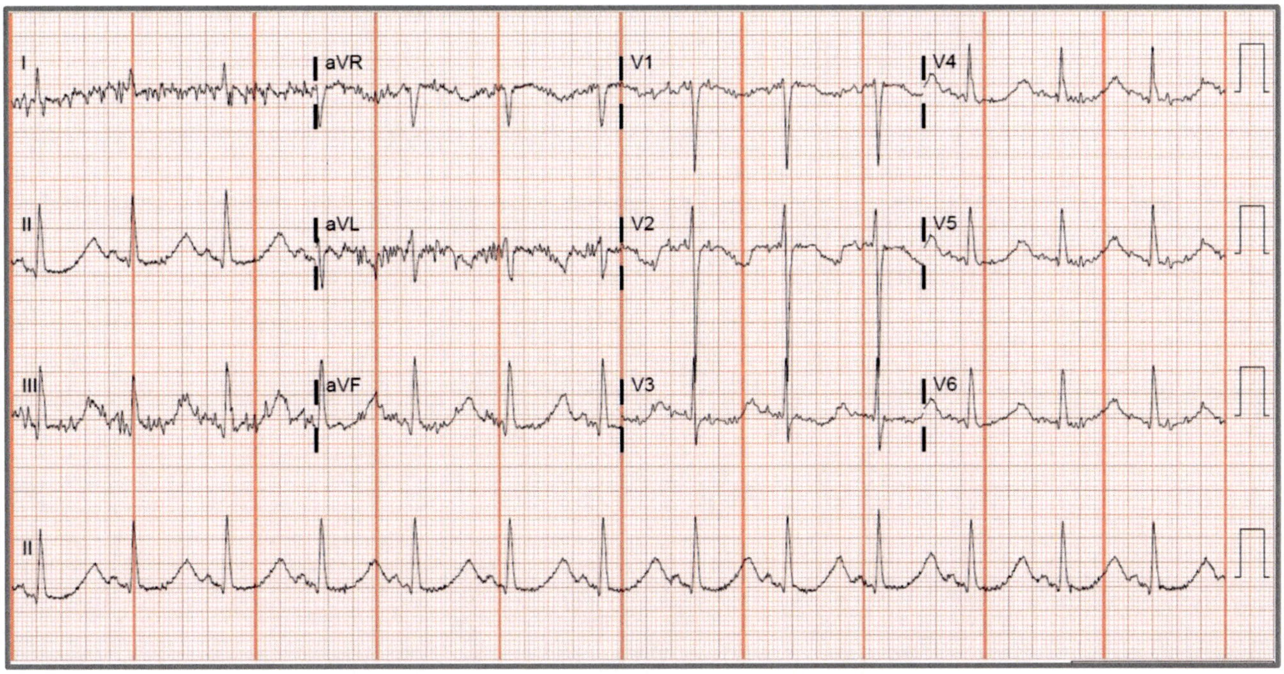

Rate:		Rhythm:		Axis:		Intervals:		Ischemia:	

#65 – 90-year-old male presents with weakness

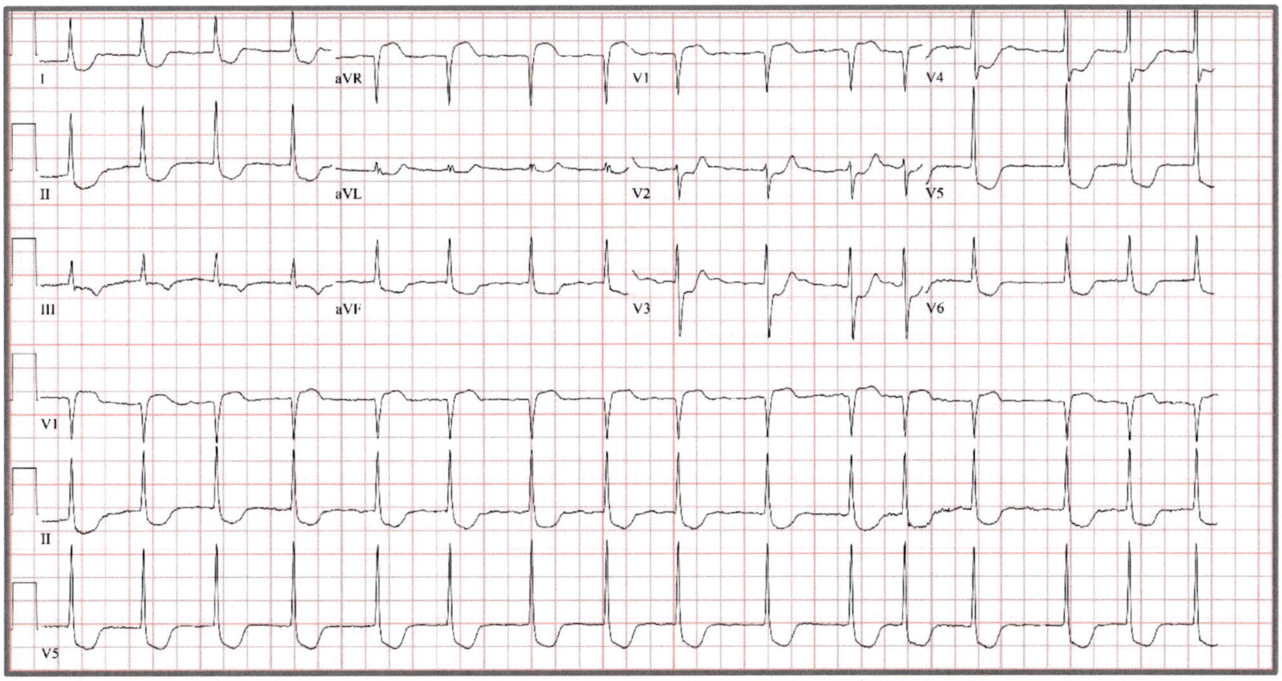

Rate:		Rhythm:		Axis:		Intervals:		Ischemia:	

#66 – 19-year-old female presents with altered mentation

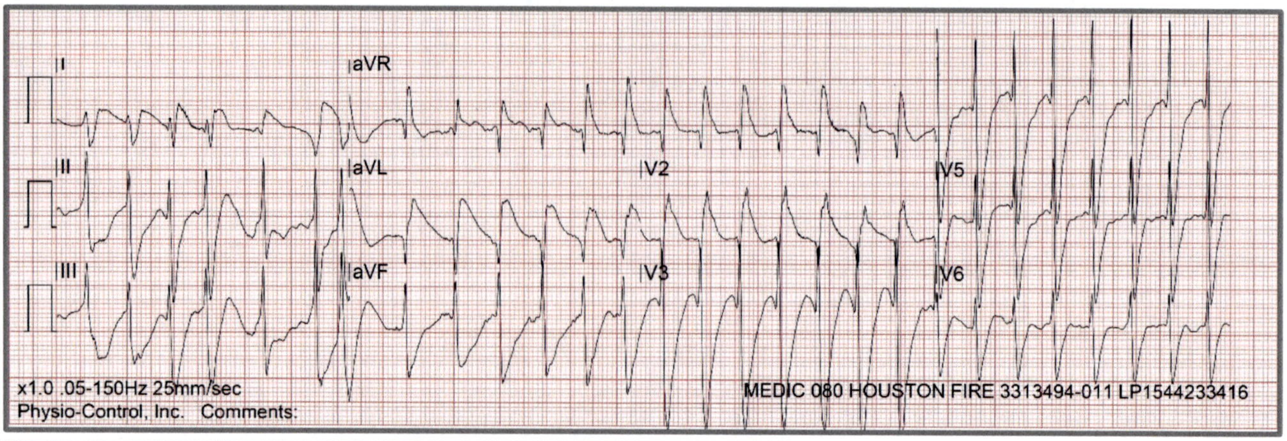

Rate: **Rhythm:** **Axis:** **Intervals:** **Ischemia:**

#67 – 44-year-old female presents with chest pain

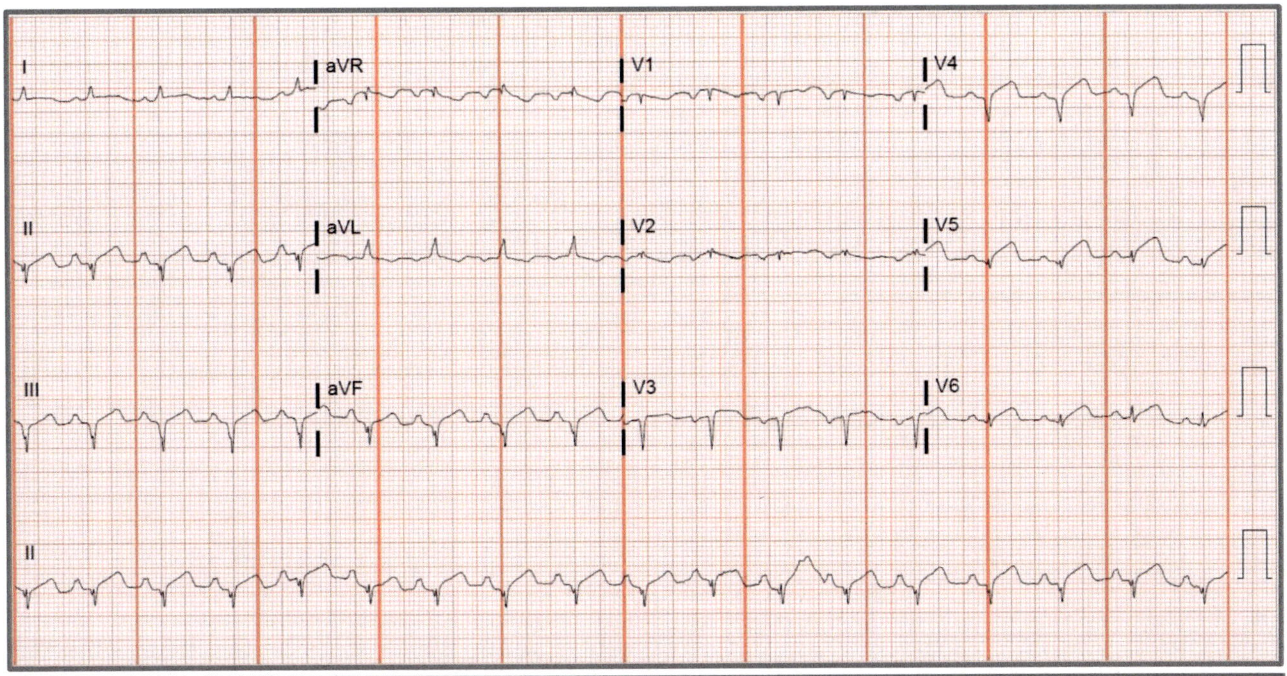

Rate: Rhythm: Axis: Intervals: Ischemia:

⇩ Repeat ECG ⇩

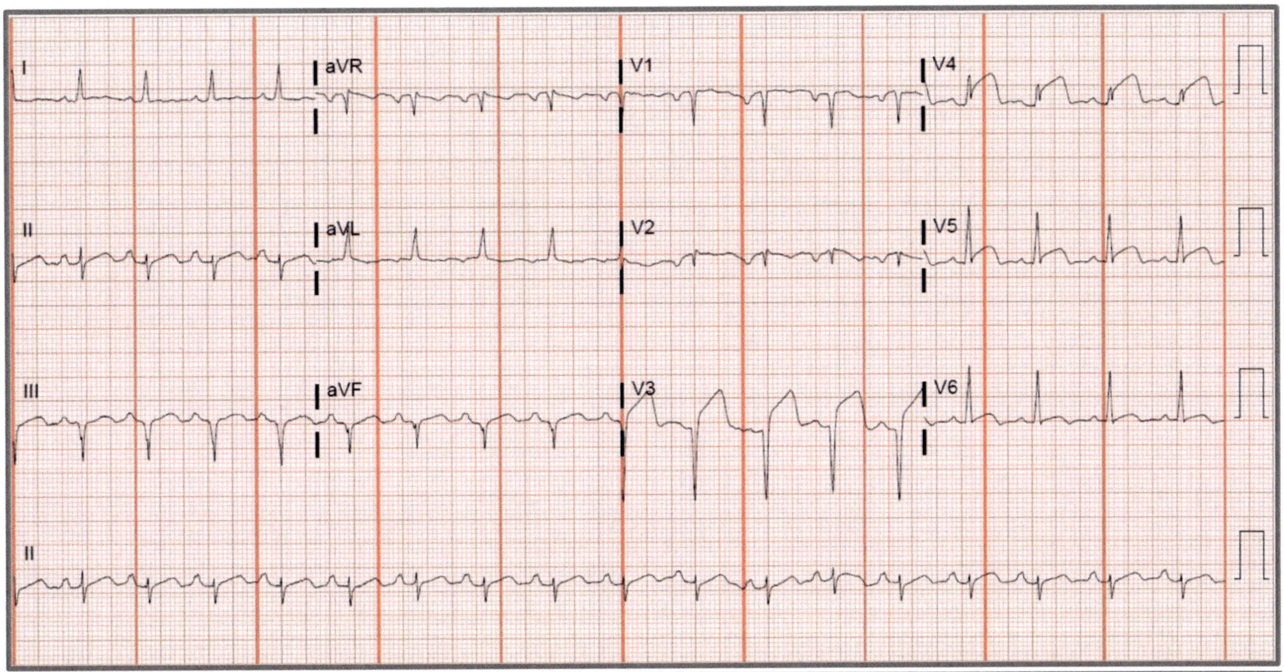

Rate: Rhythm: Axis: Intervals: Ischemia:

#68 – 48-year-old male presents status post cardiac arrest

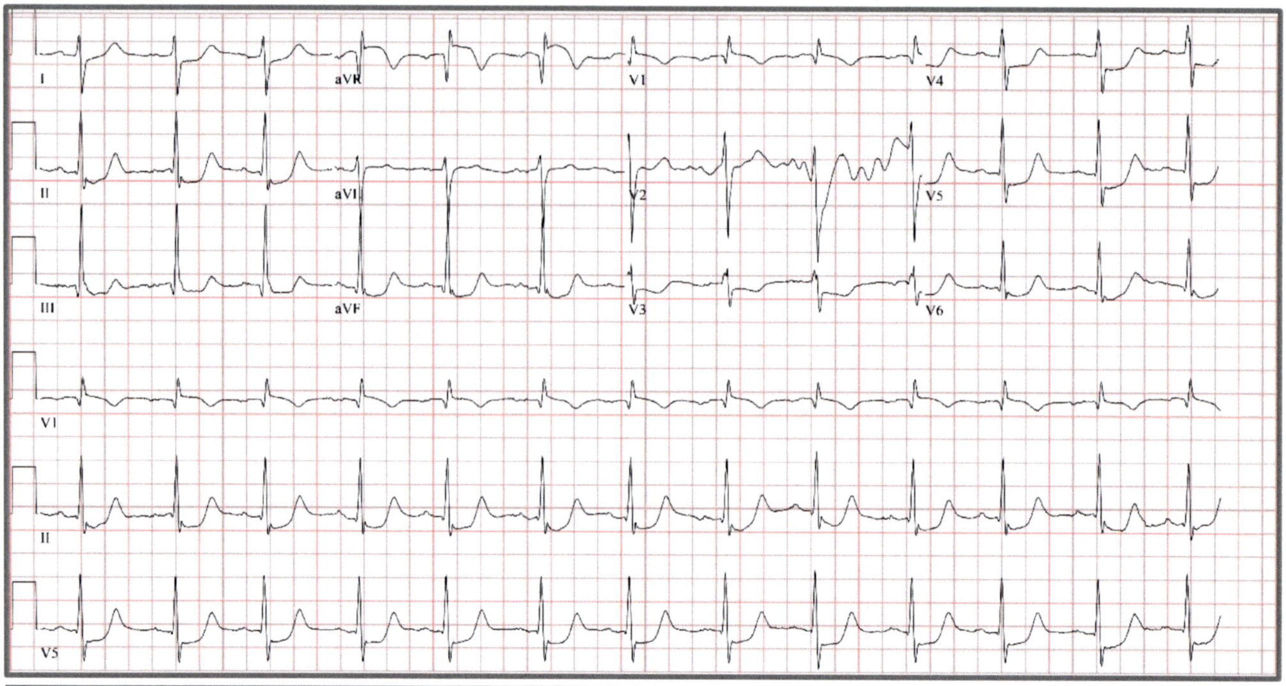

Rate: **Rhythm:** **Axis:** **Intervals:** **Ischemia:**

#69 – 31-year-old male presents with chest pain

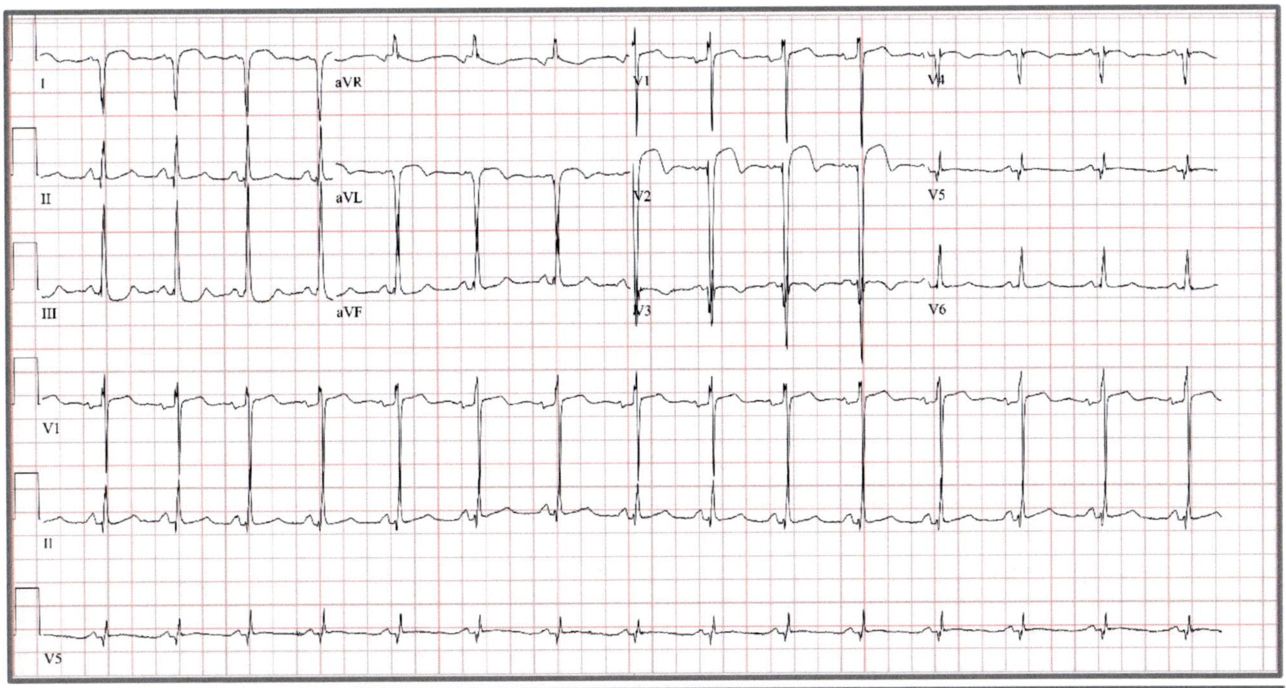

Rate: **Rhythm:** **Axis:** **Intervals:** **Ischemia:**

⇩ Prior ECG ⇩

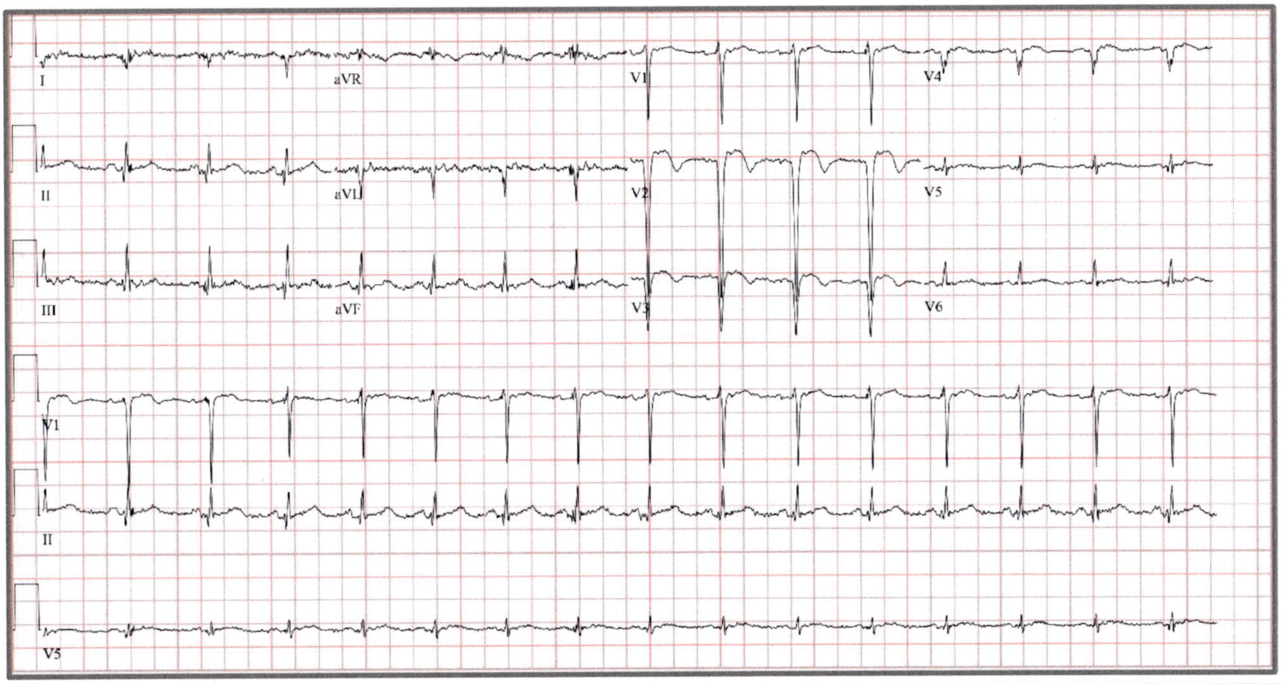

Rate: **Rhythm:** **Axis:** **Intervals:** **Ischemia:**

#70 – 9-month-old female presents with cough

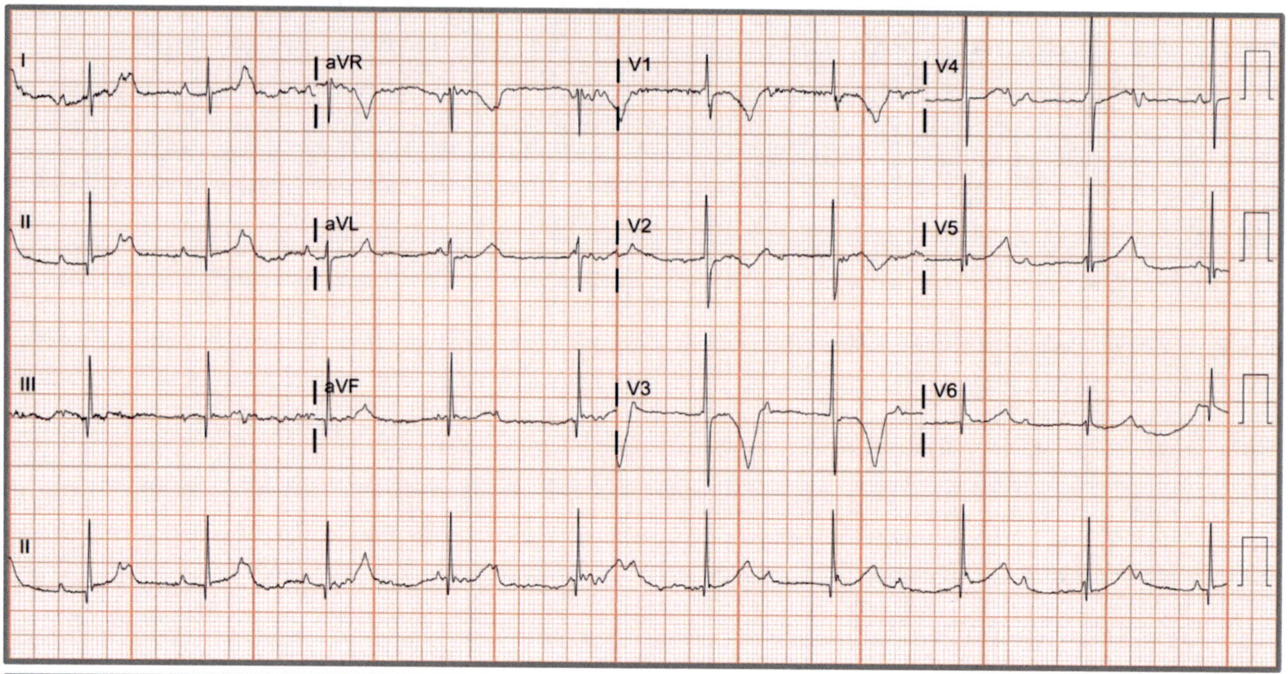

Rate:	**Rhythm:**	**Axis:**	**Intervals:**	**Ischemia:**

#71 – 41-year-old male presents with chest pain

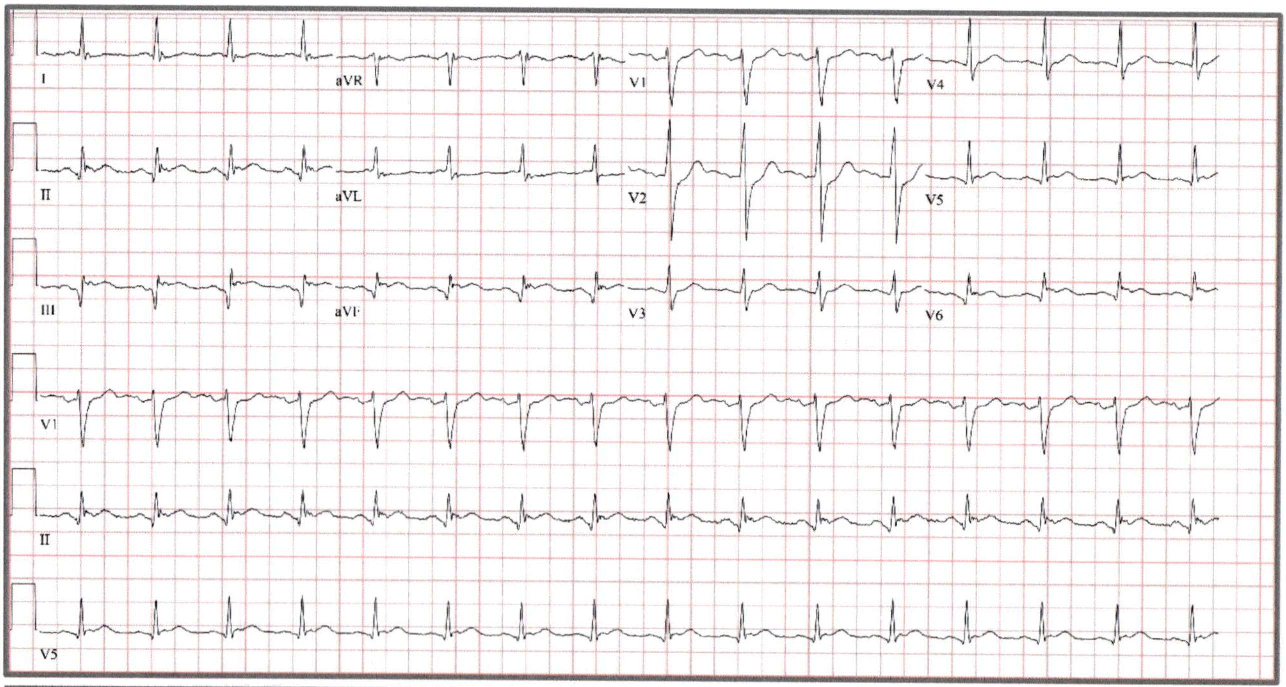

Rate:	**Rhythm:**	**Axis:**	**Intervals:**	**Ischemia:**

#72 – 63-year-old male presents with dyspnea

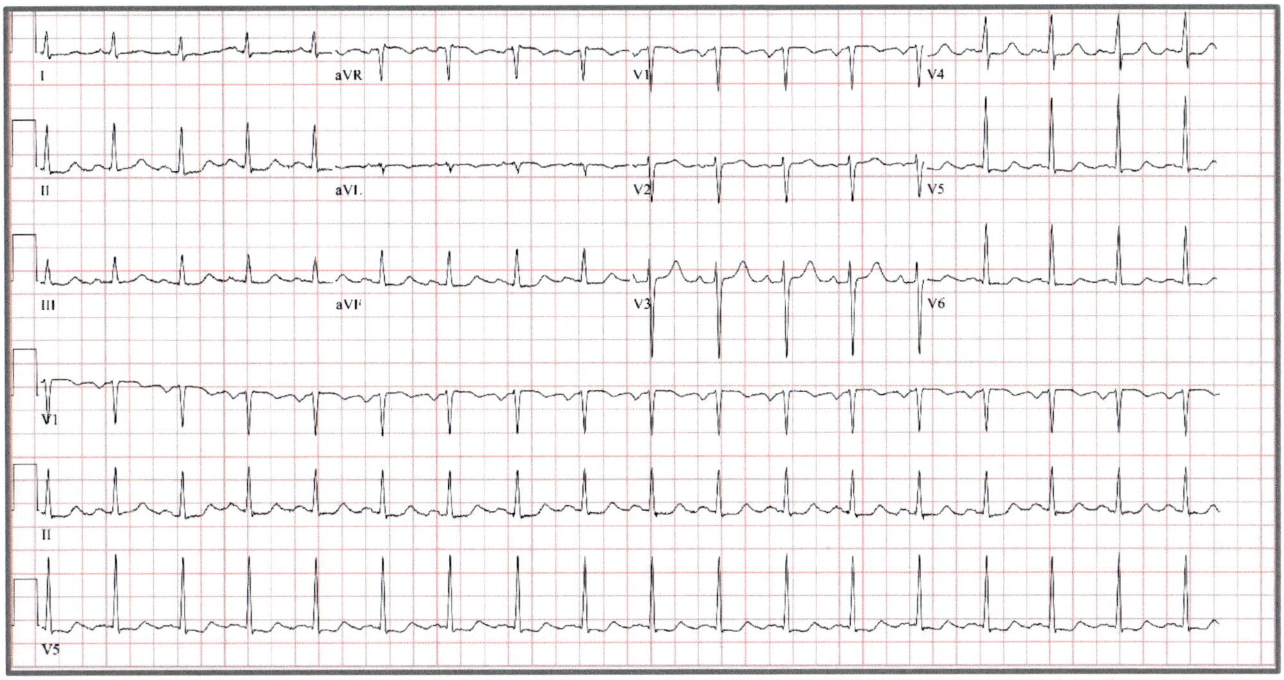

Rate:		Rhythm:		Axis:		Intervals:		Ischemia:	

#73 – 89-year-old male presents with episodic dizziness

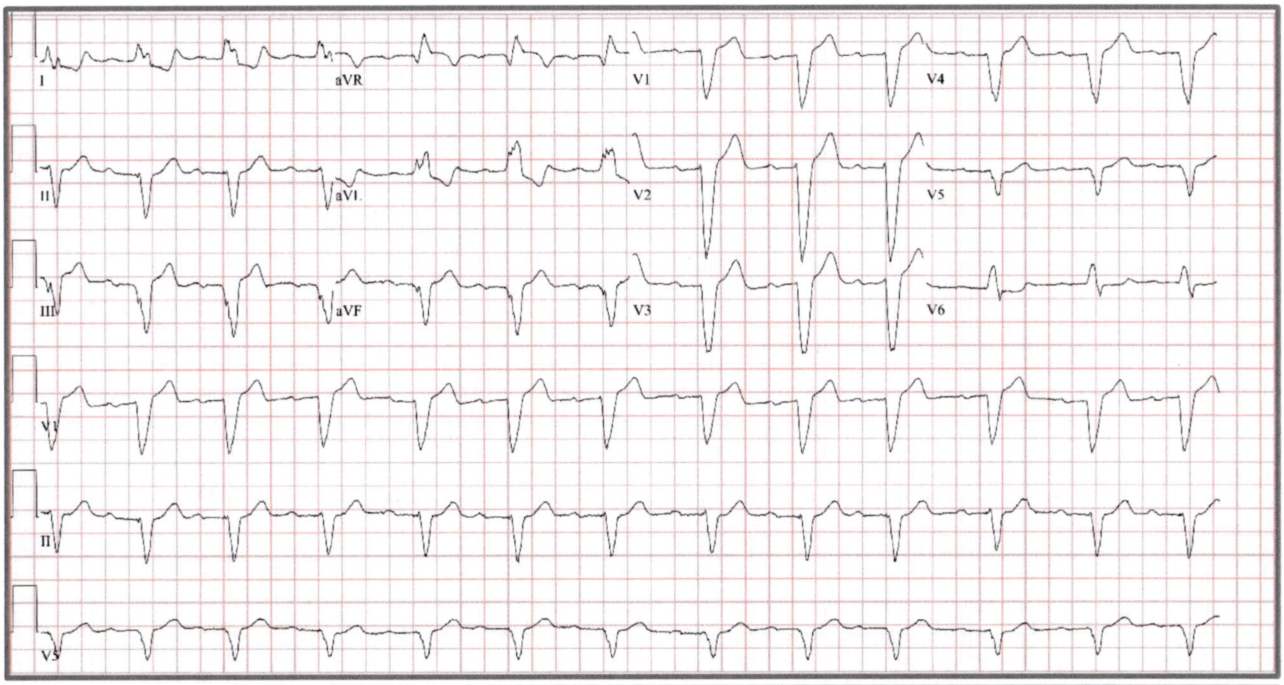

Rate:		Rhythm:		Axis:		Intervals:		Ischemia:	

#74 – 70-year-old male presents with altered mental status

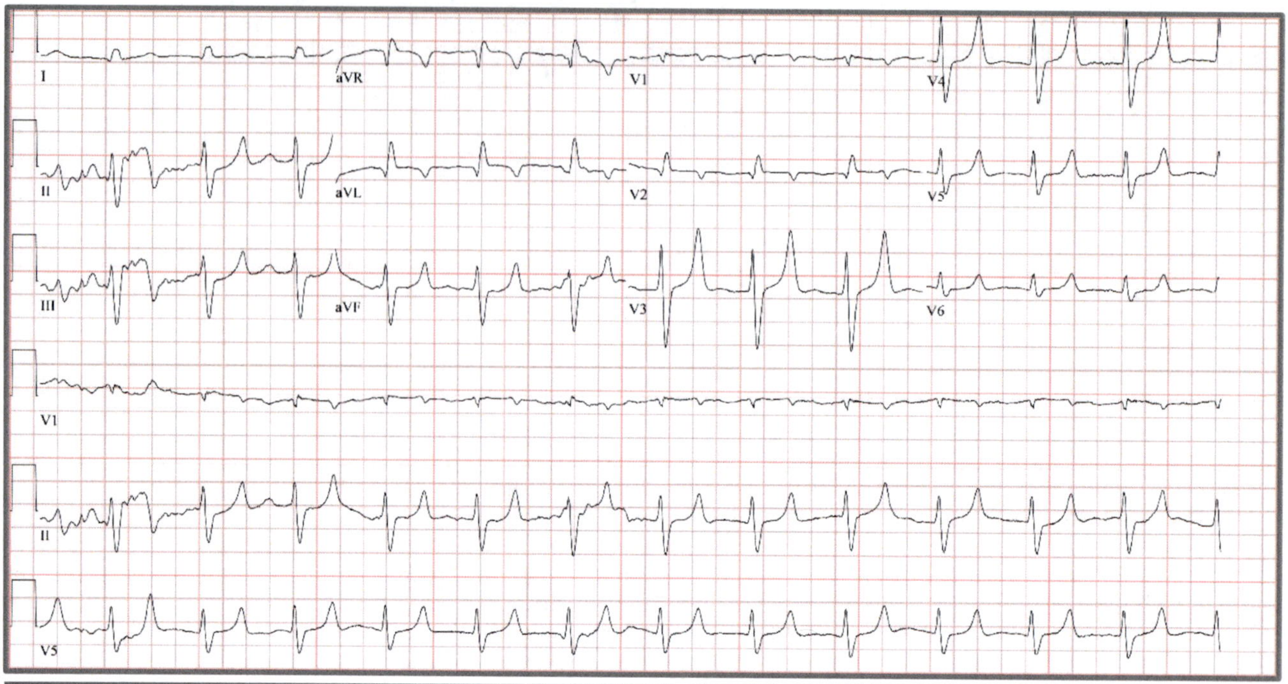

Rate:	**Rhythm:**	**Axis:**	**Intervals:**	**Ischemia:**

#75 – 30-year-old male presents with altered mental status

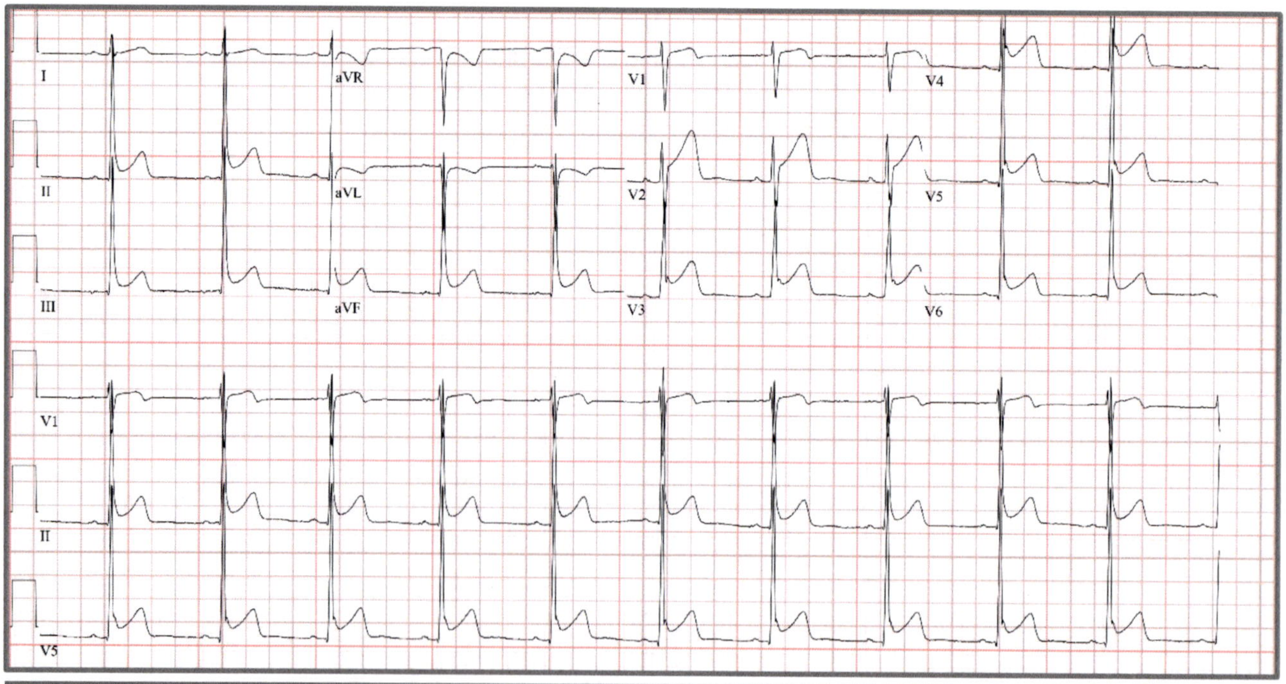

Rate:	**Rhythm:**	**Axis:**	**Intervals:**	**Ischemia:**

#76 – 74-year-old male presents with altered mental status

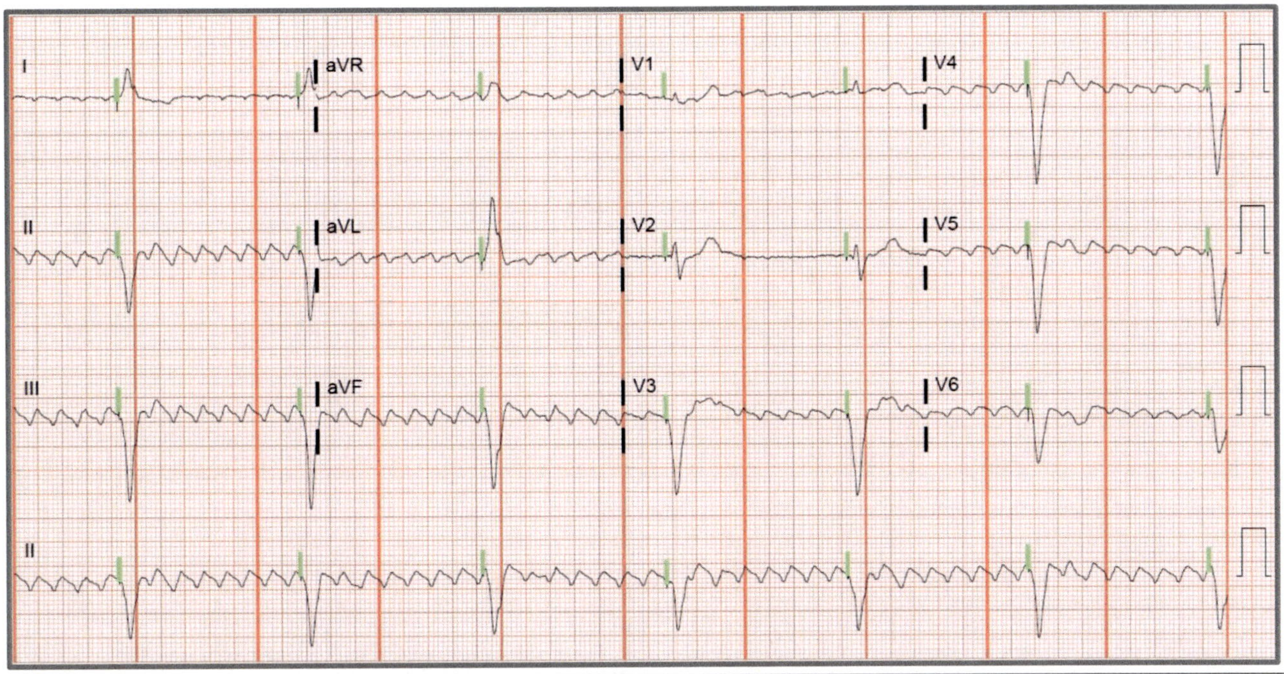

Rate: Rhythm: Axis: Intervals: Ischemia:

#77 – 83-year-old female presents with dizziness

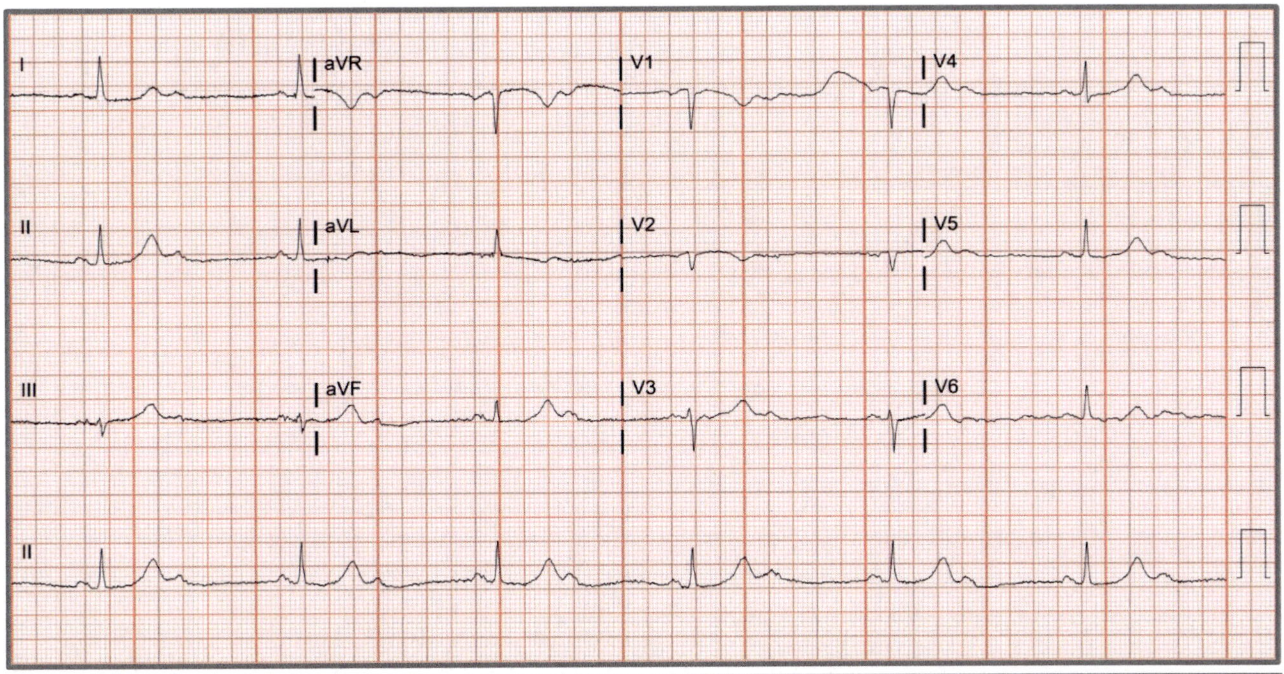

Rate: Rhythm: Axis: Intervals: Ischemia:

#78 – 58-year-old female presents with chest pain

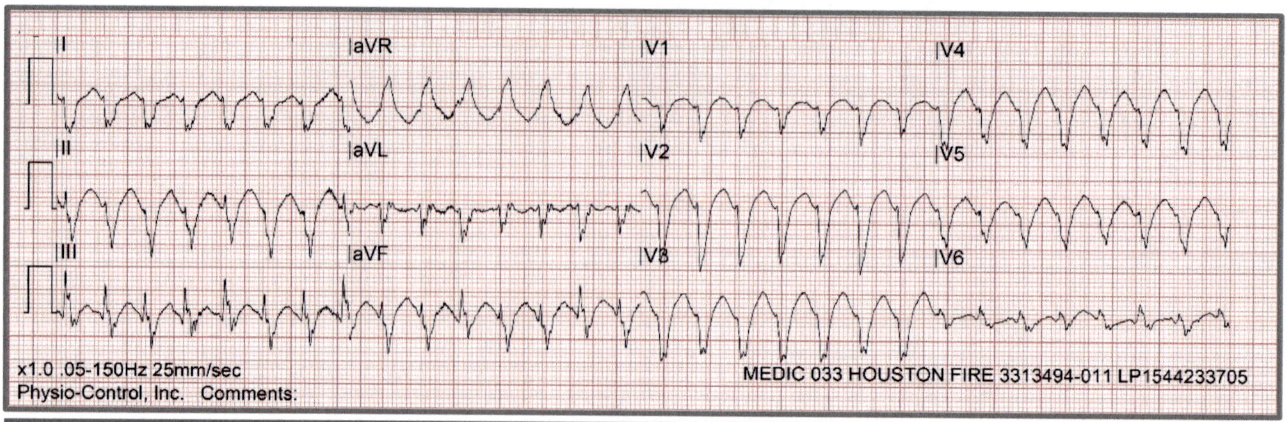

Rate: Rhythm: Axis: Intervals: Ischemia:

#79 – 59-year-old male presents with chest pain

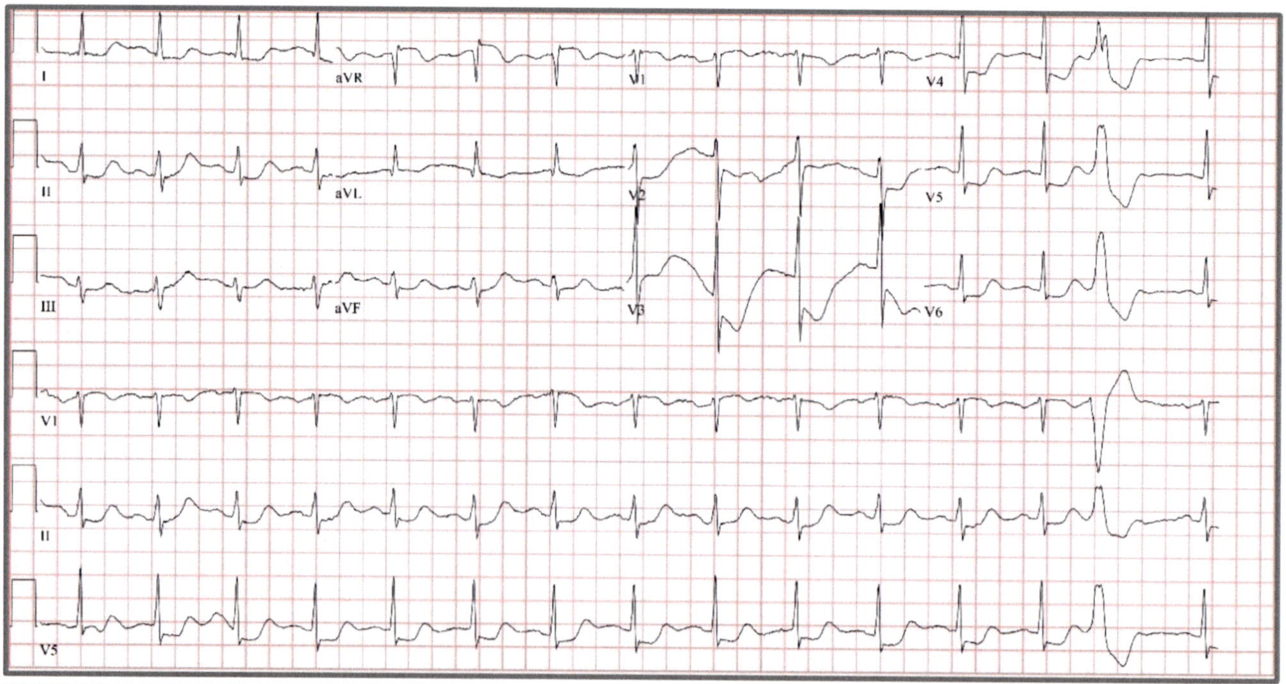

Rate: Rhythm: Axis: Intervals: Ischemia:

#80 – 79-year-old male presents with left shoulder pain

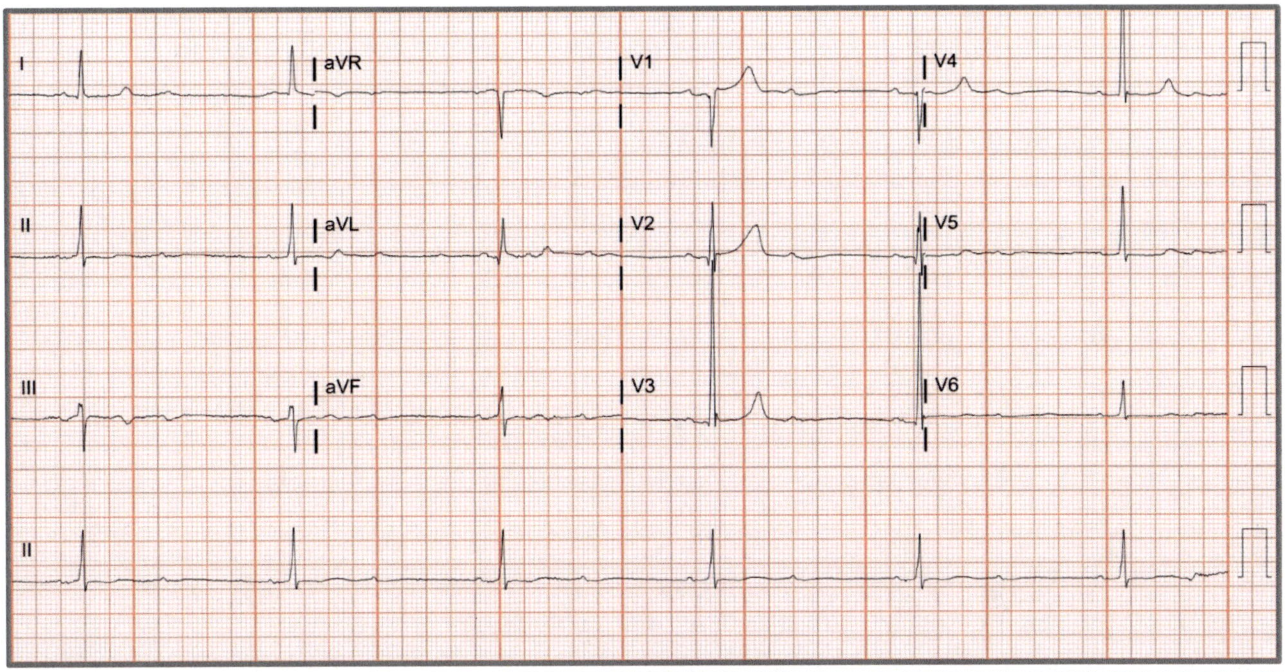

Rate:	Rhythm:	Axis:	Intervals:	Ischemia:

⇩ Repeat ECG ⇩

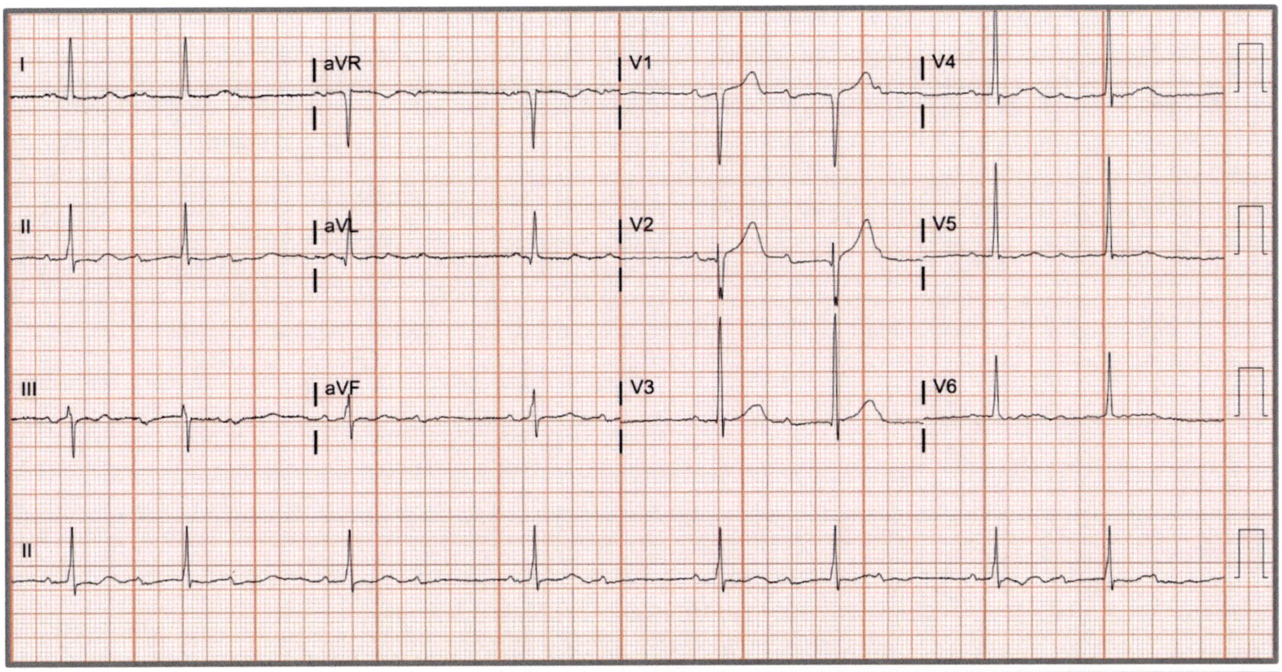

Rate:	Rhythm:	Axis:	Intervals:	Ischemia:

#81 – 65-year-old male presents with altered mental status

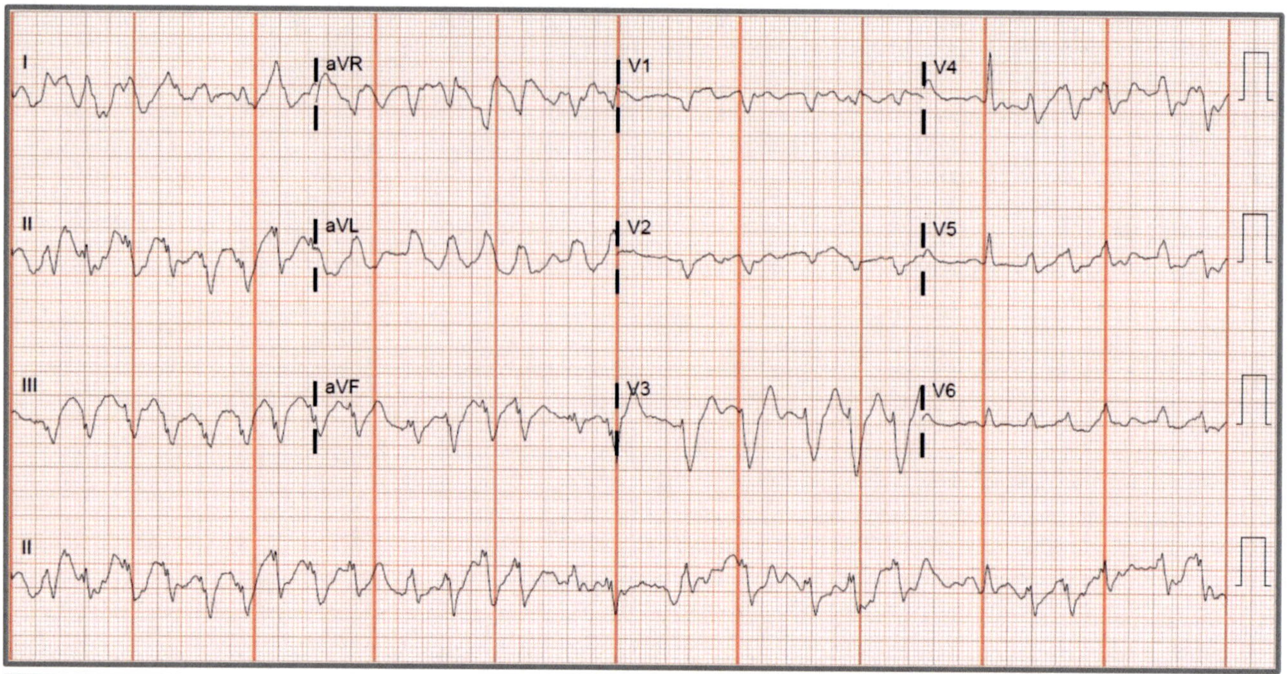

Rate: **Rhythm:** **Axis:** **Intervals:** **Ischemia:**

#82 – 39-year-old female presents with abdominal pain

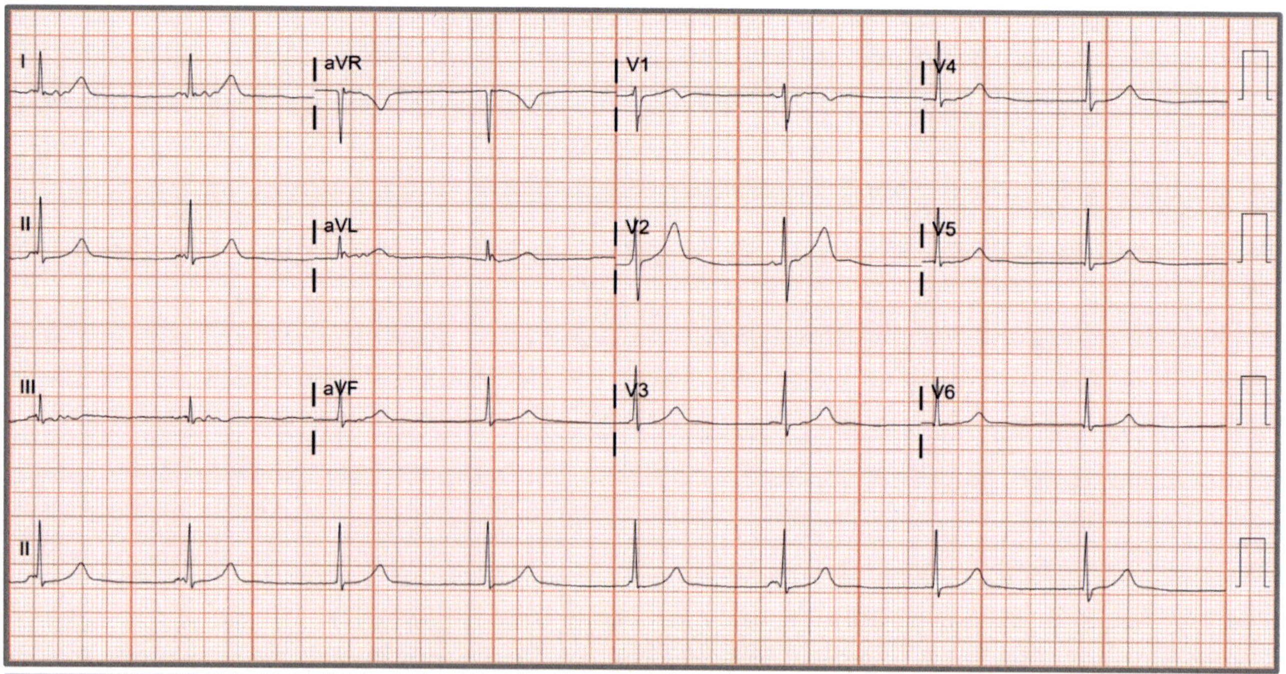

Rate: **Rhythm:** **Axis:** **Intervals:** **Ischemia:**

#83 – 47-year-old male presents with dizziness

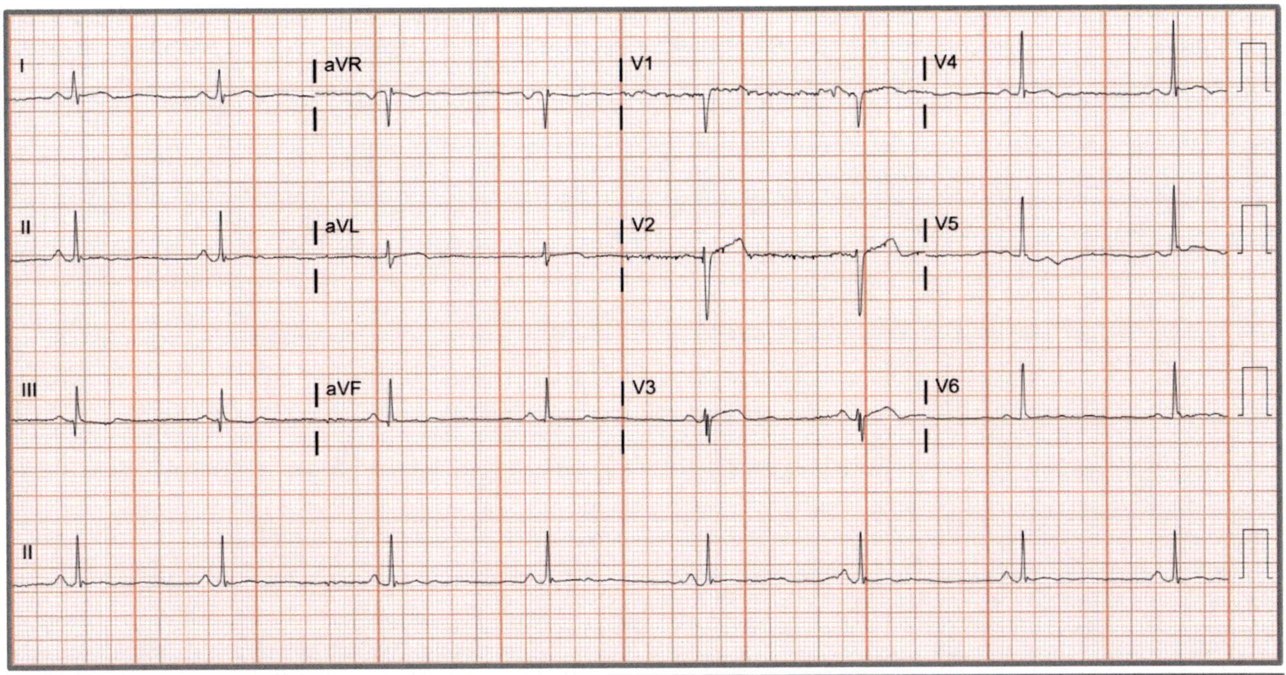

Rate: Rhythm: Axis: Intervals: Ischemia:

#84 – 50-year-old male presents with chest pain

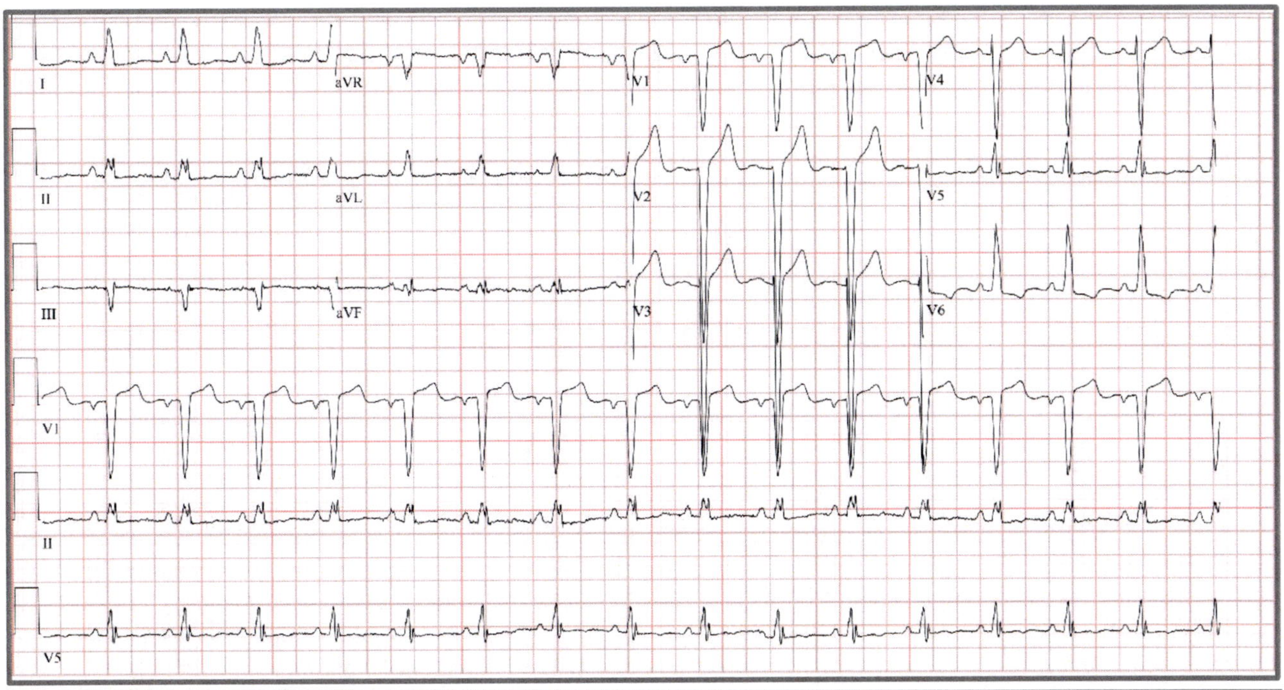

Rate: Rhythm: Axis: Intervals: Ischemia:

#85 – 83-year-old female presents with confusion

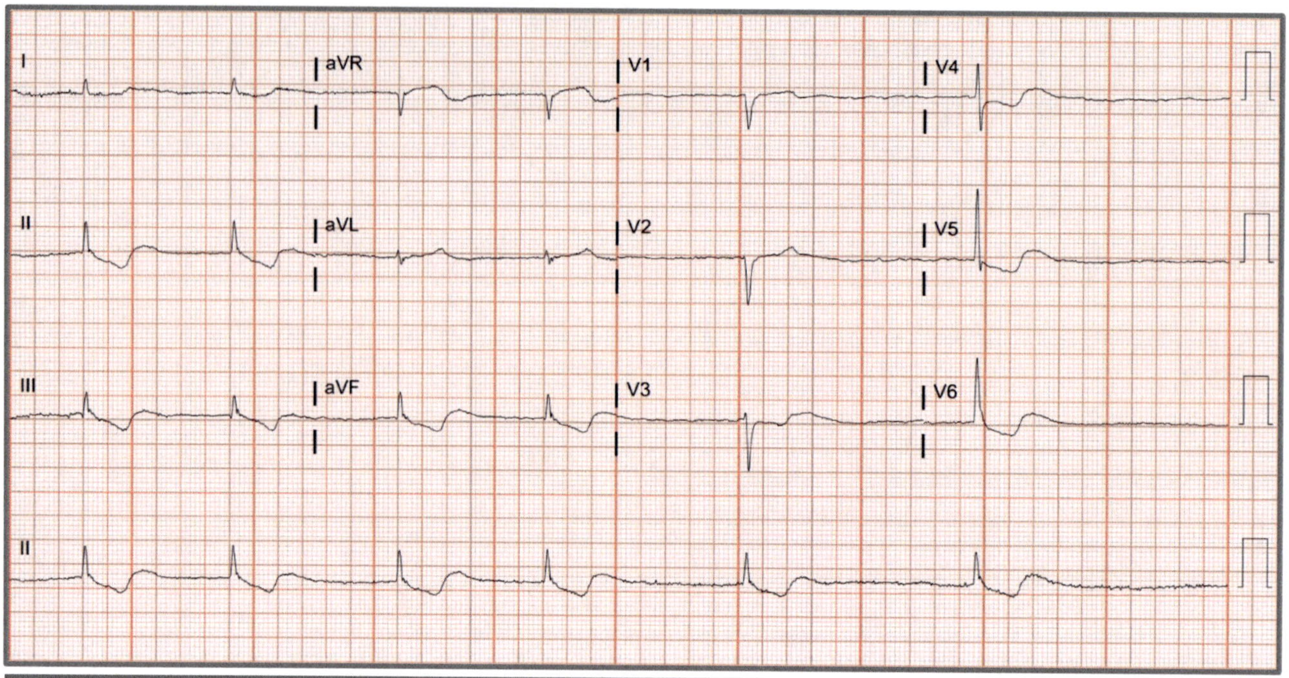

Rate: Rhythm: Axis: Intervals: Ischemia:

#86 – 57-year-old male presents with dyspnea

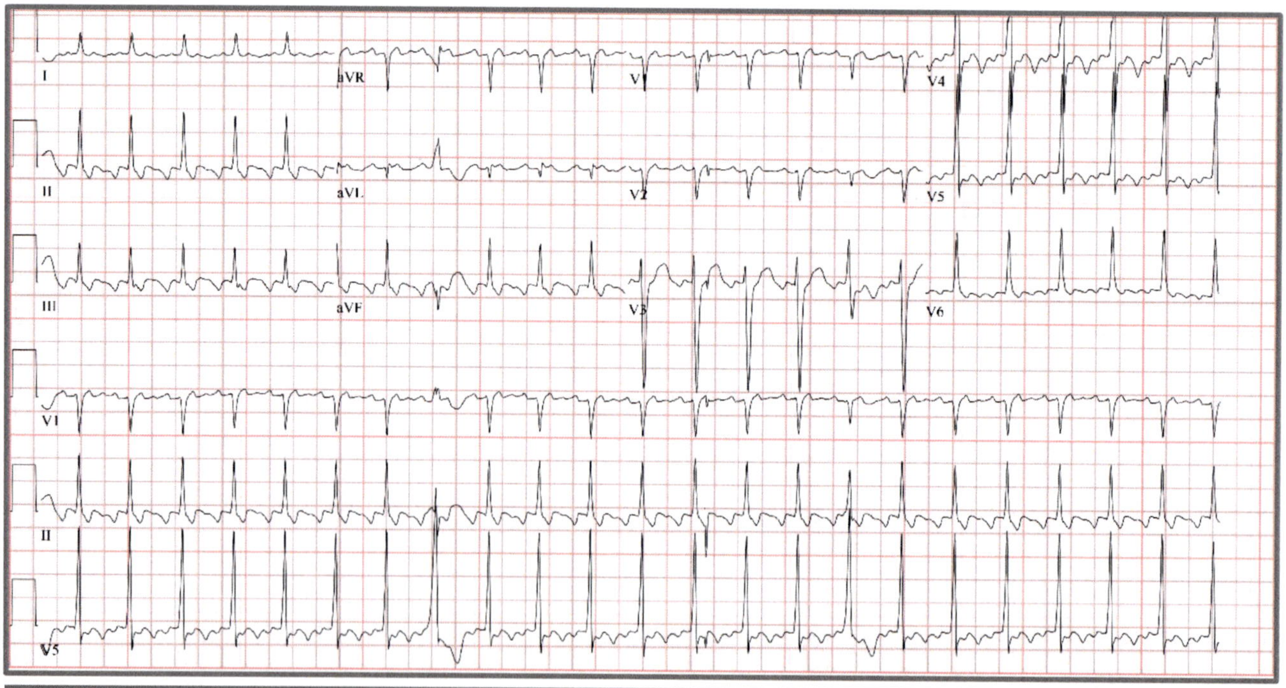

Rate: Rhythm: Axis: Intervals: Ischemia:

#87 – 65-year-old female presents with chest pain

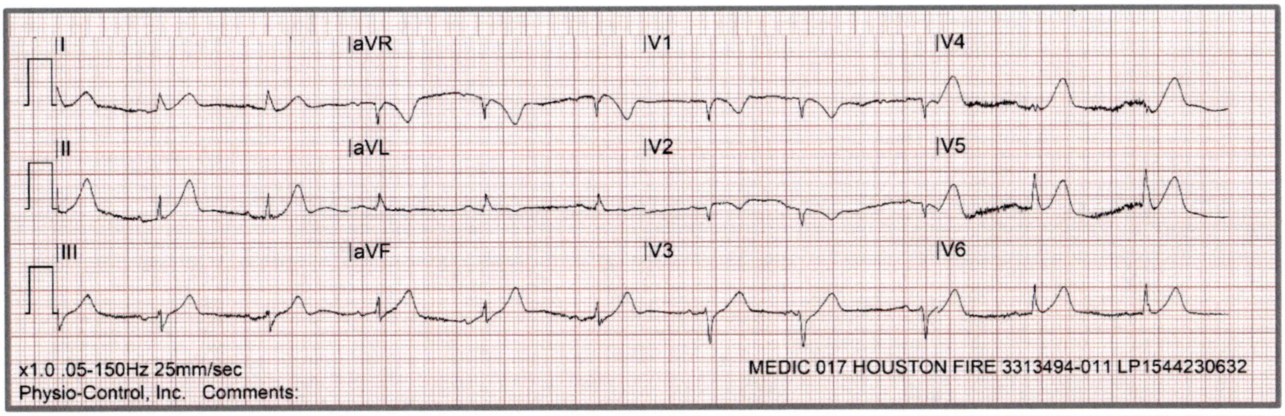

Rate: Rhythm: Axis: Intervals: Ischemia:

#88 – 77-year-old male presents with syncope

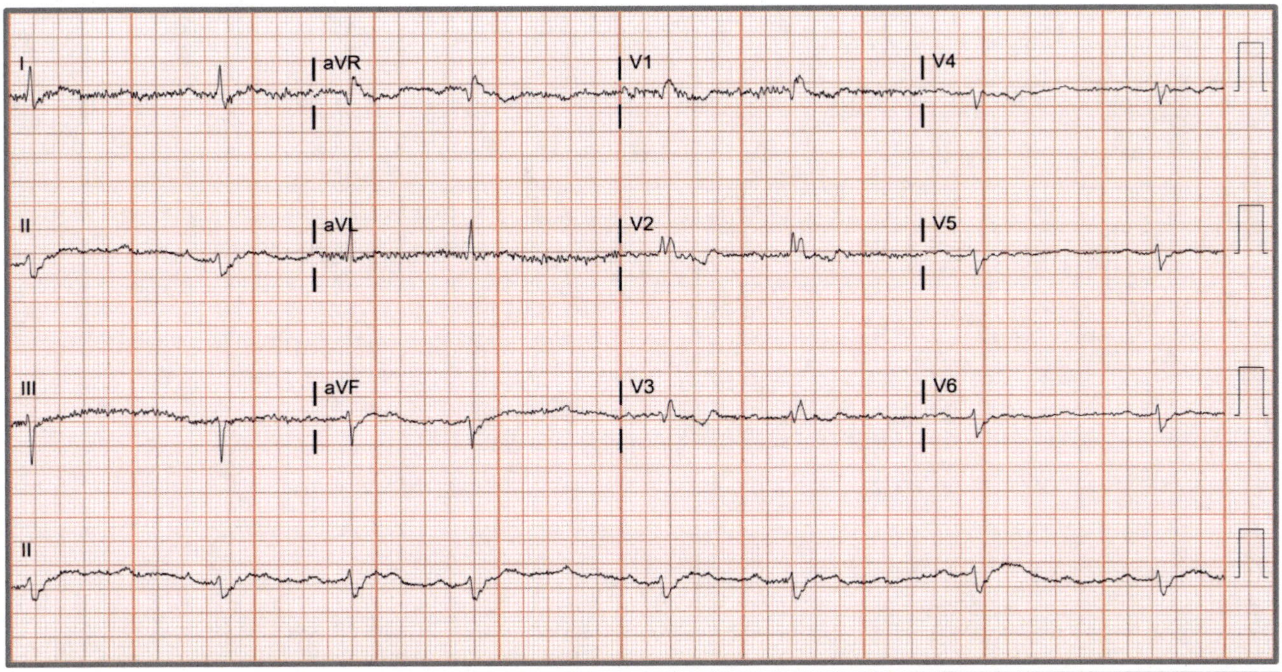

Rate: Rhythm: Axis: Intervals: Ischemia:

#89 – 63-year-old male presents with chest pain

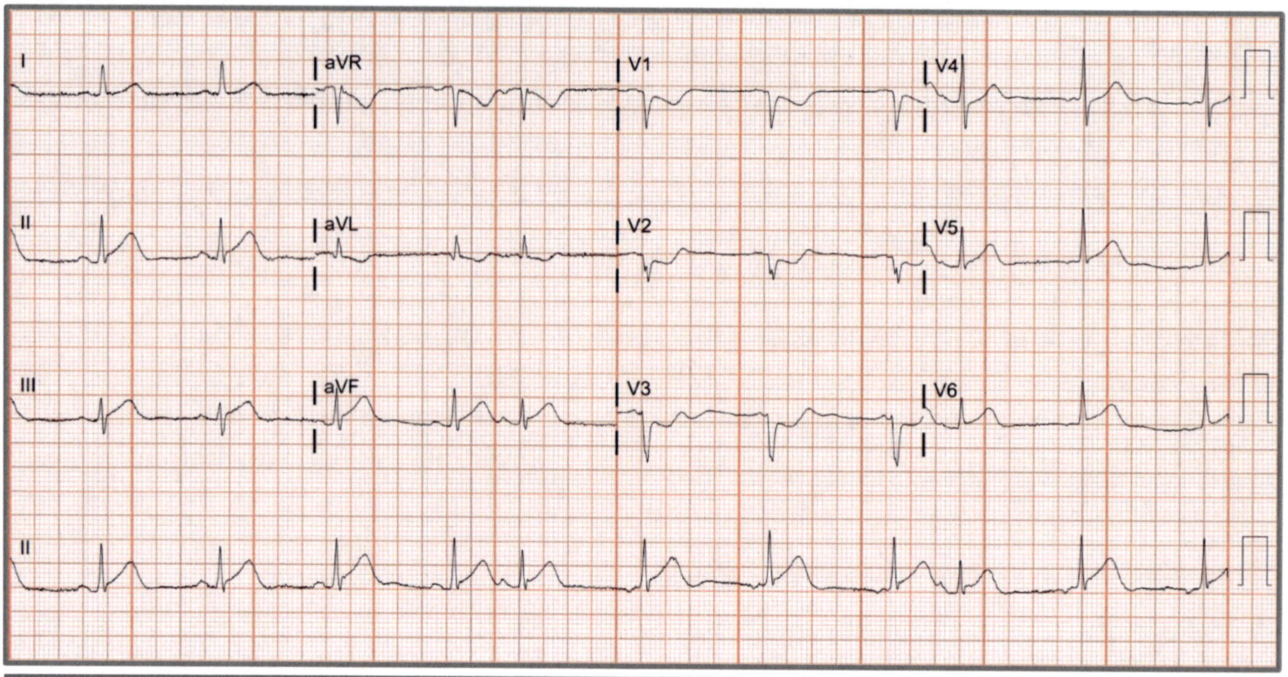

Rate: Rhythm: Axis: Intervals: Ischemia:

#90 – 87-year-old male presents with chest pain and dyspnea

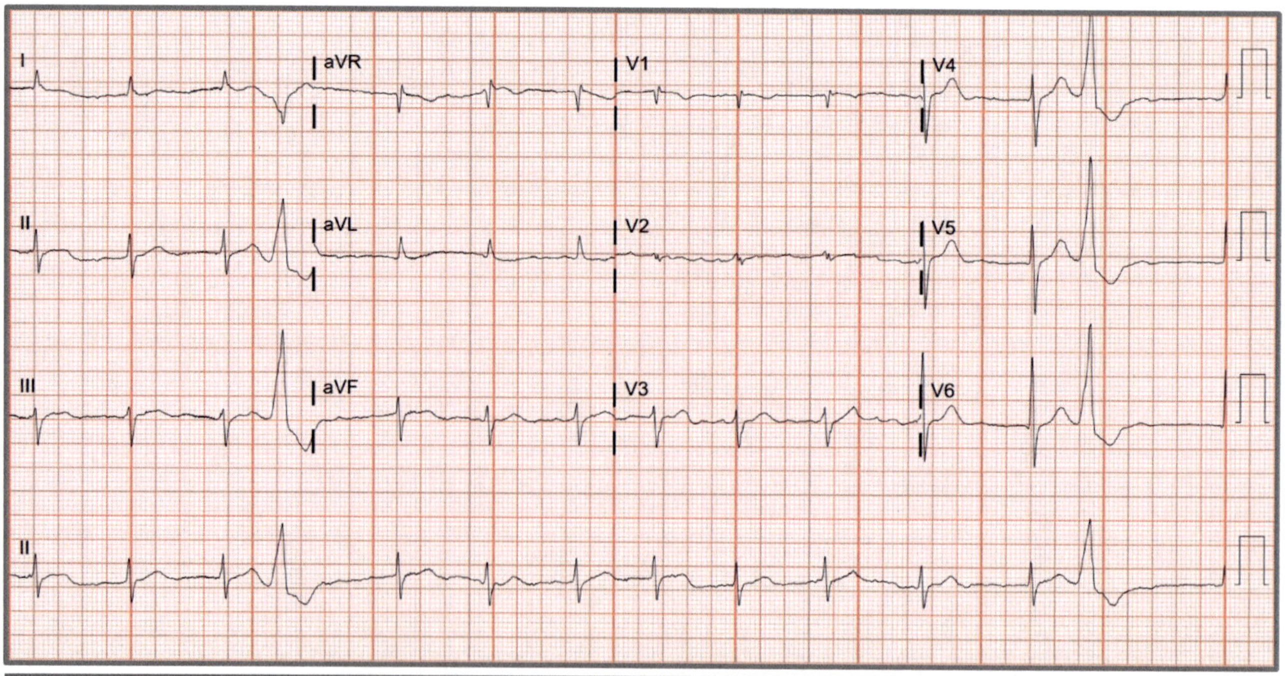

Rate: Rhythm: Axis: Intervals: Ischemia:

#91 – 58-year-old male presents with dizziness

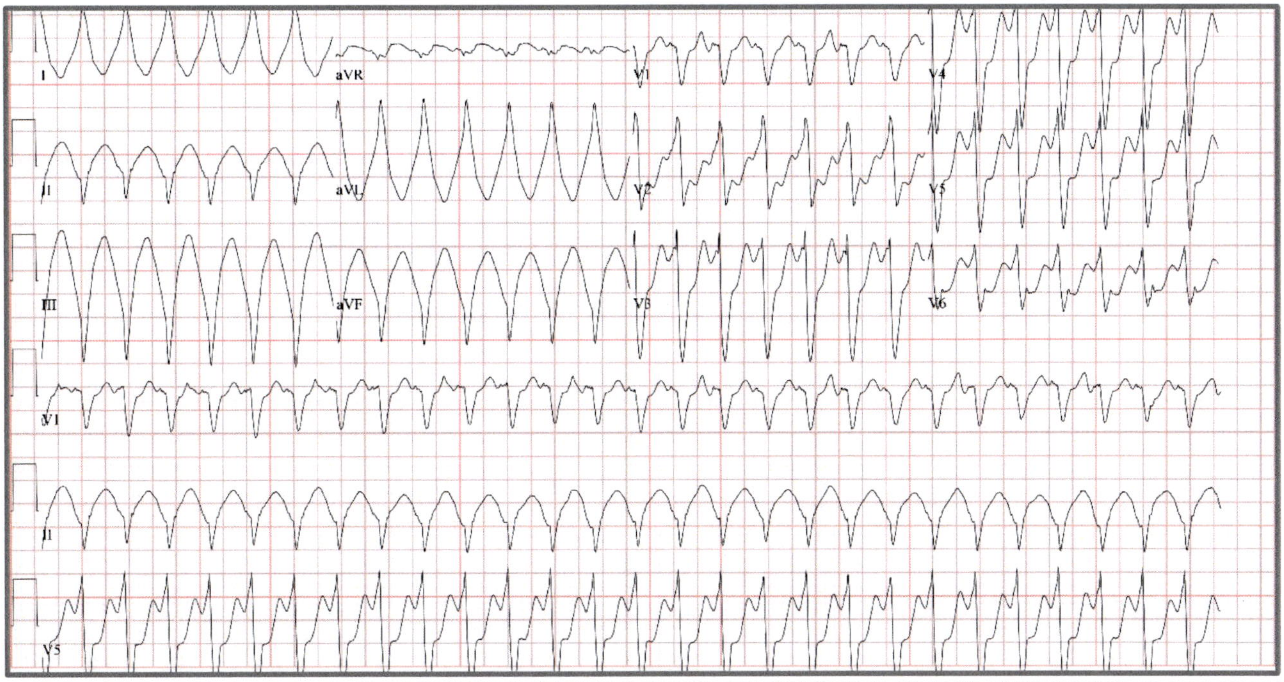

Rate: **Rhythm:** **Axis:** **Intervals:** **Ischemia:**

#92 – 63-year-old male presents with syncope

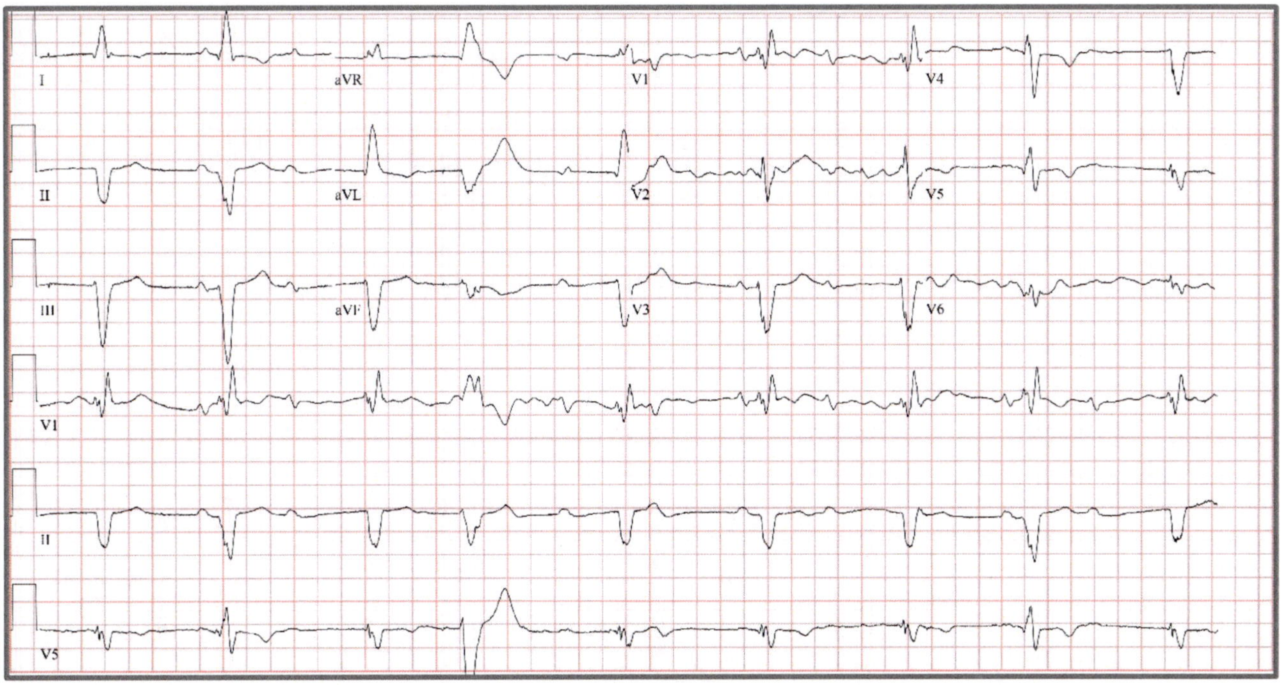

Rate: **Rhythm:** **Axis:** **Intervals:** **Ischemia:**

#93 – 57-year-old female presents with dyspnea

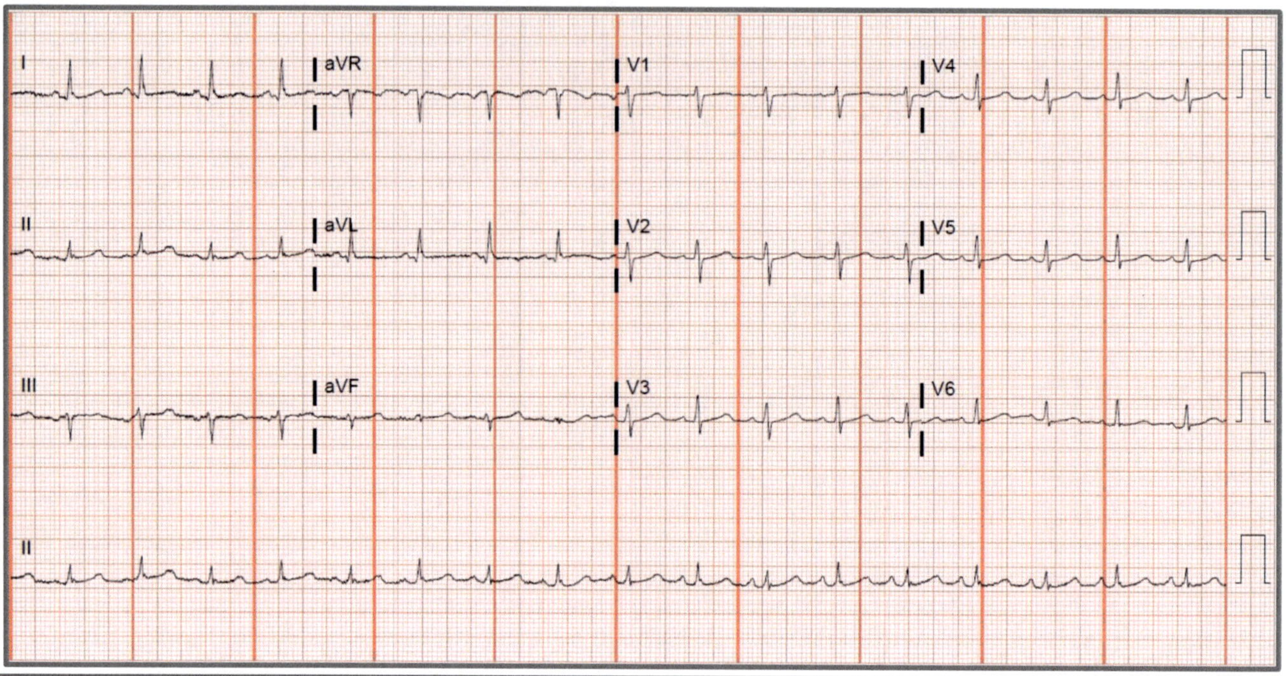

Rate: **Rhythm:** **Axis:** **Intervals:** **Ischemia:**

#94 – 58-year-old male presents with palpitations

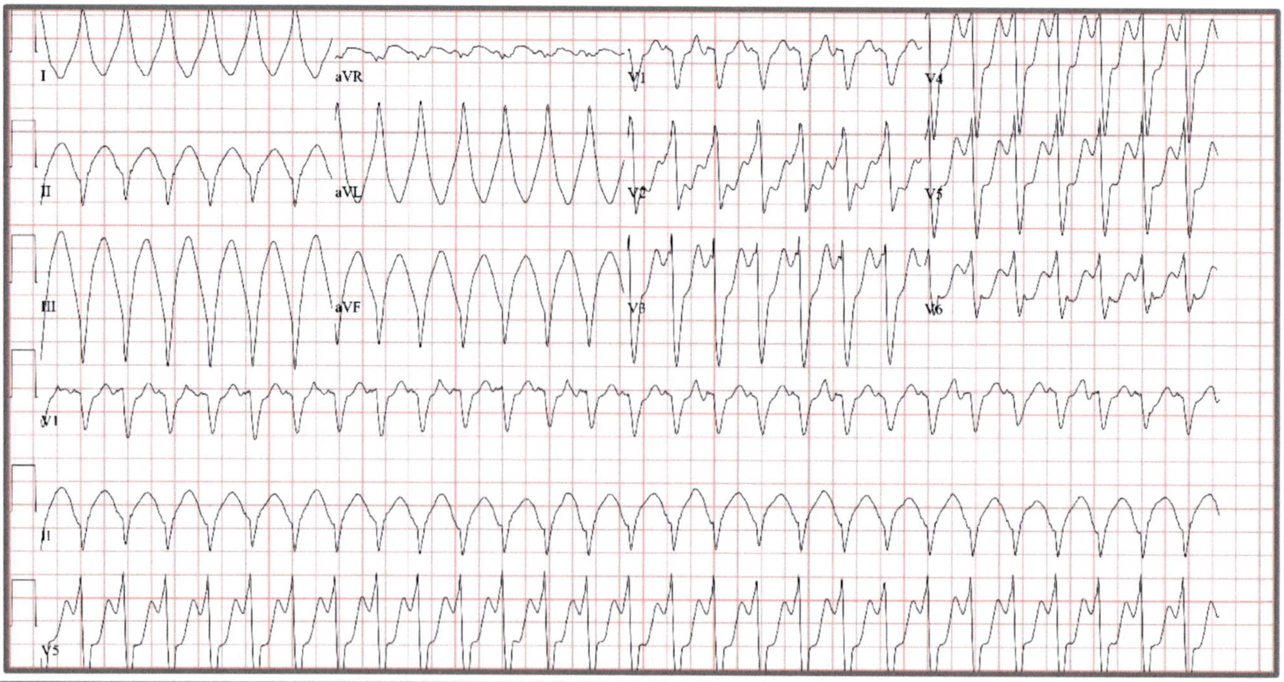

Rate: **Rhythm:** **Axis:** **Intervals:** **Ischemia:**

#95 – 64-year-old male presents with chest pain

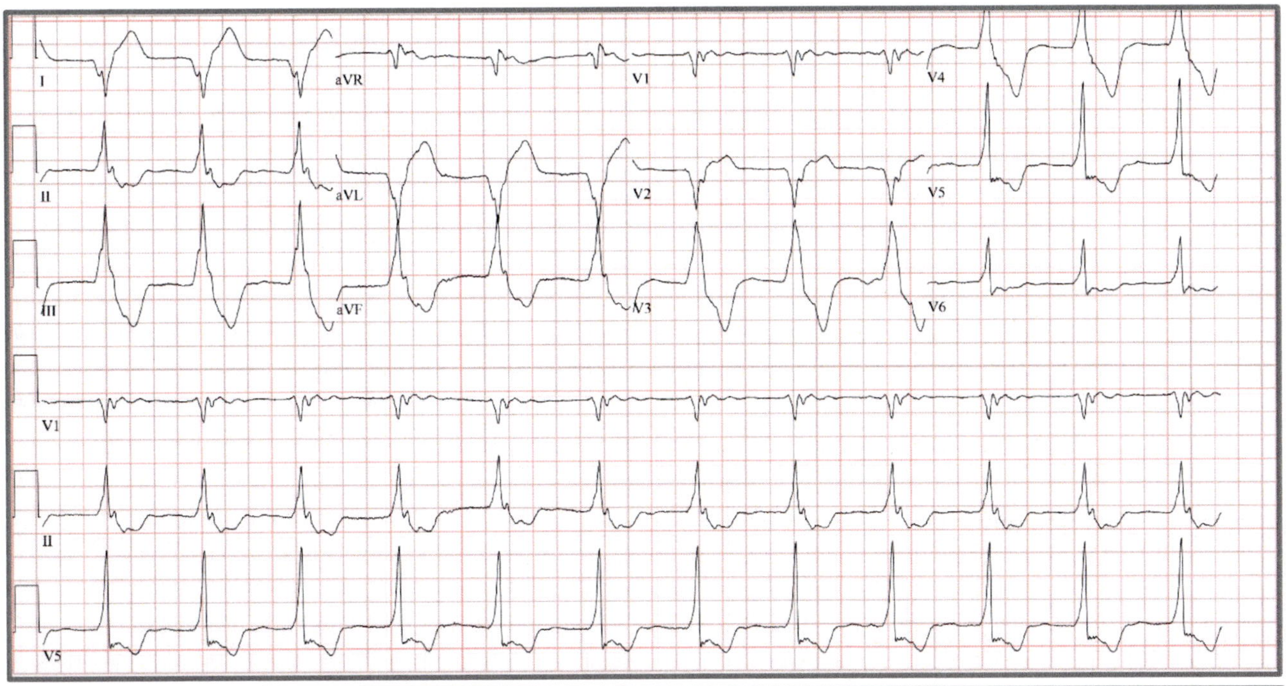

Rate: Rhythm: Axis: Intervals: Ischemia:

#96 – 63-year-old female presents with weakness

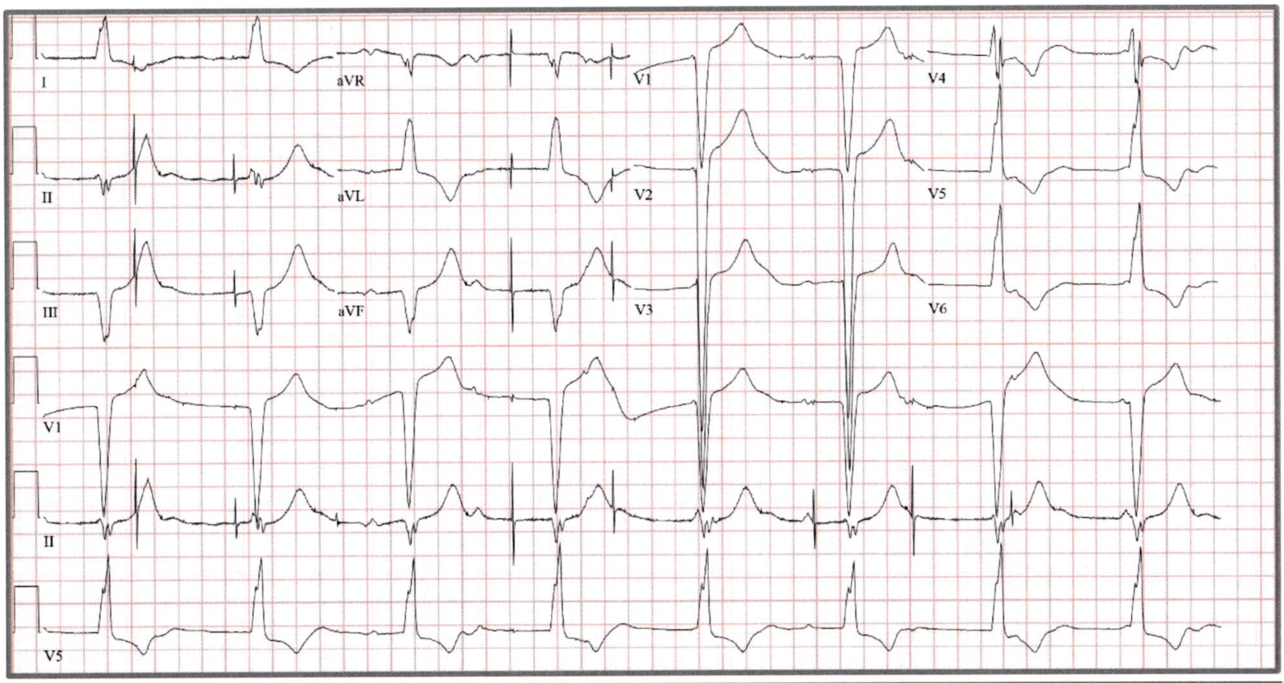

Rate: Rhythm: Axis: Intervals: Ischemia:

#97 – 42-year-old male presents with dyspnea

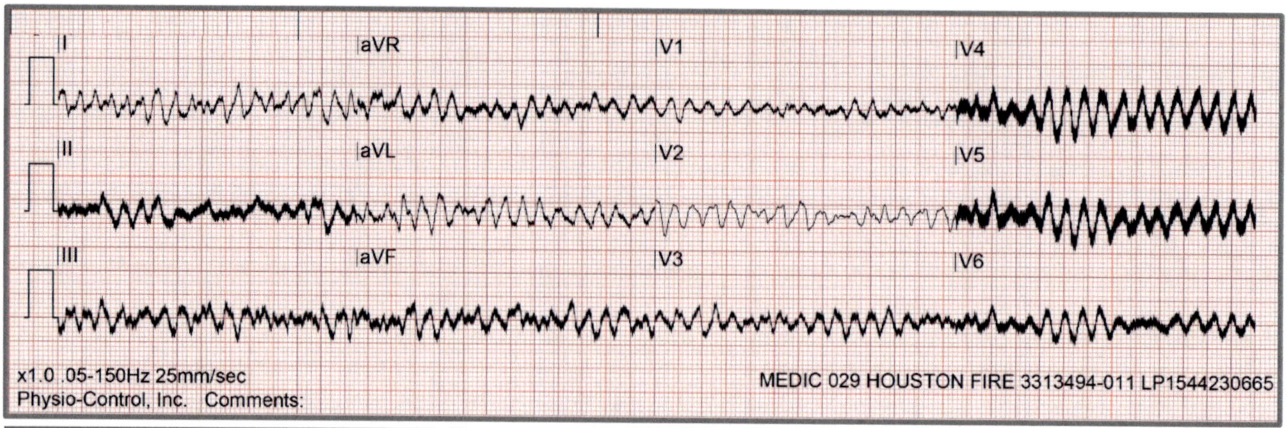

Rate: **Rhythm:** **Axis:** **Intervals:** **Ischemia:**

#98 – 58-year-old male presents with abdominal pain

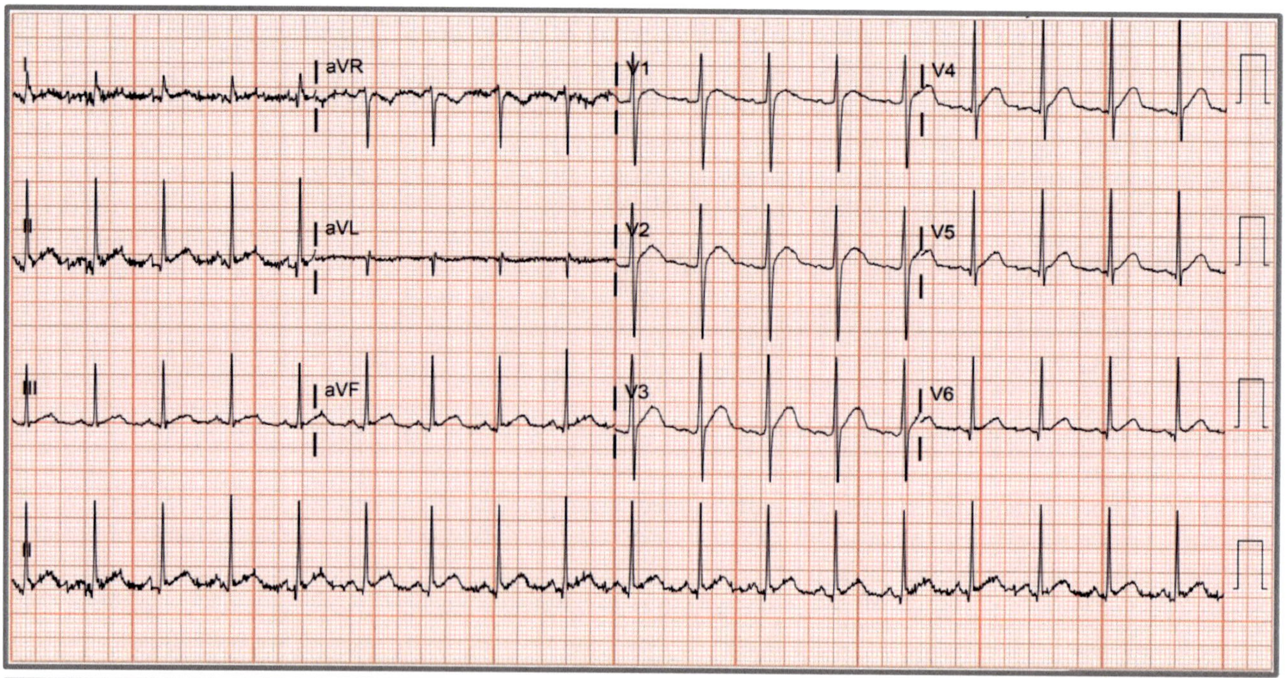

Rate: **Rhythm:** **Axis:** **Intervals:** **Ischemia:**

#99 – 58-year-old male presents with chest pain

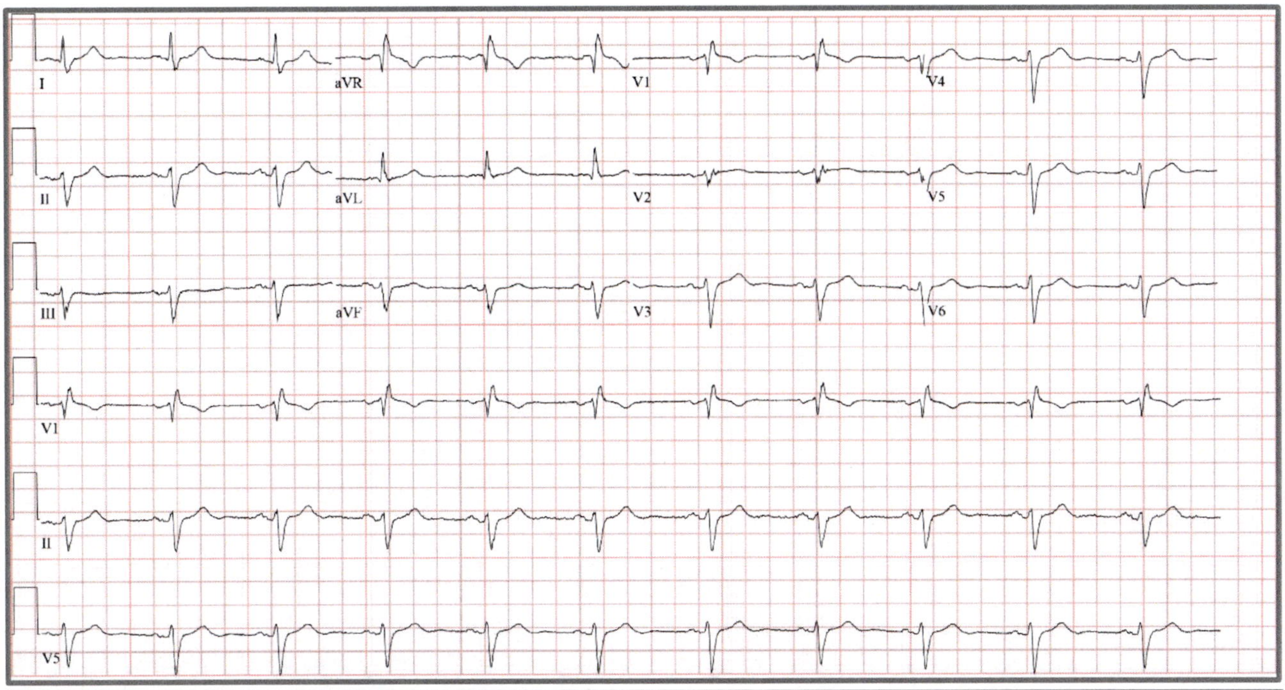

Rate: **Rhythm:** **Axis:** **Intervals:** **Ischemia:**

#100 – 39-year-old male presents with chest pain

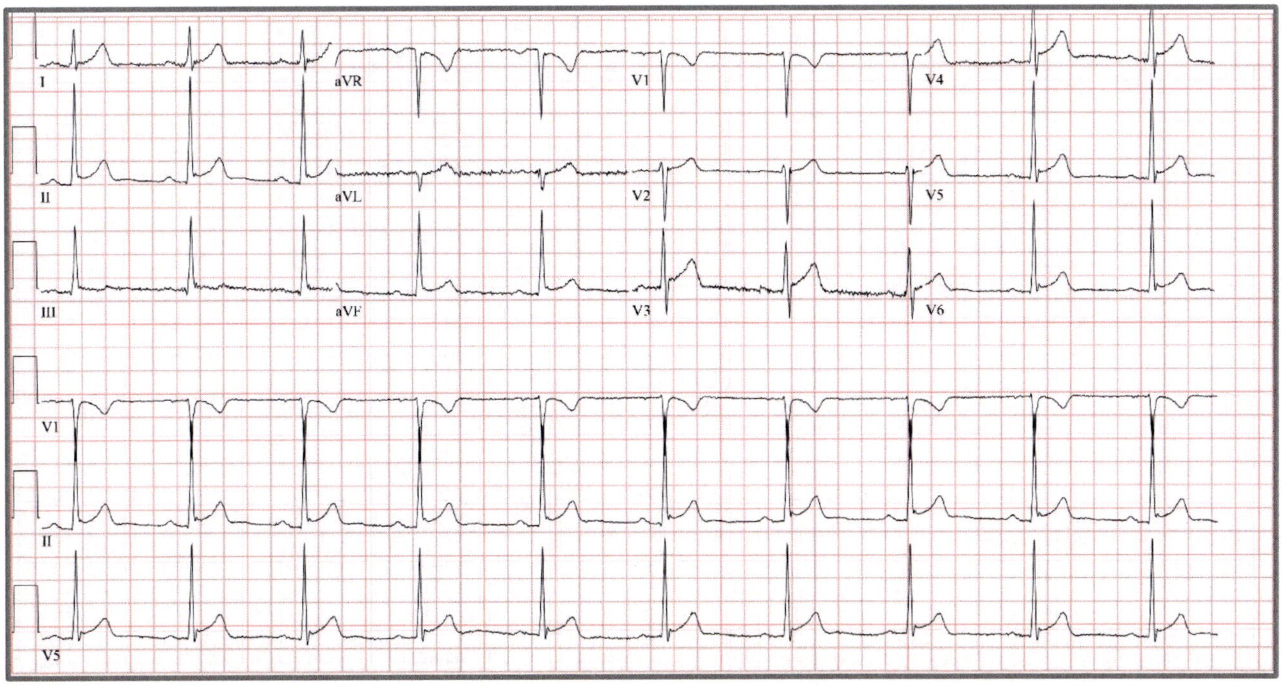

Rate: **Rhythm:** **Axis:** **Intervals:** **Ischemia:**

#101 – 45-year-old male presents with dyspnea

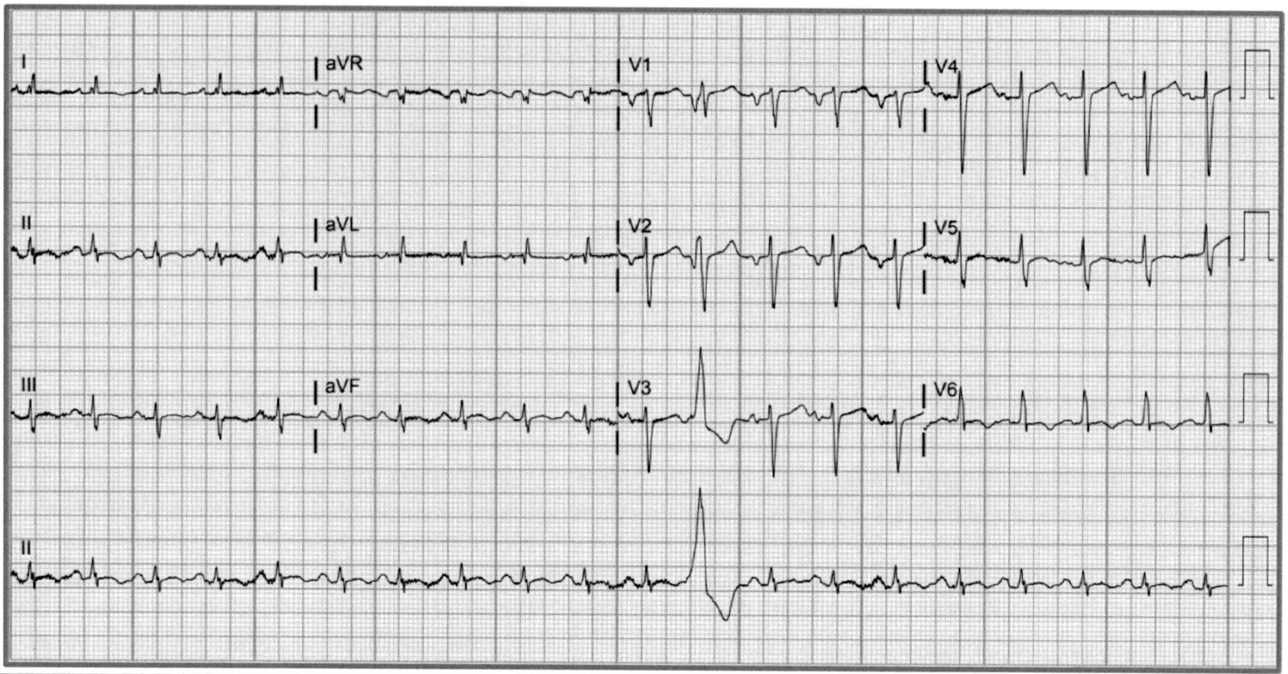

Rate: Rhythm: Axis: Intervals: Ischemia:

#102 – 20-year-old female presents with palpitations

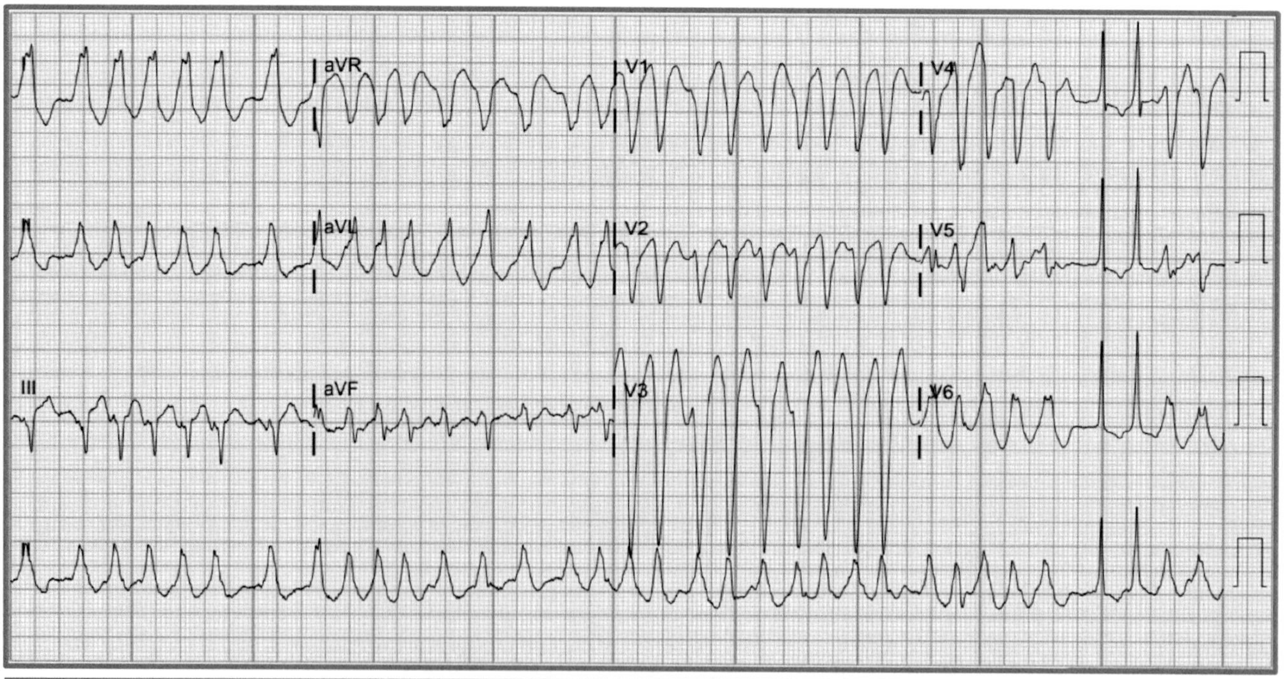

Rate: Rhythm: Axis: Intervals: Ischemia:

#103 – 64-year-old male presents with chest pain

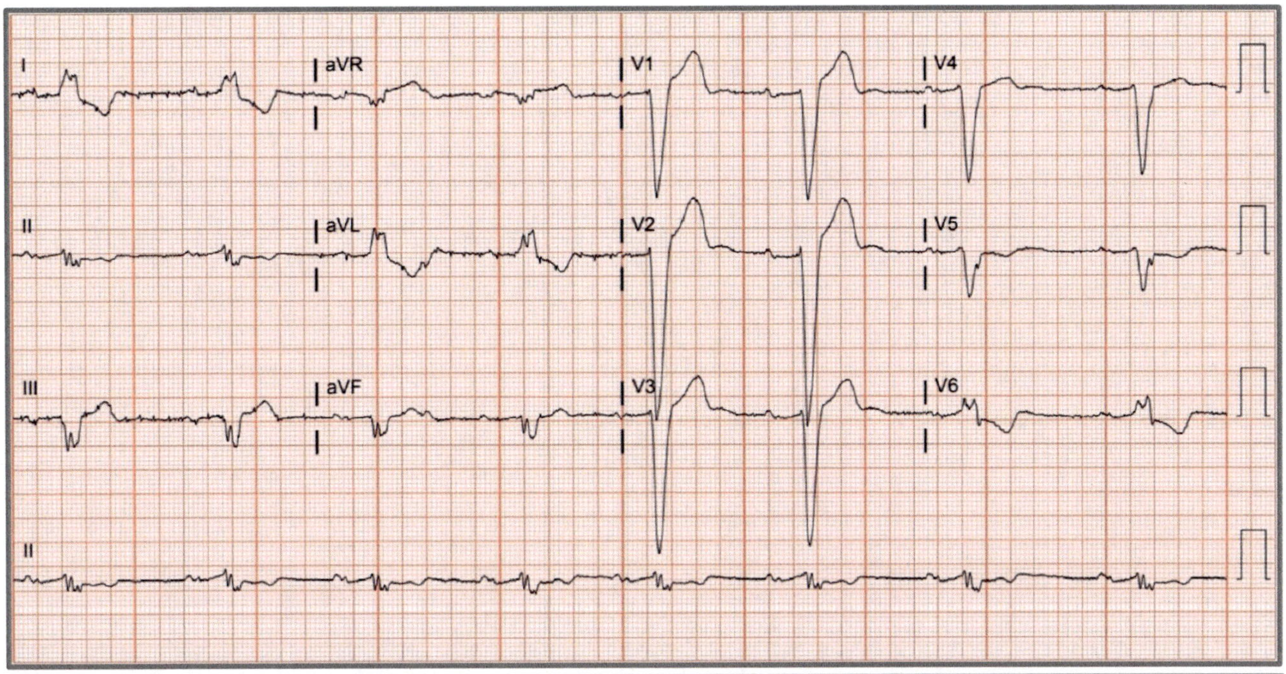

Rate: Rhythm: Axis: Intervals: Ischemia:

#104 – 80-year-old male presents with dyspnea

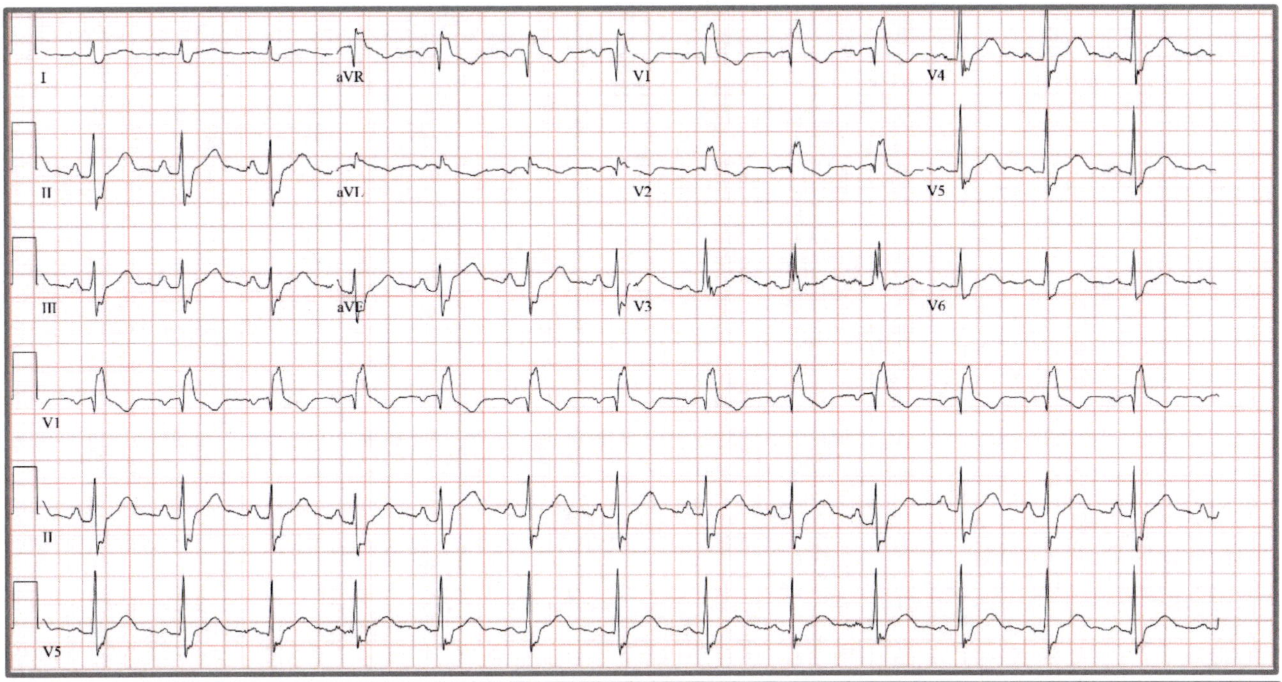

Rate: Rhythm: Axis: Intervals: Ischemia:

#105 – 18-year-old male presents with chest pain

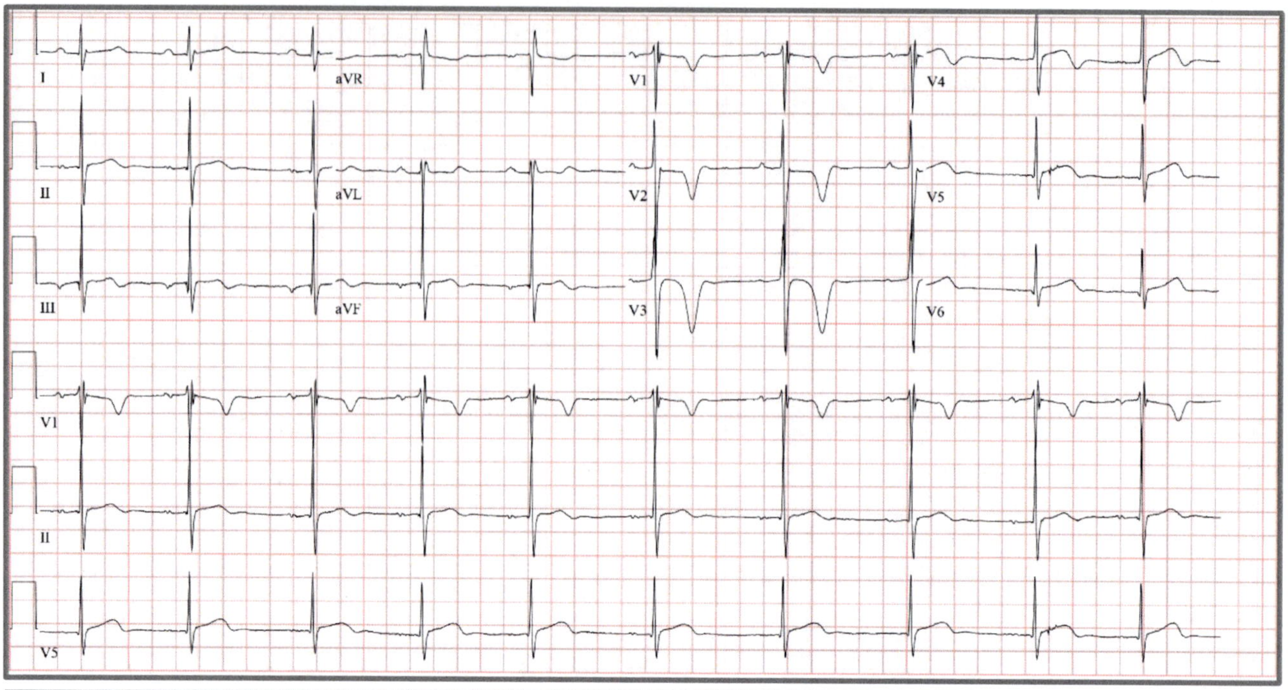

Rate: **Rhythm:** **Axis:** **Intervals:** **Ischemia:**

#106 – 43-year-old male presents with episodic chest pain

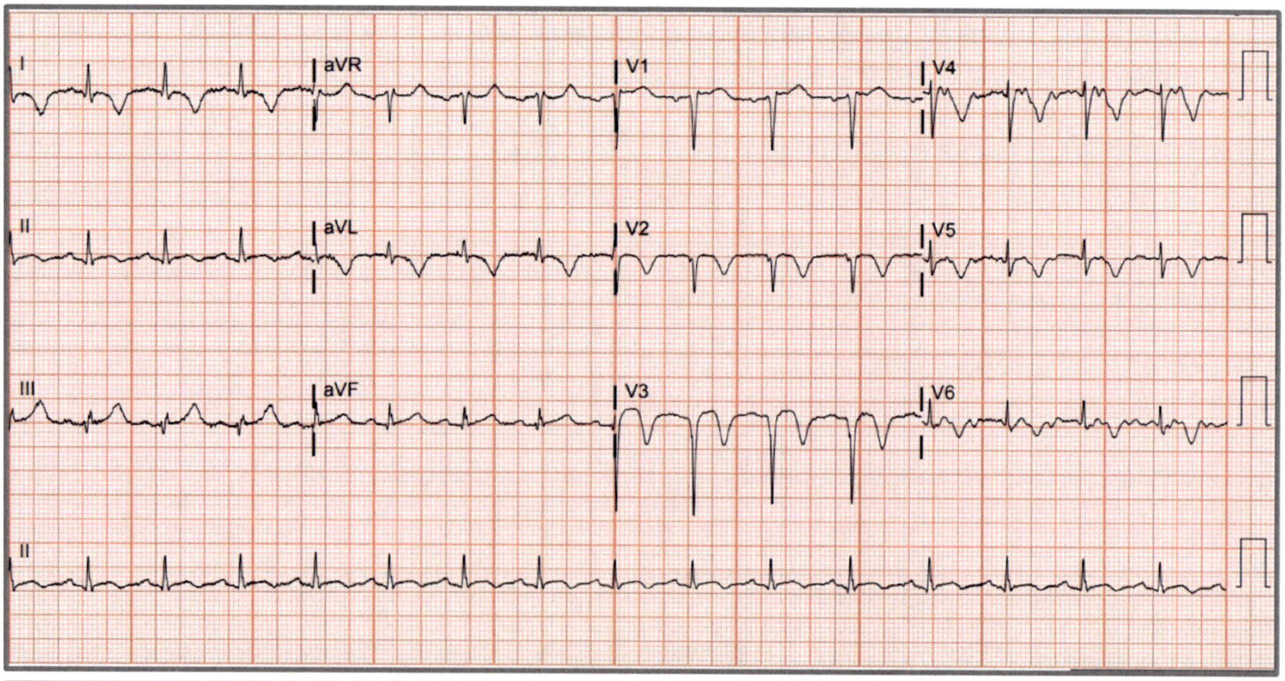

Rate: **Rhythm:** **Axis:** **Intervals:** **Ischemia:**

#107 – 90-year-old male presents with dyspnea

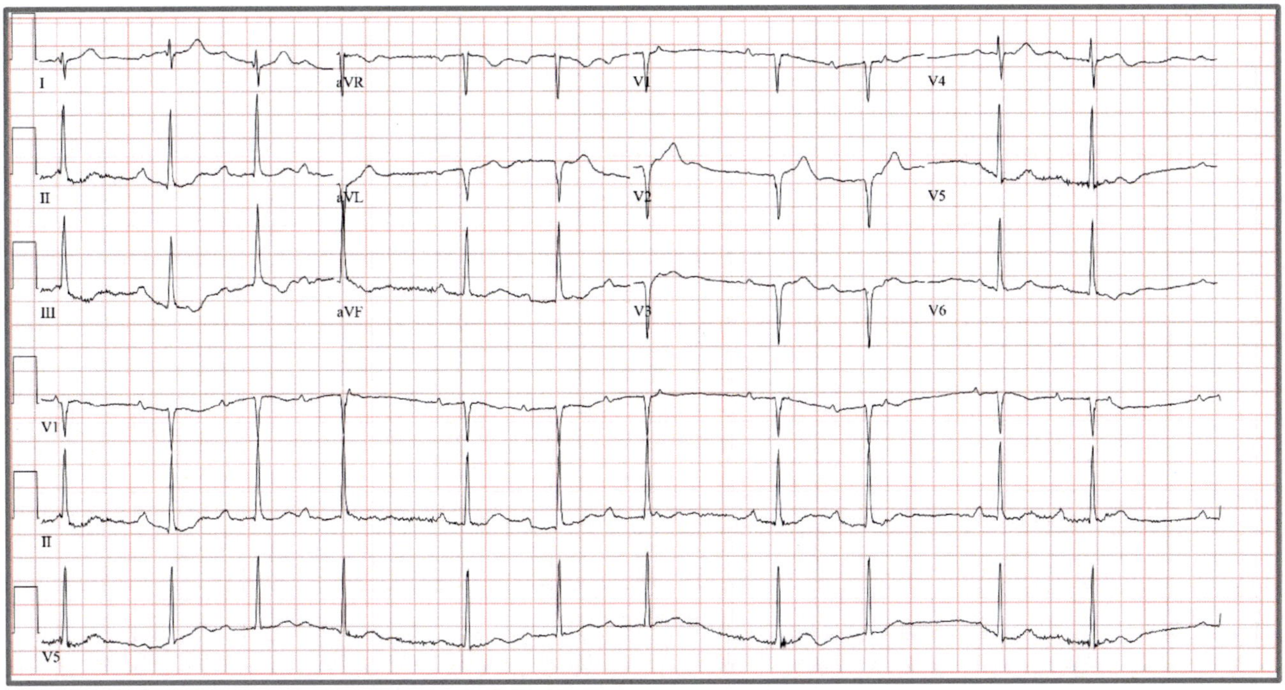

Rate: Rhythm: Axis: Intervals: Ischemia:

#108 – 62-year-old male presents with chest pain

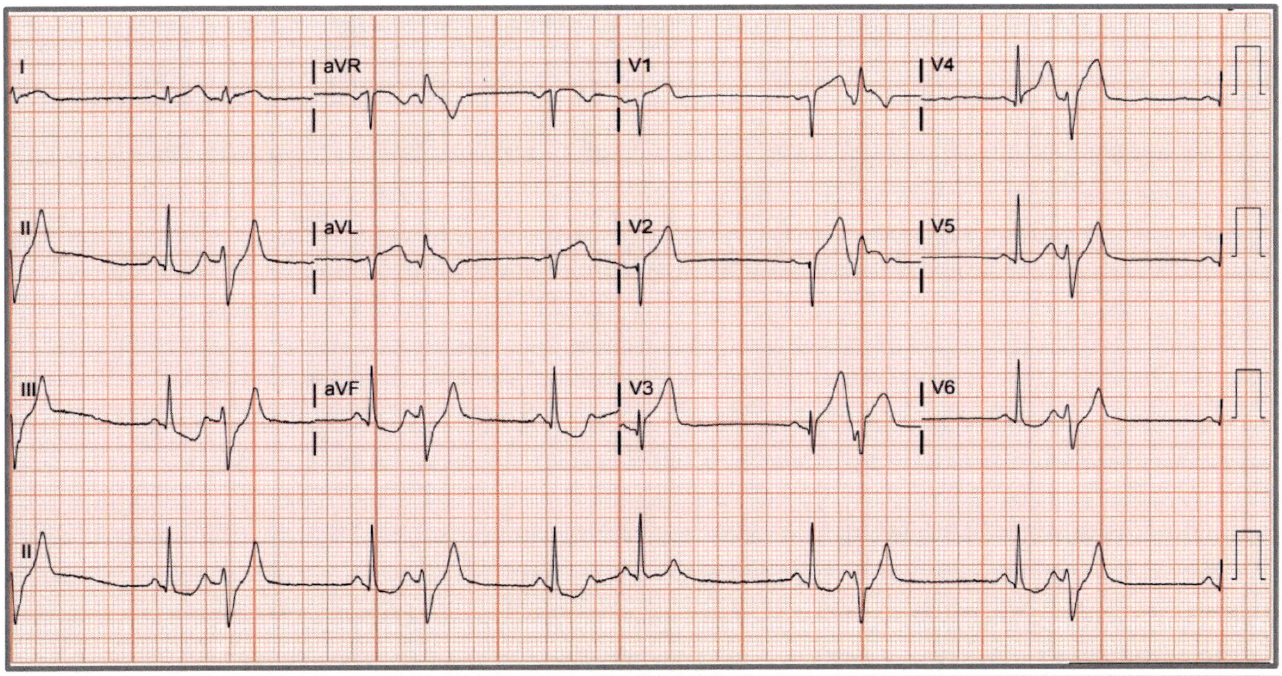

Rate: Rhythm: Axis: Intervals: Ischemia:

#109 – 59-year-old male presents with chest pain

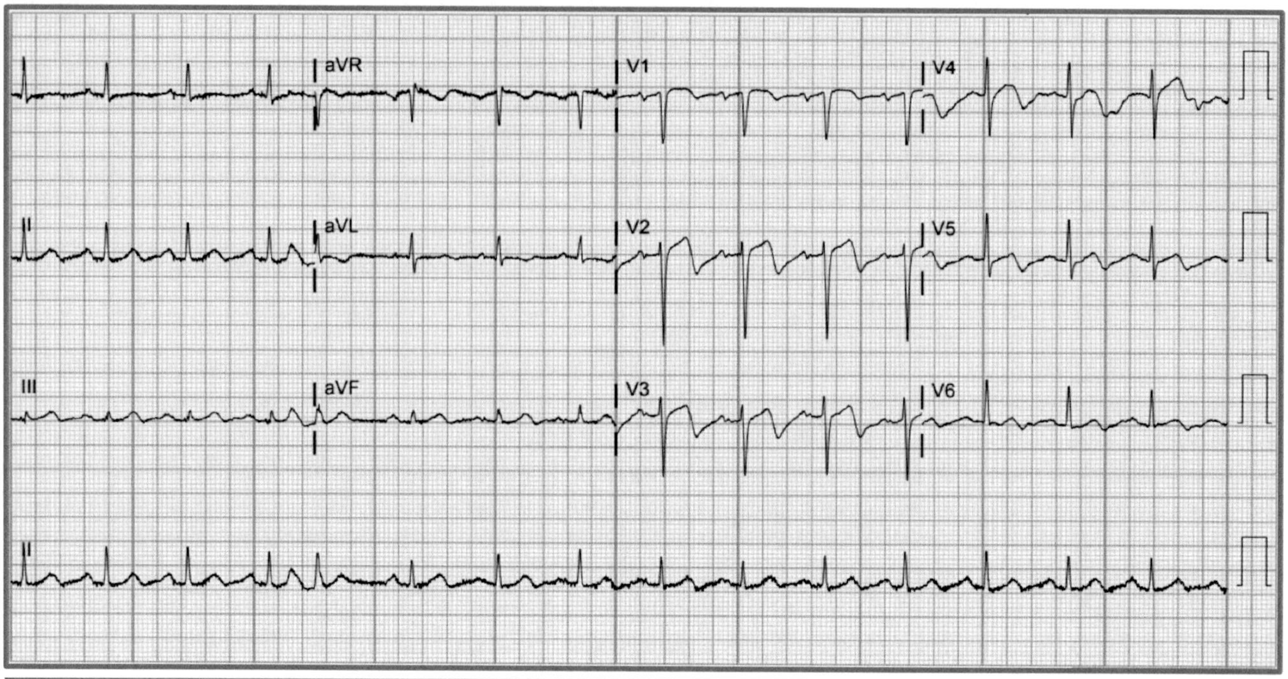

Rate: Rhythm: Axis: Intervals: Ischemia:

#110 – 48-year-old male presents with chest pain

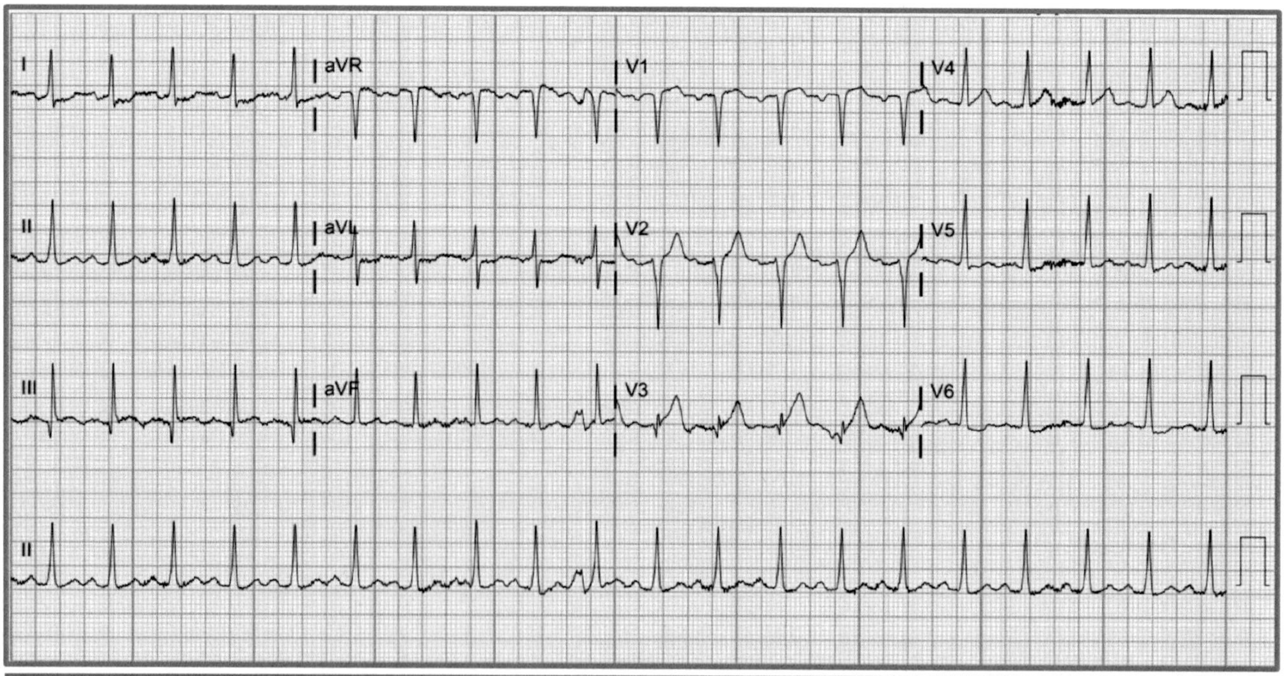

Rate: Rhythm: Axis: Intervals: Ischemia:

#111 – 75-year-old male presents with wrist pain

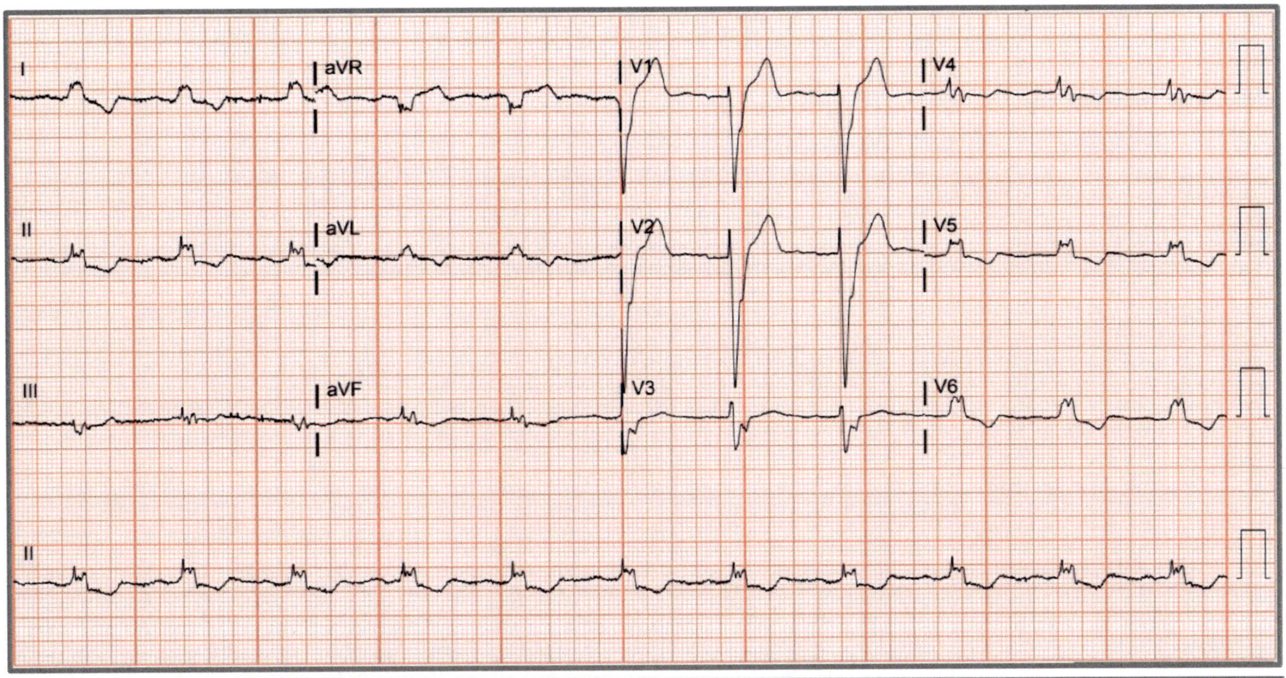

Rate:	Rhythm:	Axis:	Intervals:	Ischemia:

#112 – 21-year-old male presents with chest pain

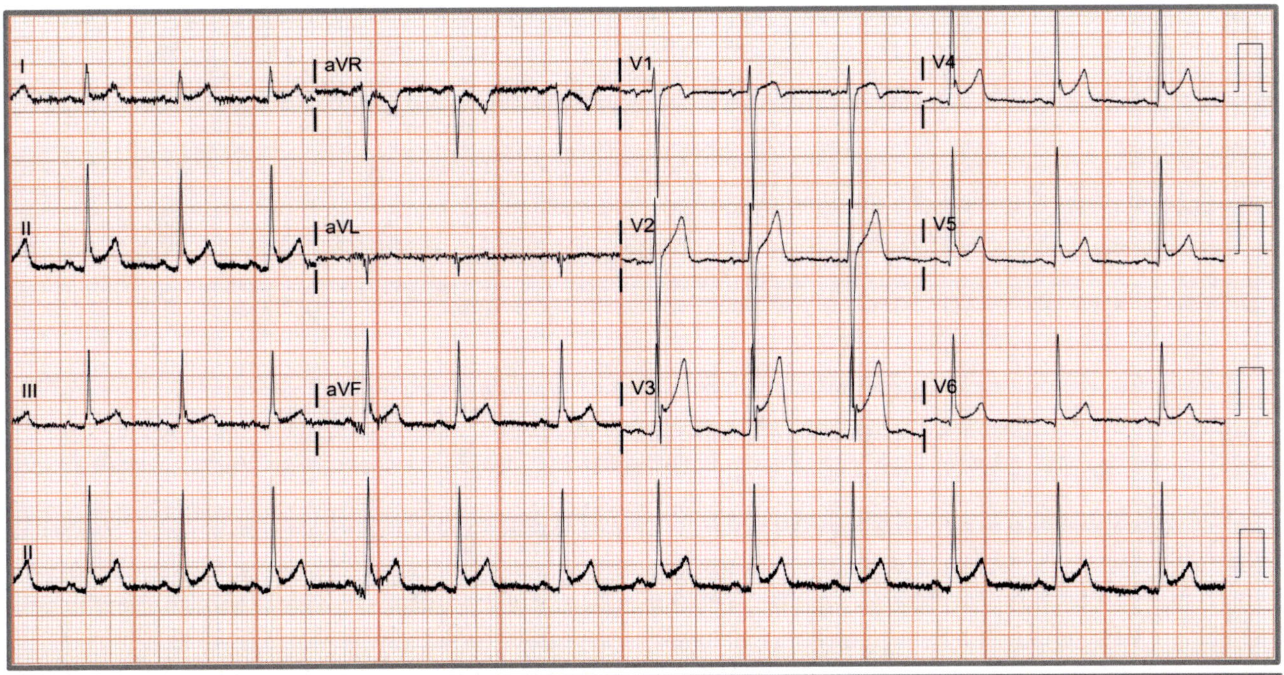

Rate:	Rhythm:	Axis:	Intervals:	Ischemia:

#113 – 36-year-old male presents with light-headedness

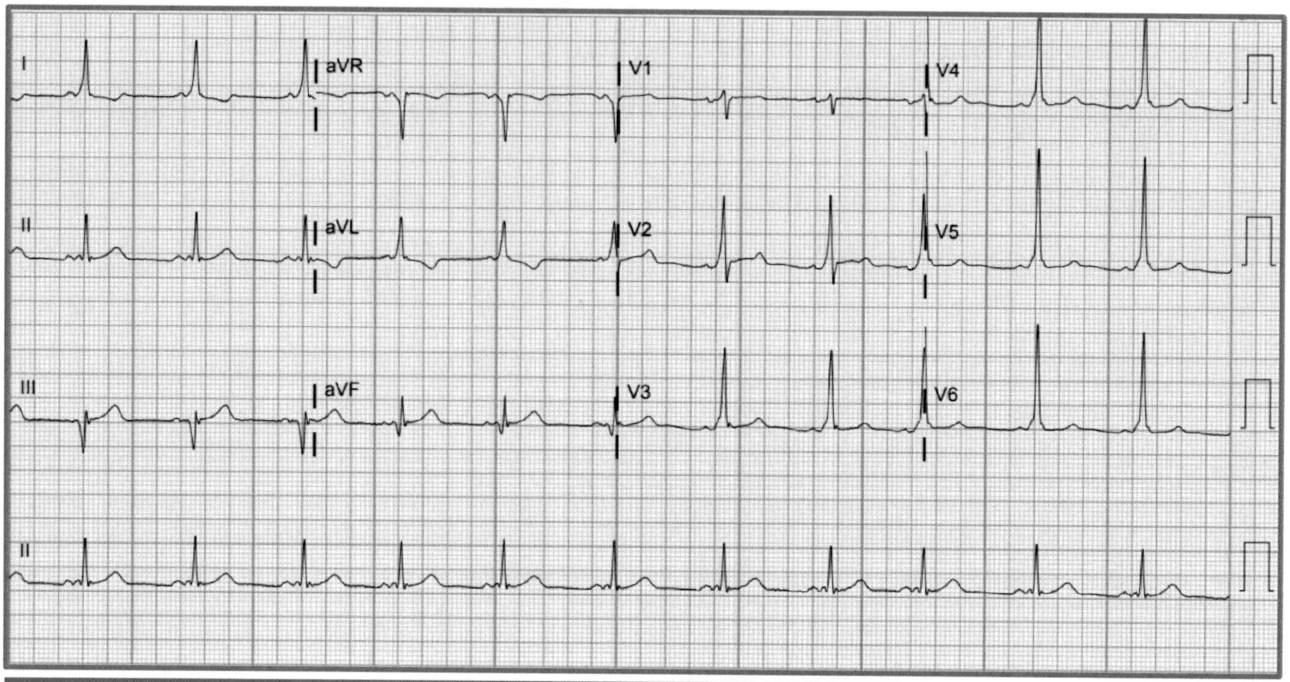

Rate:	Rhythm:	Axis:	Intervals:	Ischemia:

#114 – 60-year-old male presents with chest pain

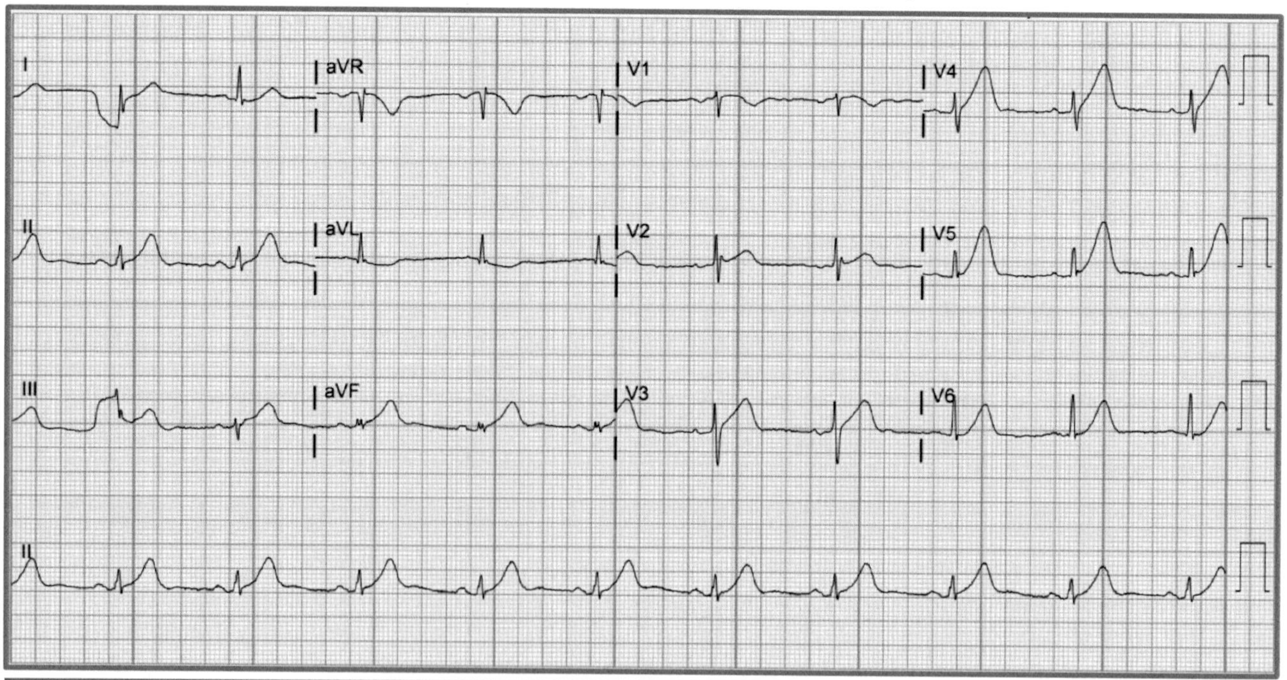

Rate:	Rhythm:	Axis:	Intervals:	Ischemia:

#115 – 33-year-old male presents with neck pain

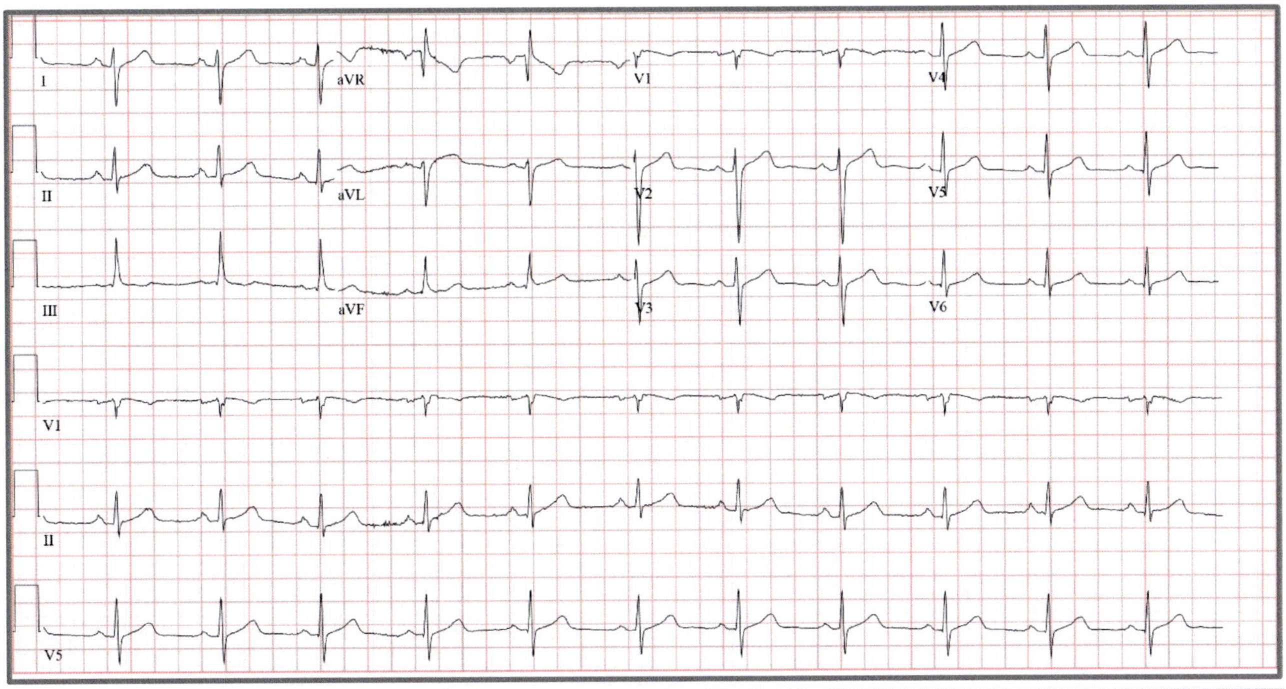

Rate: **Rhythm:** **Axis:** **Intervals:** **Ischemia:**

#116 – 68-year-old female presents with palpitations

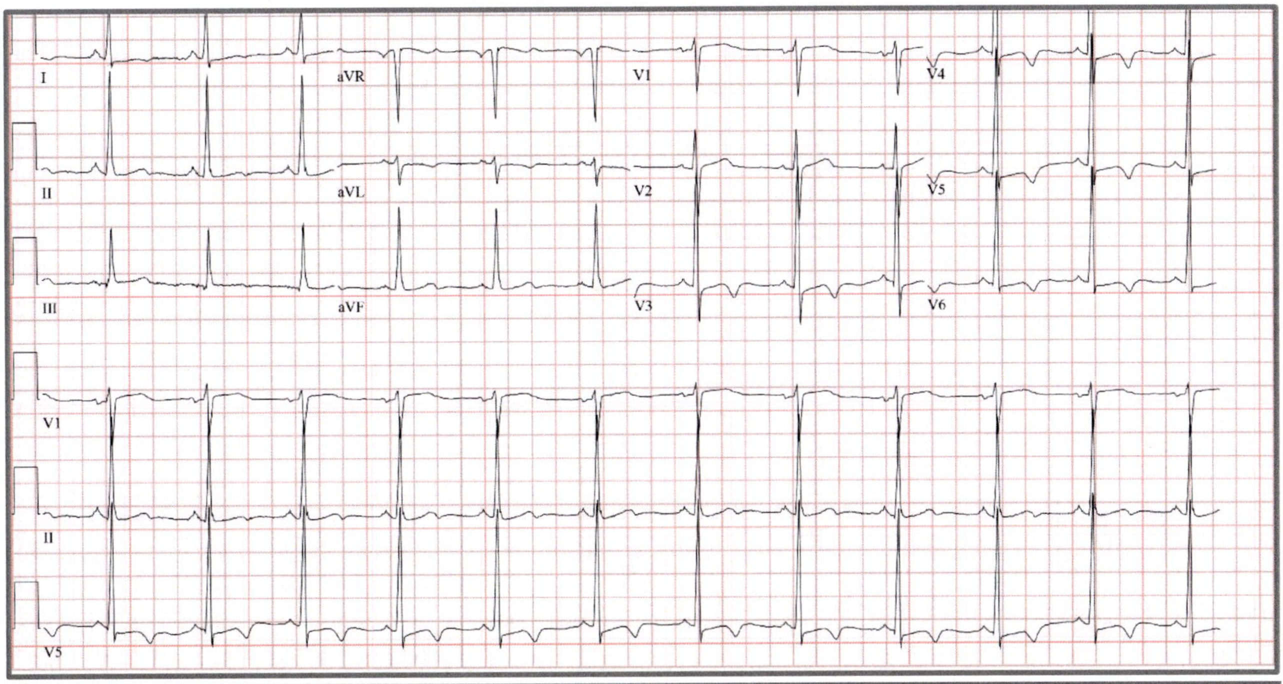

Rate: **Rhythm:** **Axis:** **Intervals:** **Ischemia:**

#117 – 68-year-old male presents with chest pain

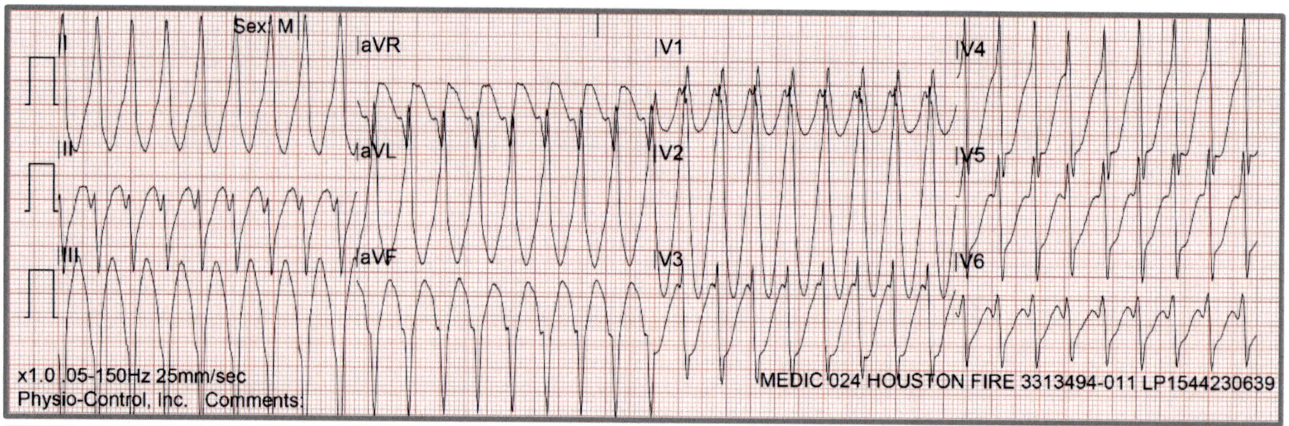

Rate: Rhythm: Axis: Intervals: Ischemia:

#118 – 38-year-old male presents with sharp chest pain

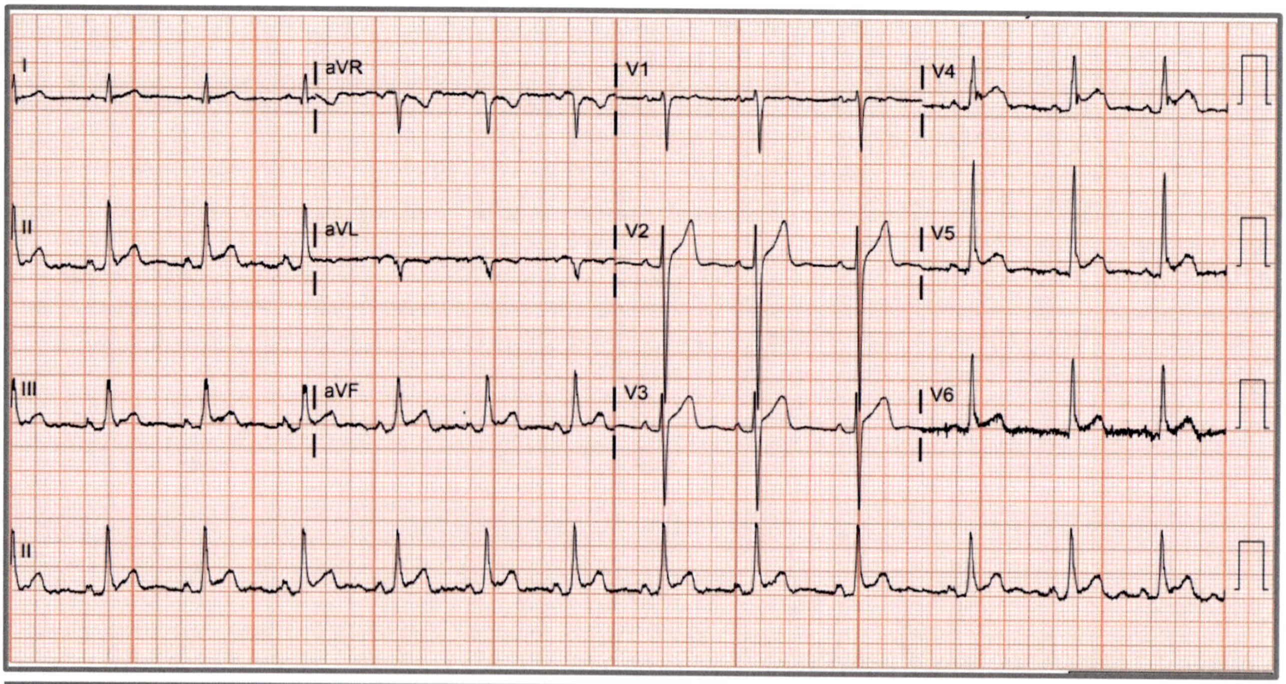

Rate: Rhythm: Axis: Intervals: Ischemia:

#119 – 55-year-old male presents with syncope

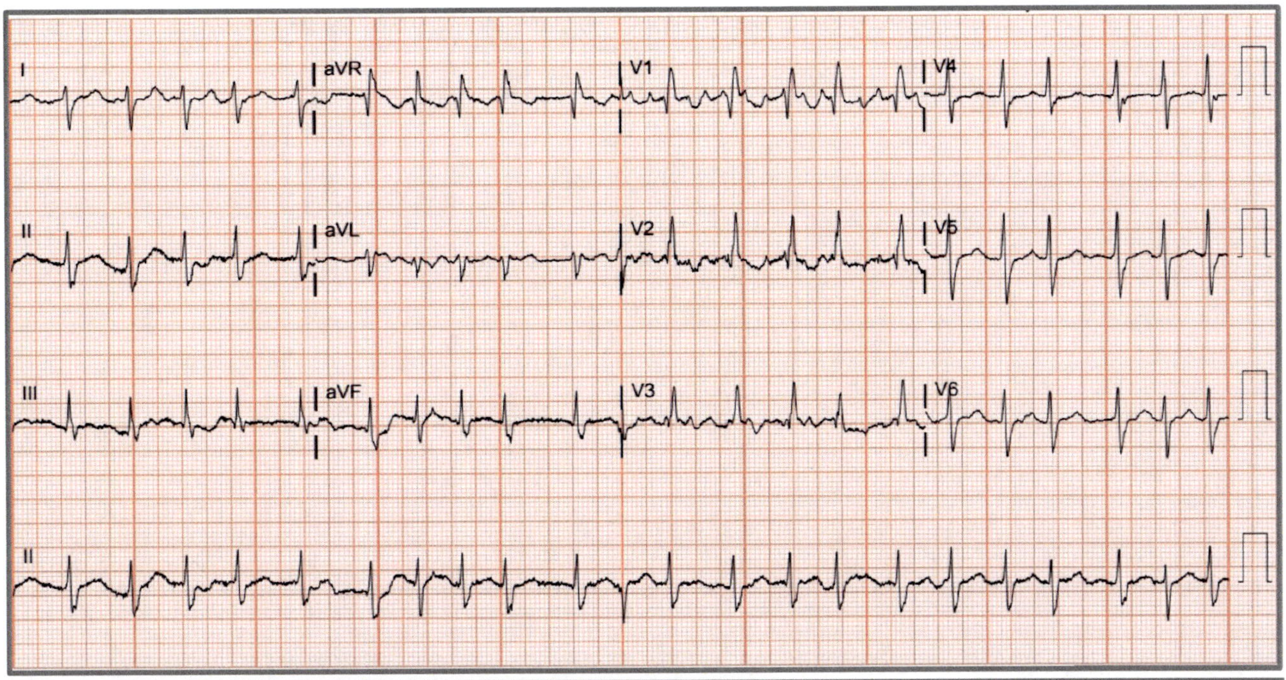

Rate:		Rhythm:		Axis:		Intervals:		Ischemia:	

#120 – 74-year-old male presents with chest pain

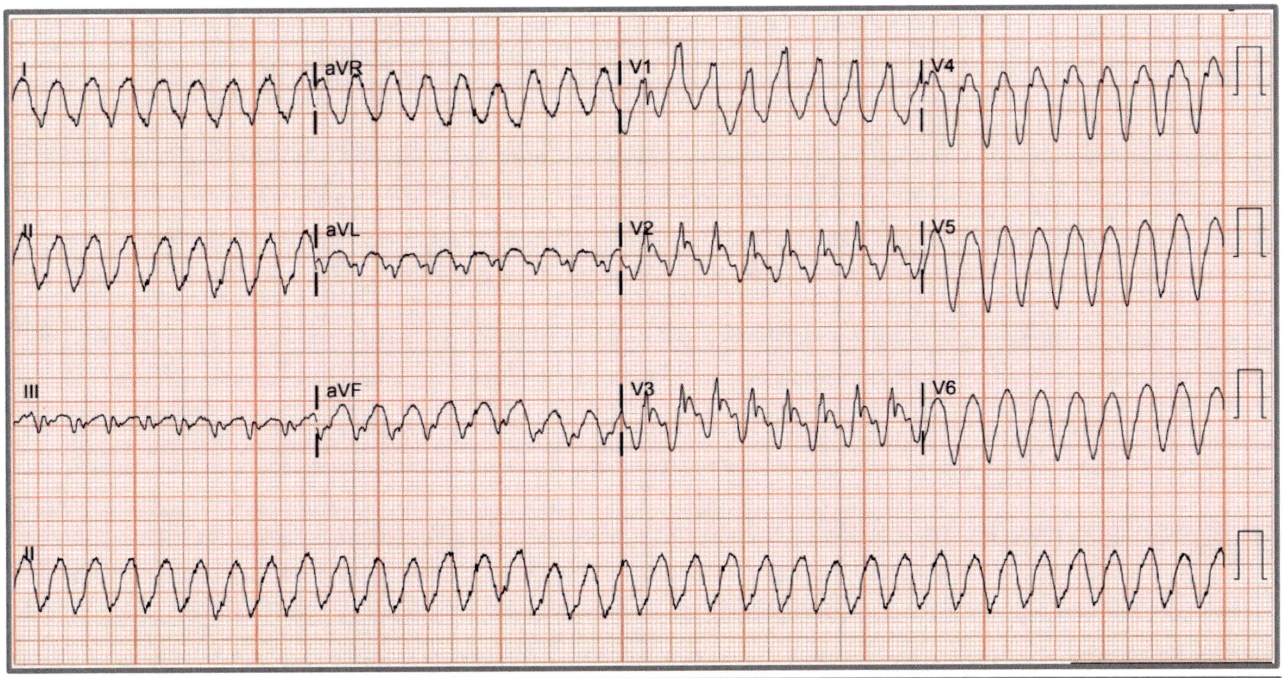

Rate:		Rhythm:		Axis:		Intervals:		Ischemia:	

#121 – 88-year-old female presents with confusion

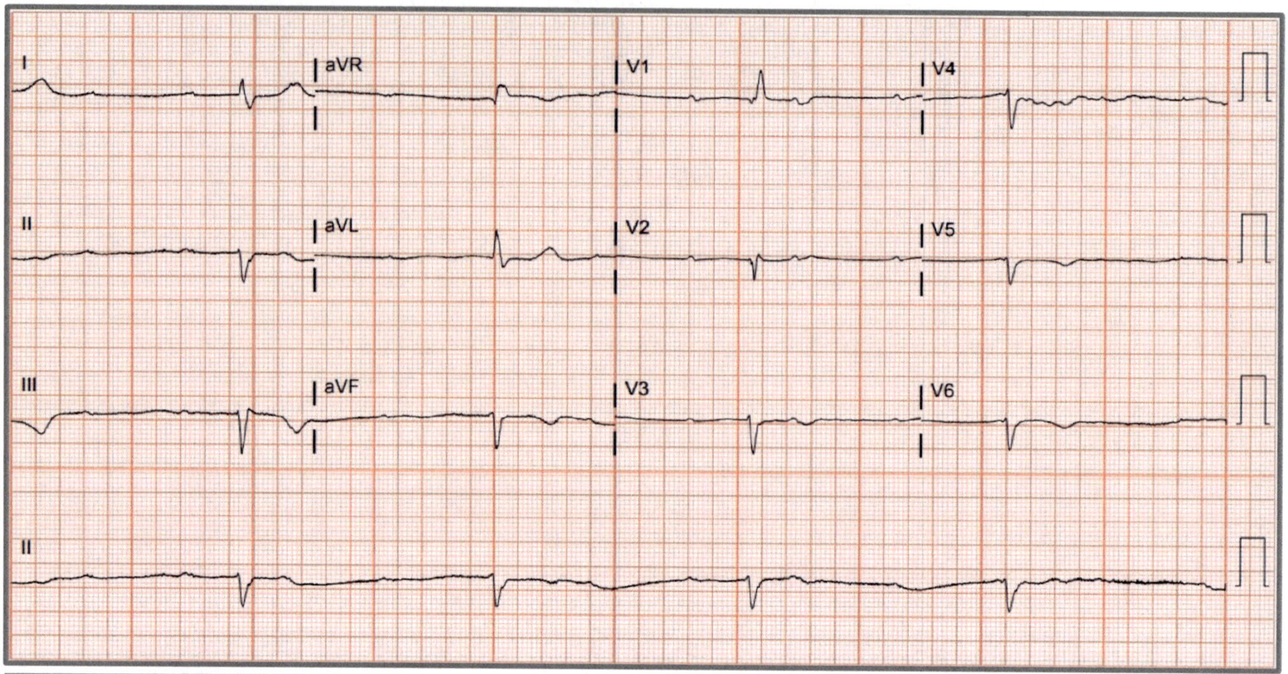

Rate: **Rhythm:** **Axis:** **Intervals:** **Ischemia:**

#122 – 75-year-old female presents with dizziness

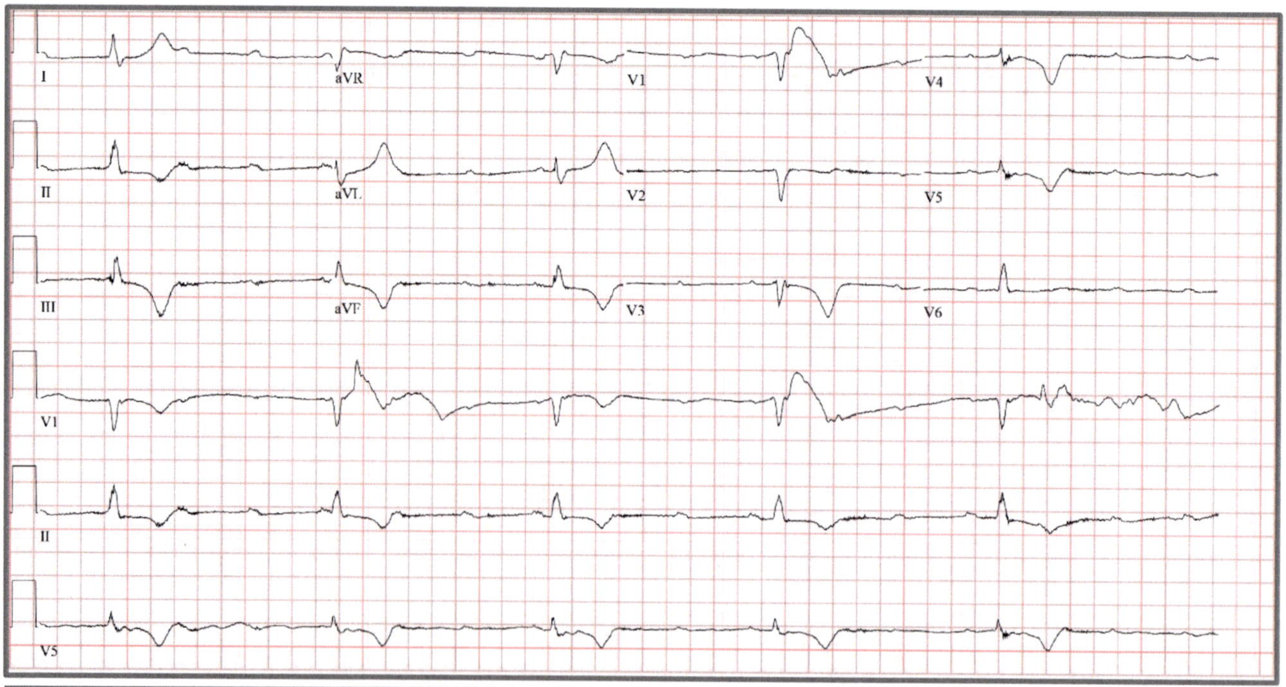

Rate: **Rhythm:** **Axis:** **Intervals:** **Ischemia:**

#123 – 45-year-old female presents with palpitations

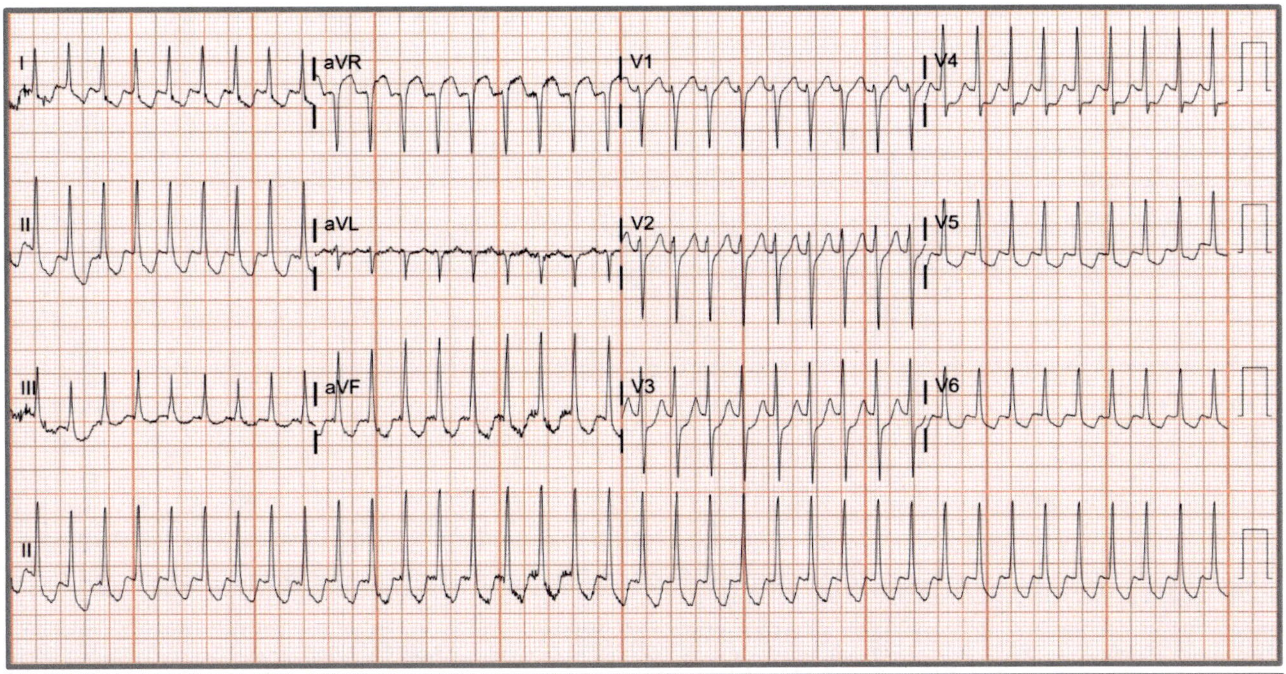

Rate:	Rhythm:	Axis:	Intervals:	Ischemia:

#124 – 55-year-old male presents with chest pain

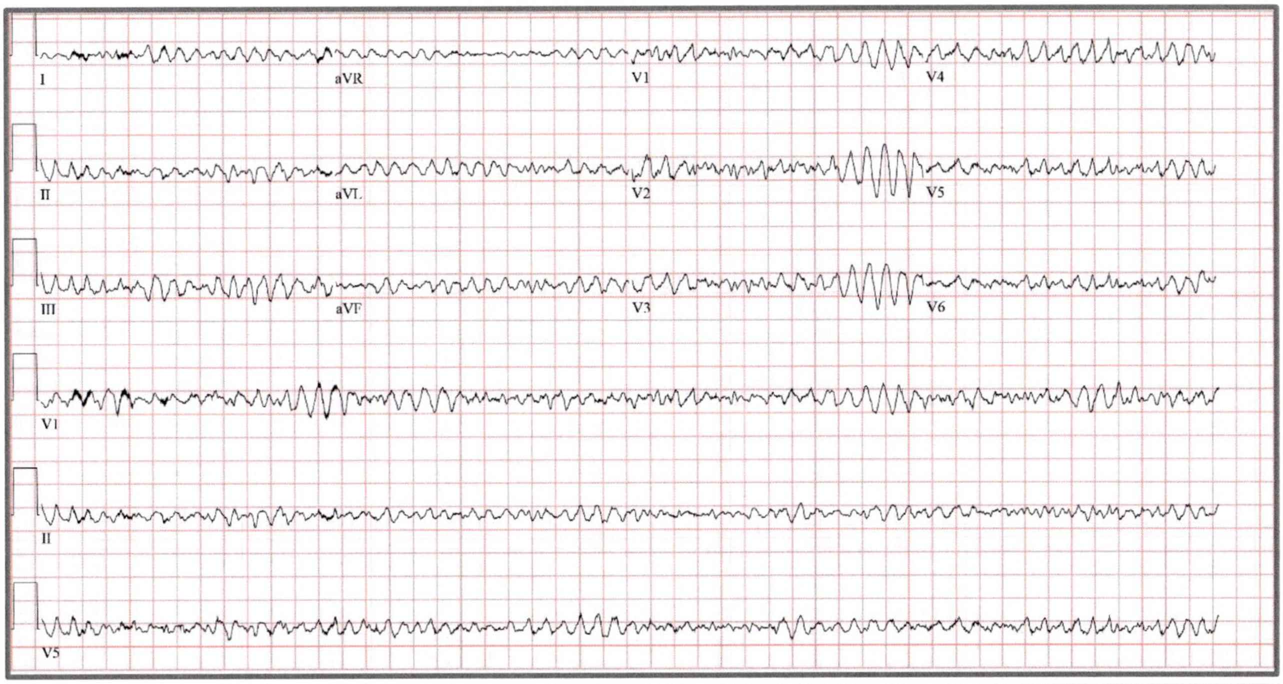

Rate:	Rhythm:	Axis:	Intervals:	Ischemia:

#125 – 13-year-old female presents with chest pain

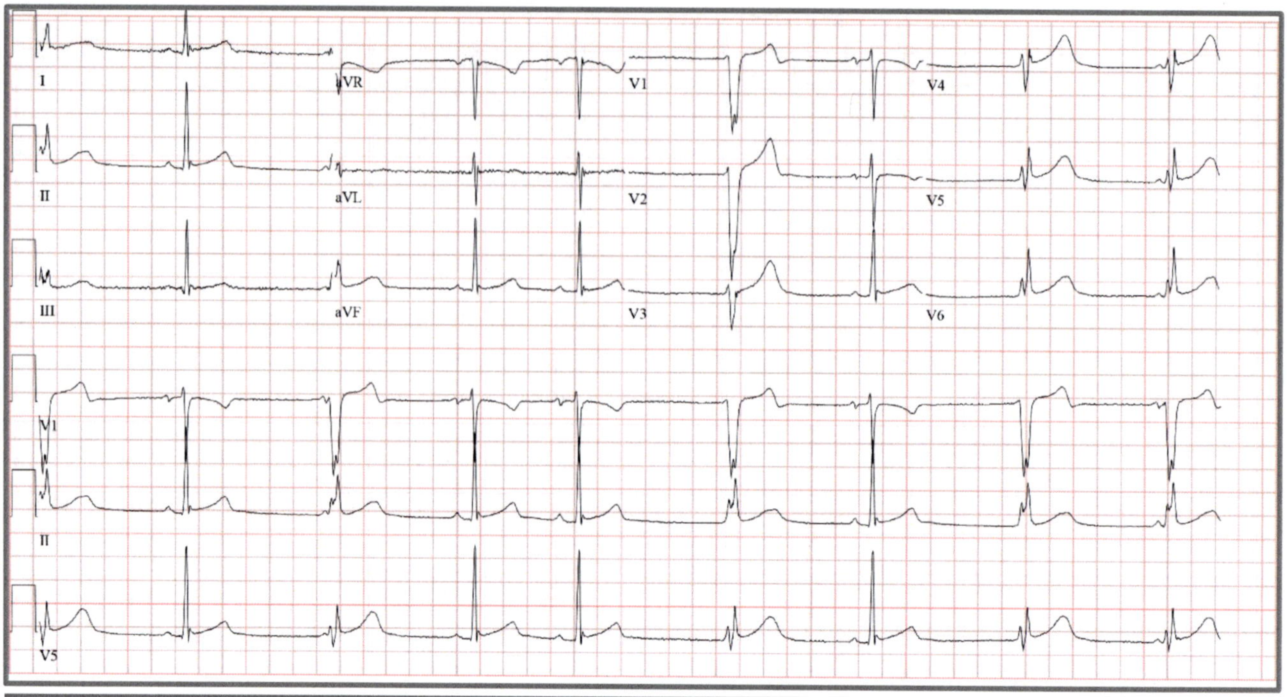

Rate:	Rhythm:	Axis:	Intervals:	Ischemia:

#126 – 17-year-old male presents with palpitations

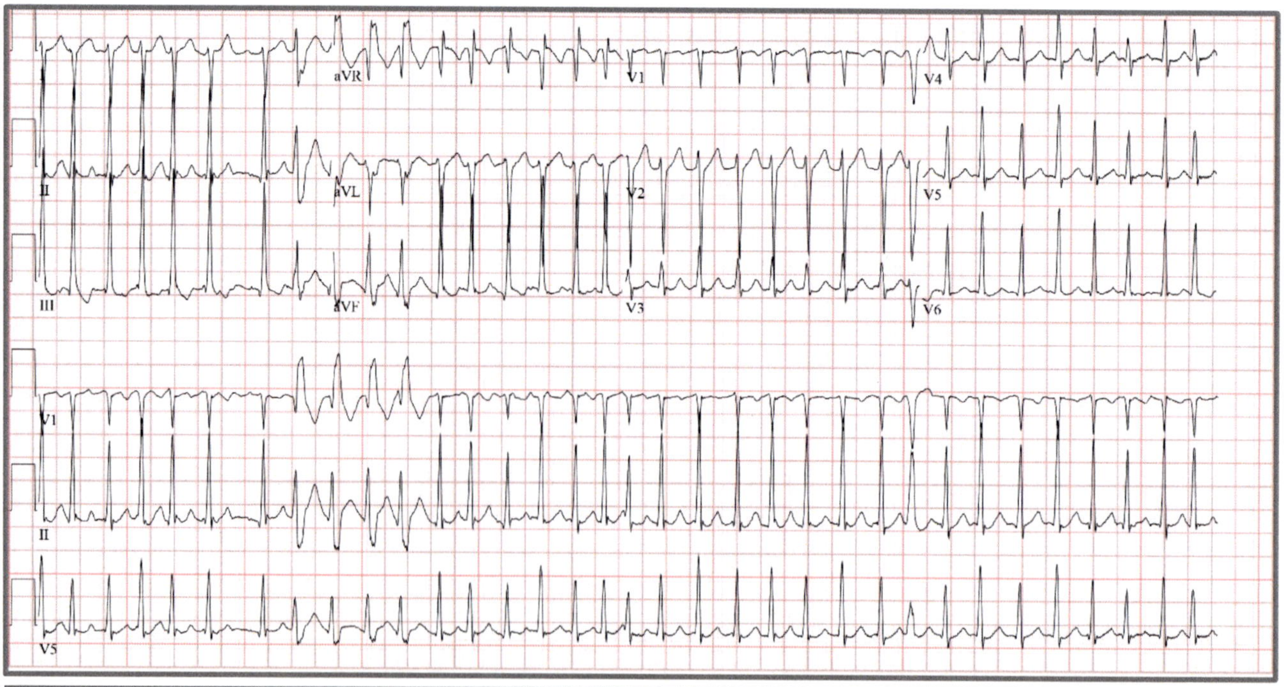

Rate:	Rhythm:	Axis:	Intervals:	Ischemia:

#127 – 83-year-old male presents with bradycardia

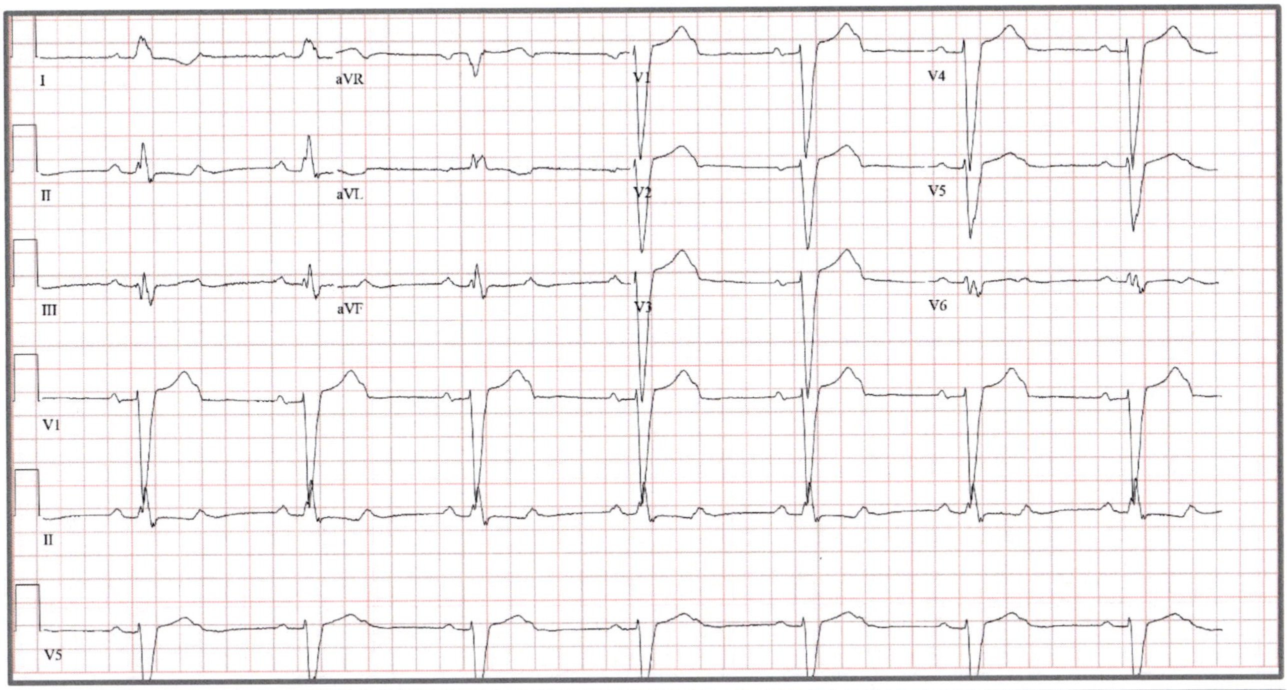

Rate: Rhythm: Axis: Intervals: Ischemia:

⇩ Repeat ECG ⇩

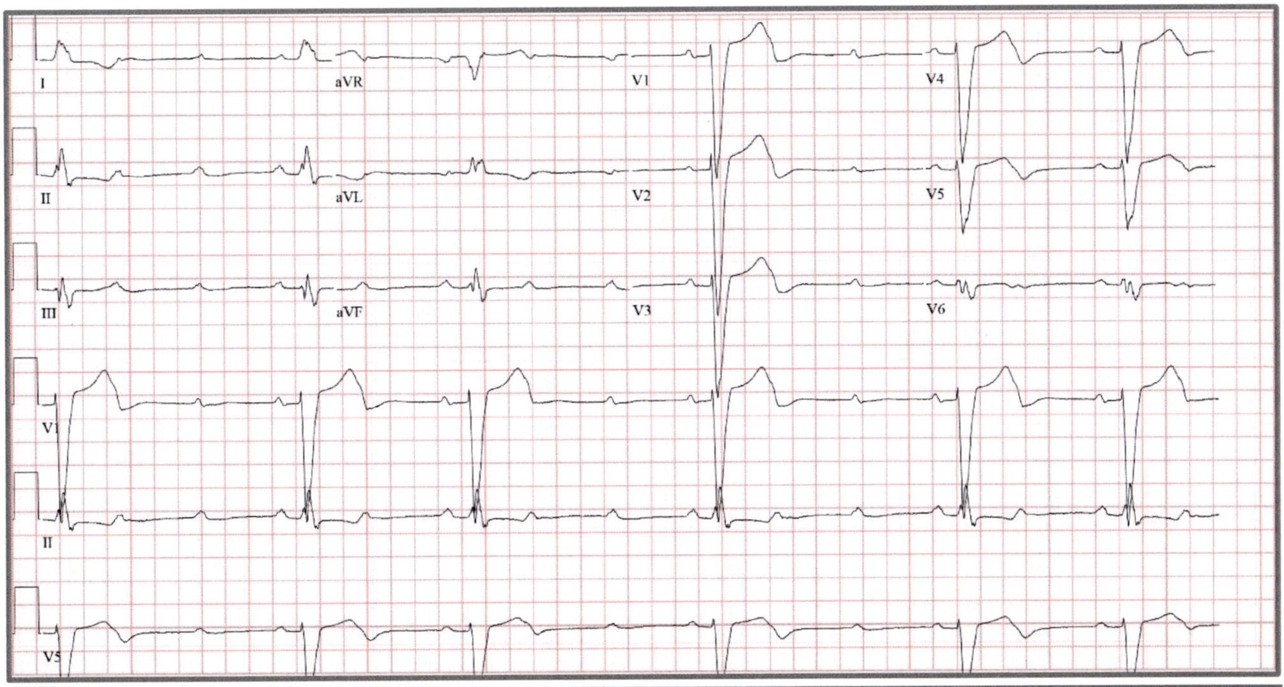

Rate: Rhythm: Axis: Intervals: Ischemia:

#128 – 57-year-old male presents with syncope

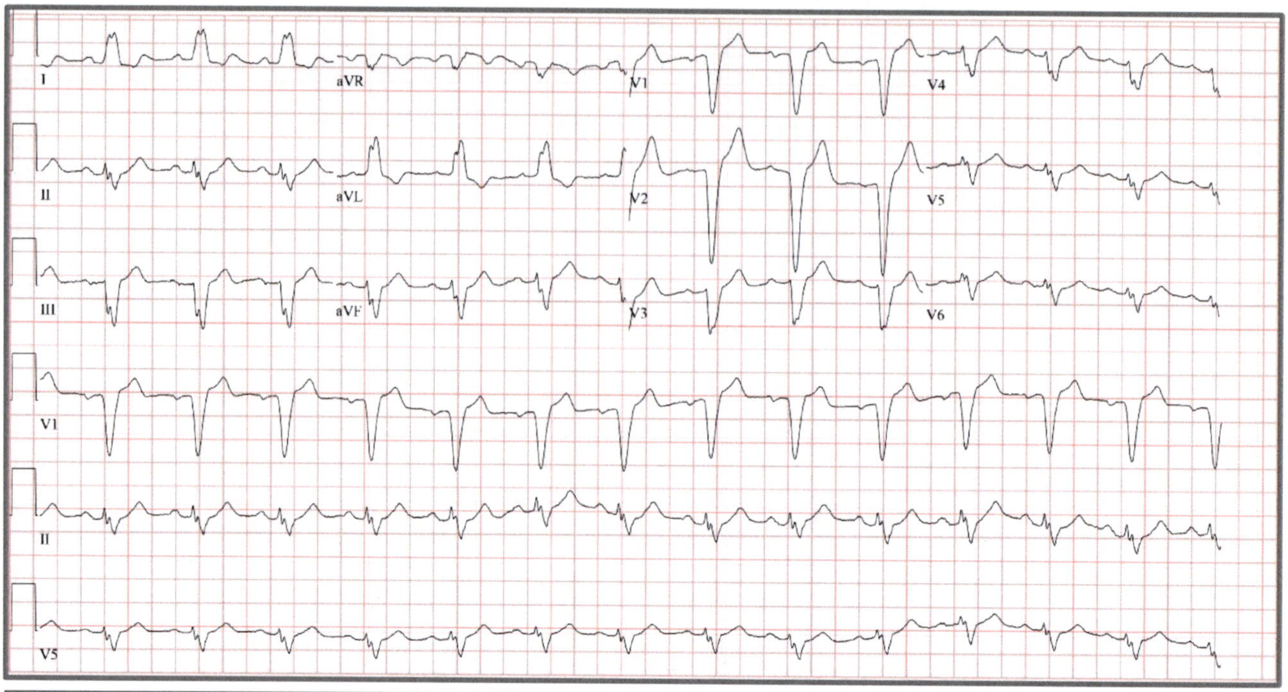

Rate:	Rhythm:	Axis:	Intervals:	Ischemia:

#129 – 81-year-old male presents with syncope

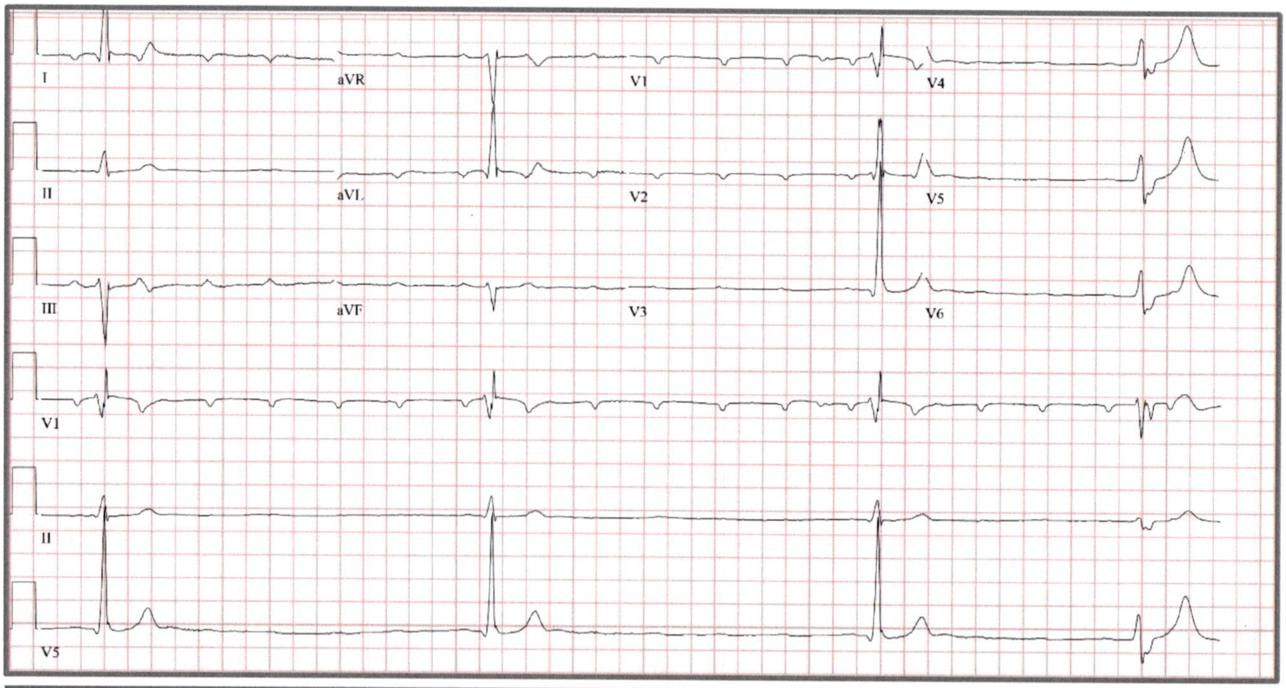

Rate:	Rhythm:	Axis:	Intervals:	Ischemia:

#130 – 26-year-old male presents with overdose

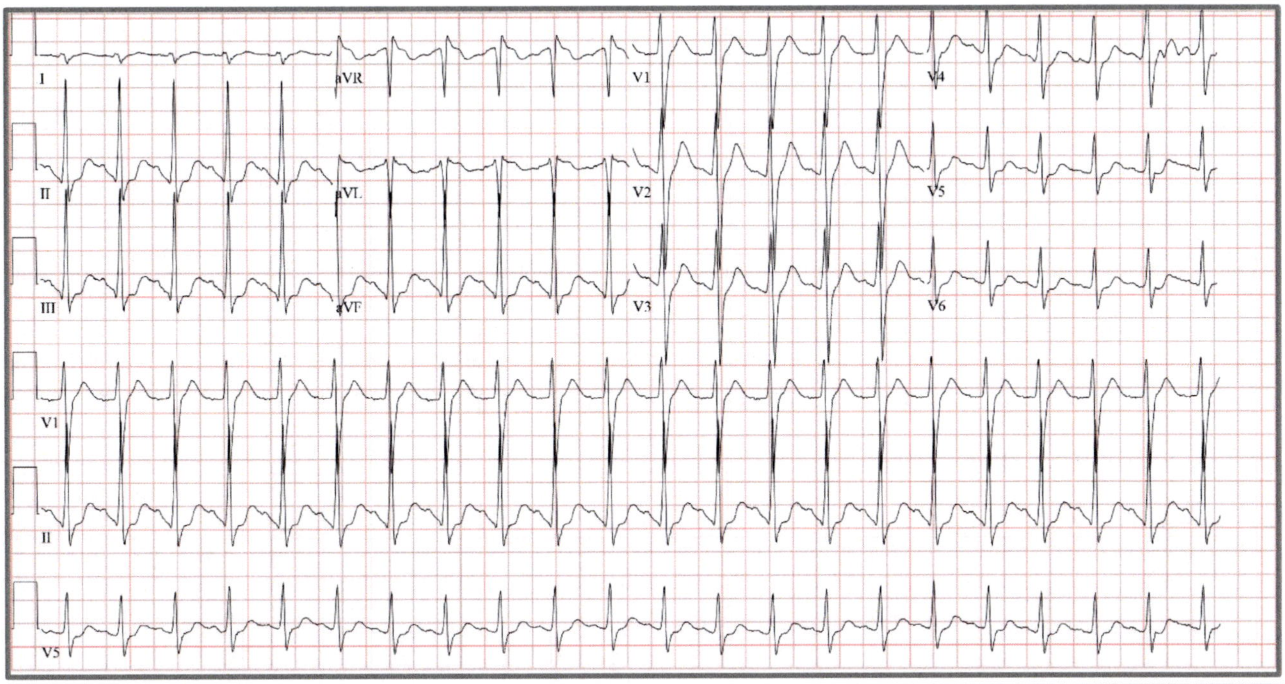

Rate:	Rhythm:	Axis:	Intervals:	Ischemia:

#131 – 27-year-old female presents with dyspnea

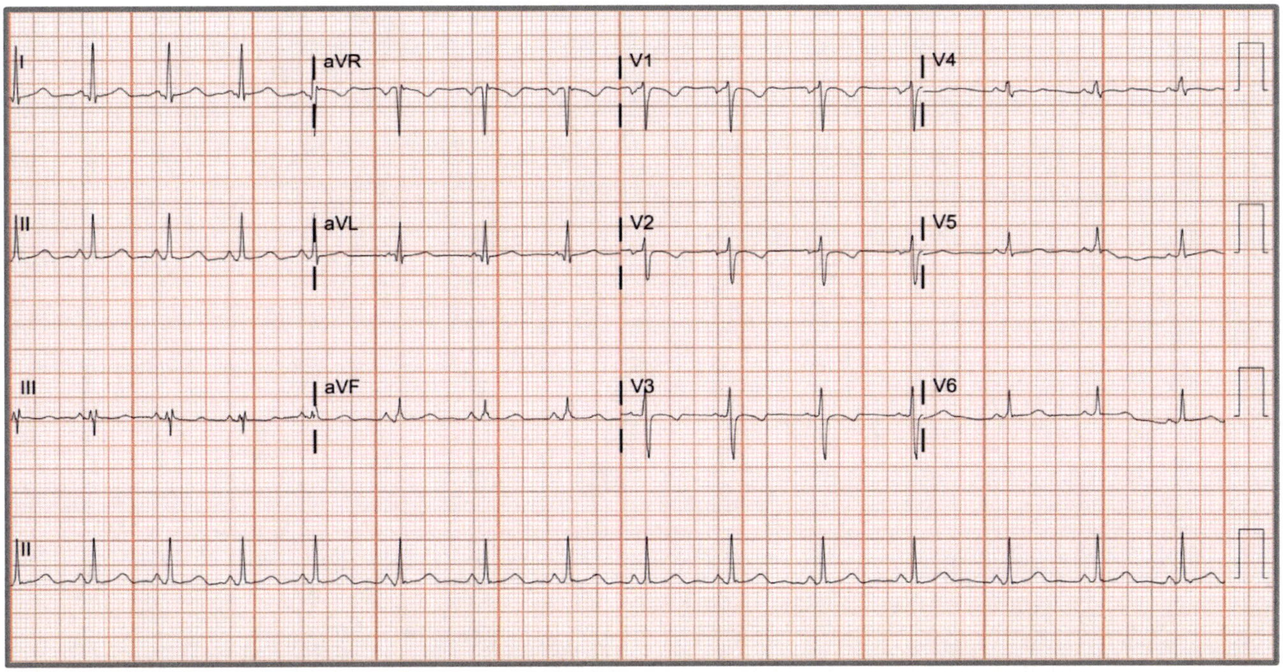

Rate:	Rhythm:	Axis:	Intervals:	Ischemia:

#132 – 75-year-old male presents with confusion

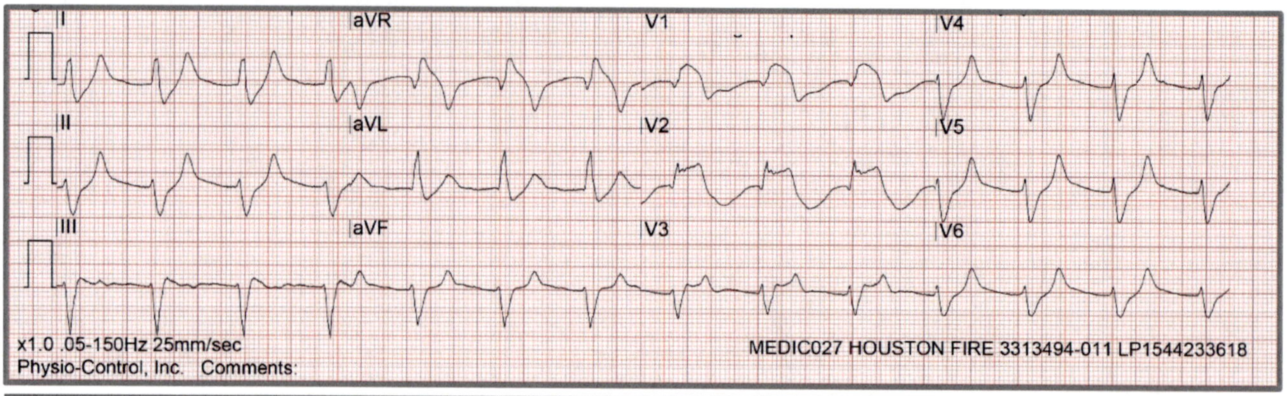

Rate: **Rhythm:** **Axis:** **Intervals:** **Ischemia:**

#133 – 65-year-old female presents with chest pain

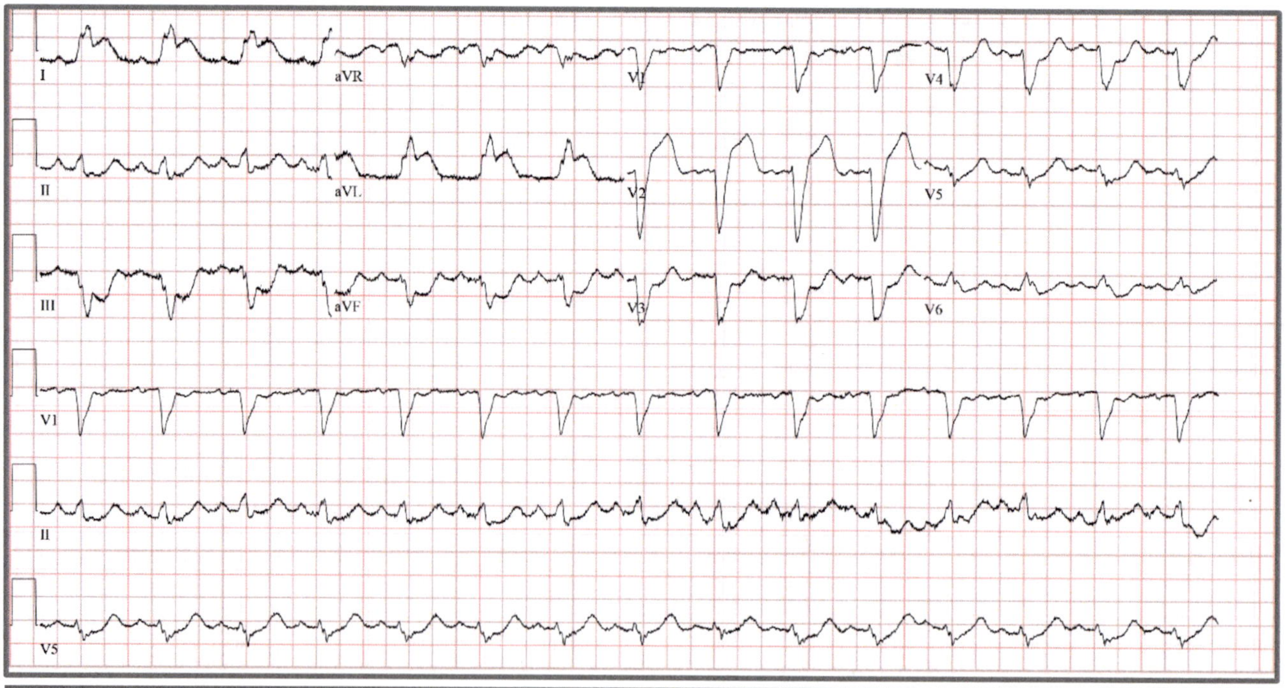

Rate: **Rhythm:** **Axis:** **Intervals:** **Ischemia:**

#134 – 46-year-old male presents with chest pain

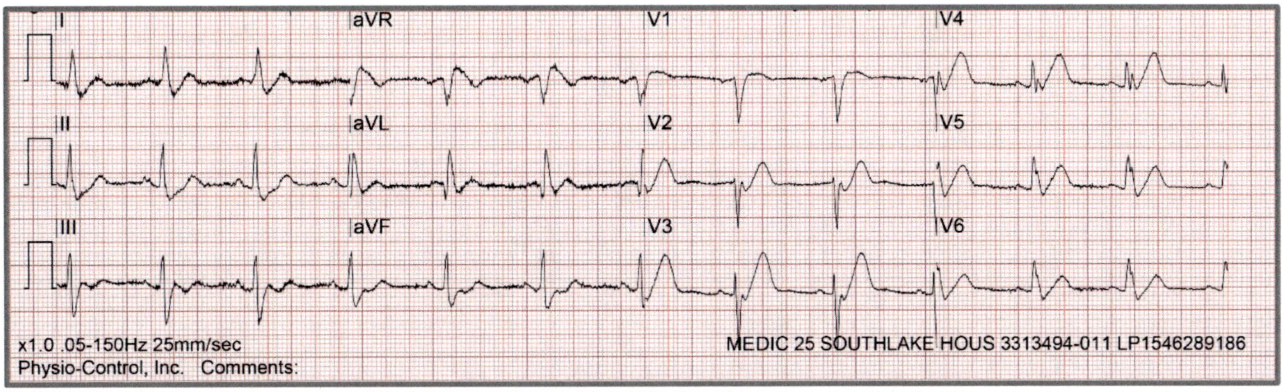

Rate: **Rhythm:** **Axis:** **Intervals:** **Ischemia:**

⇩ Repeat ECG ⇩

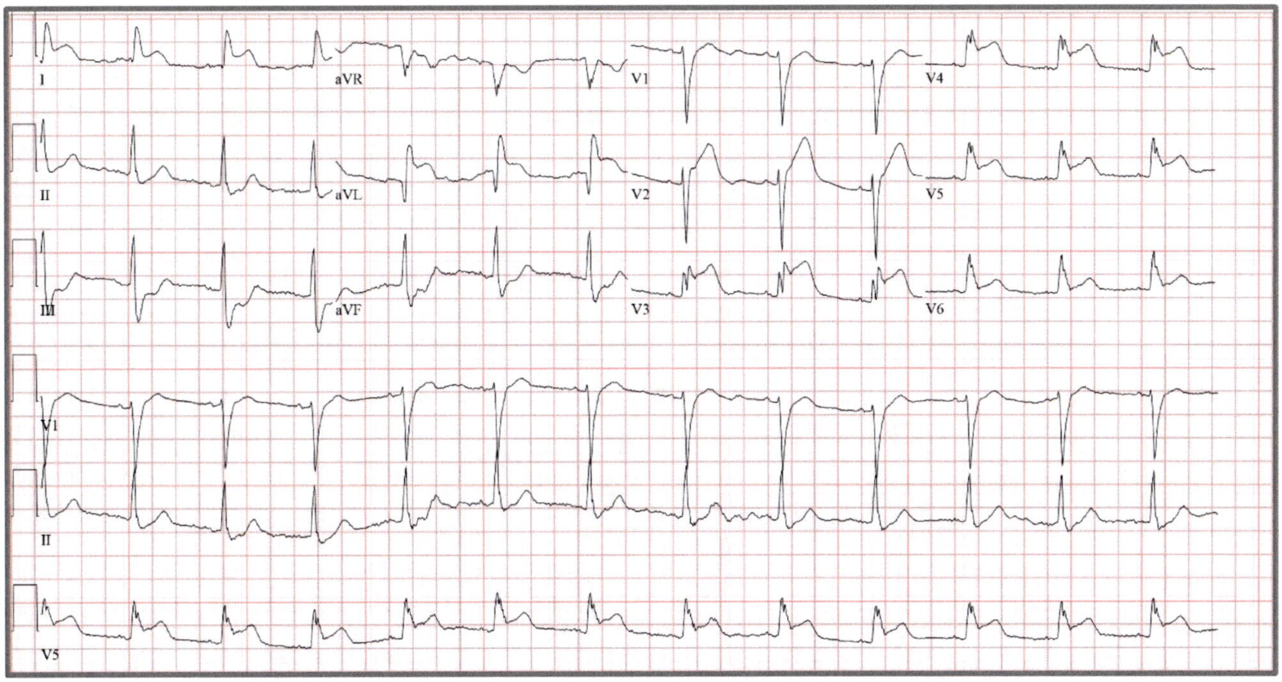

Rate: **Rhythm:** **Axis:** **Intervals:** **Ischemia:**

#135 – 3-month-old male presents with cough

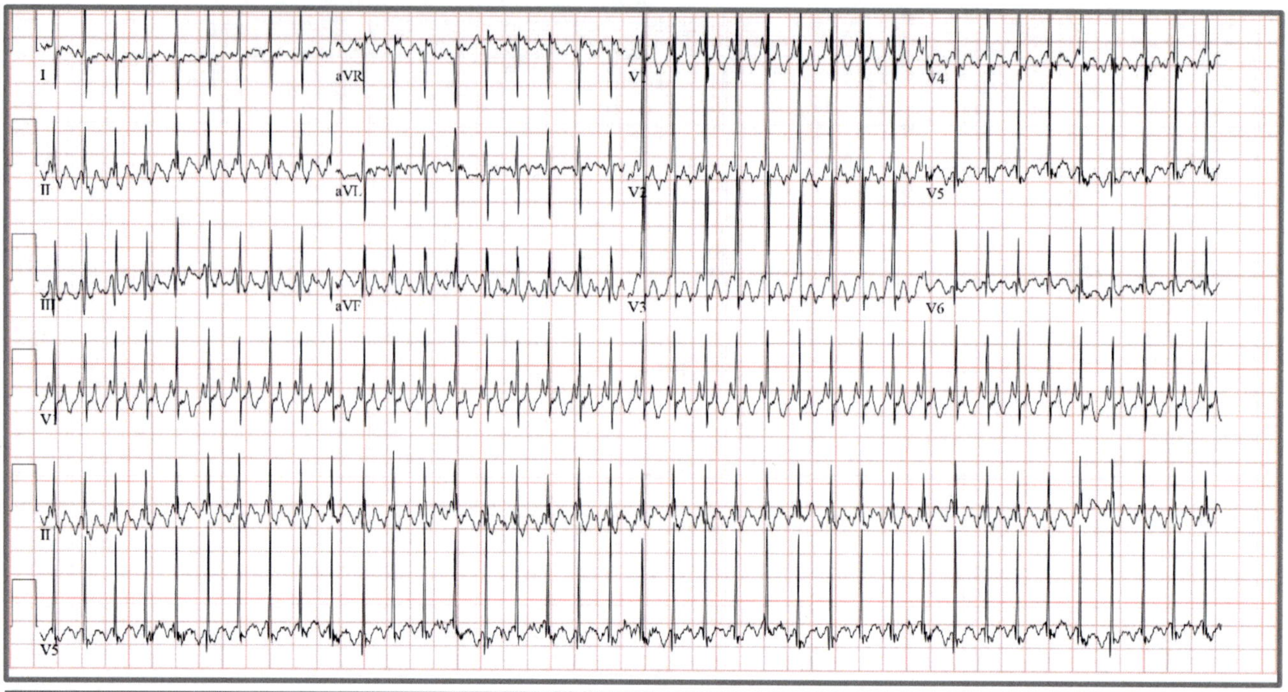

Rate: **Rhythm:** **Axis:** **Intervals:** **Ischemia:**

#136 – 15-year-old male presents with syncope

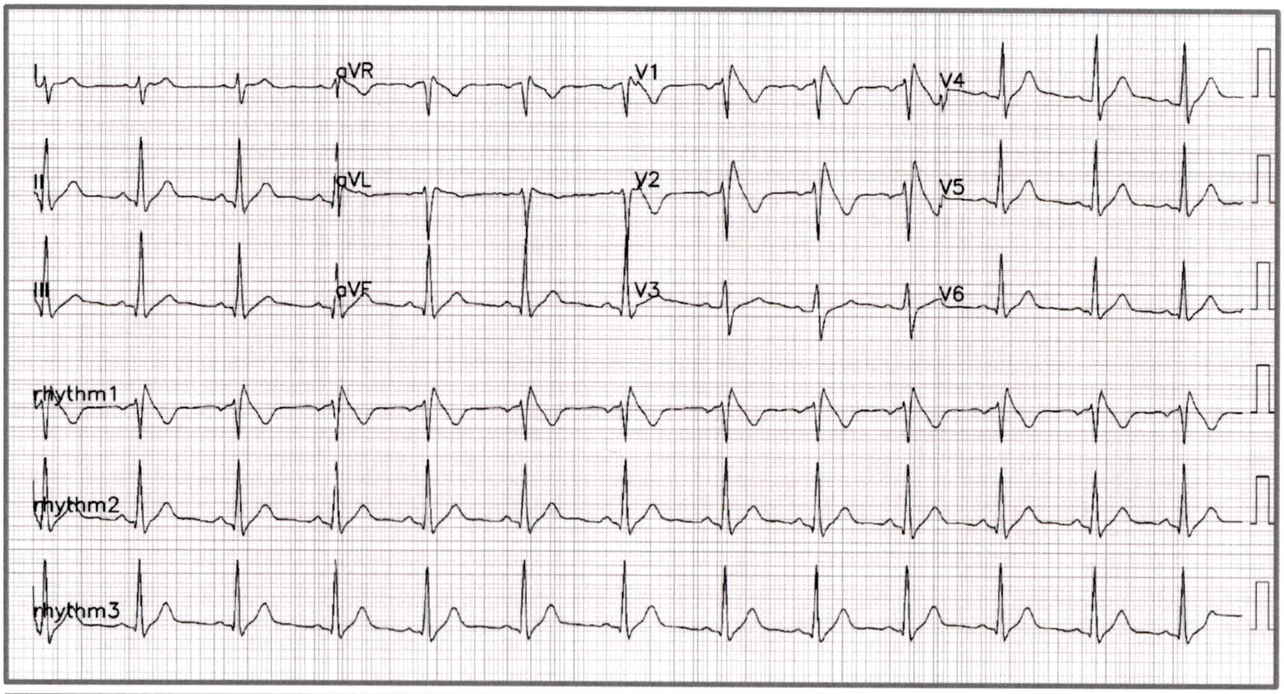

Rate: **Rhythm:** **Axis:** **Intervals:** **Ischemia:**

#137 – 53-year-old male presents with chest pain

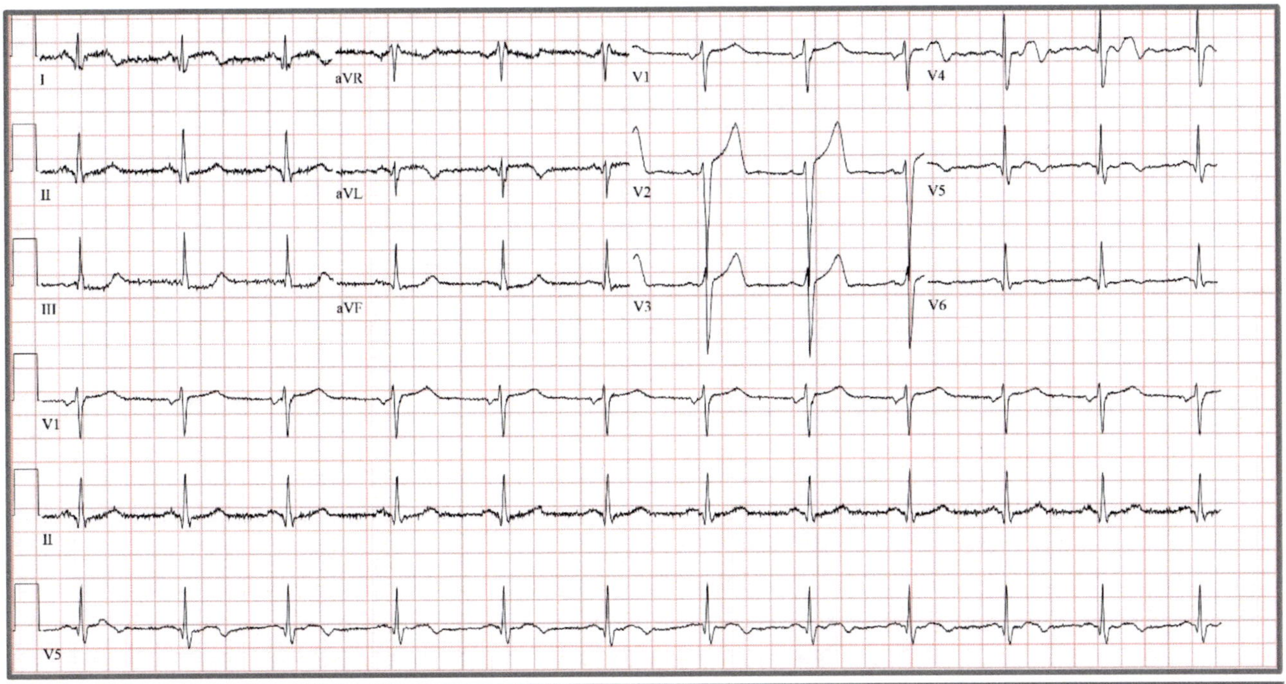

Rate: | **Rhythm:** | **Axis:** | **Intervals:** | **Ischemia:**

⇩ Repeat ECG ⇩

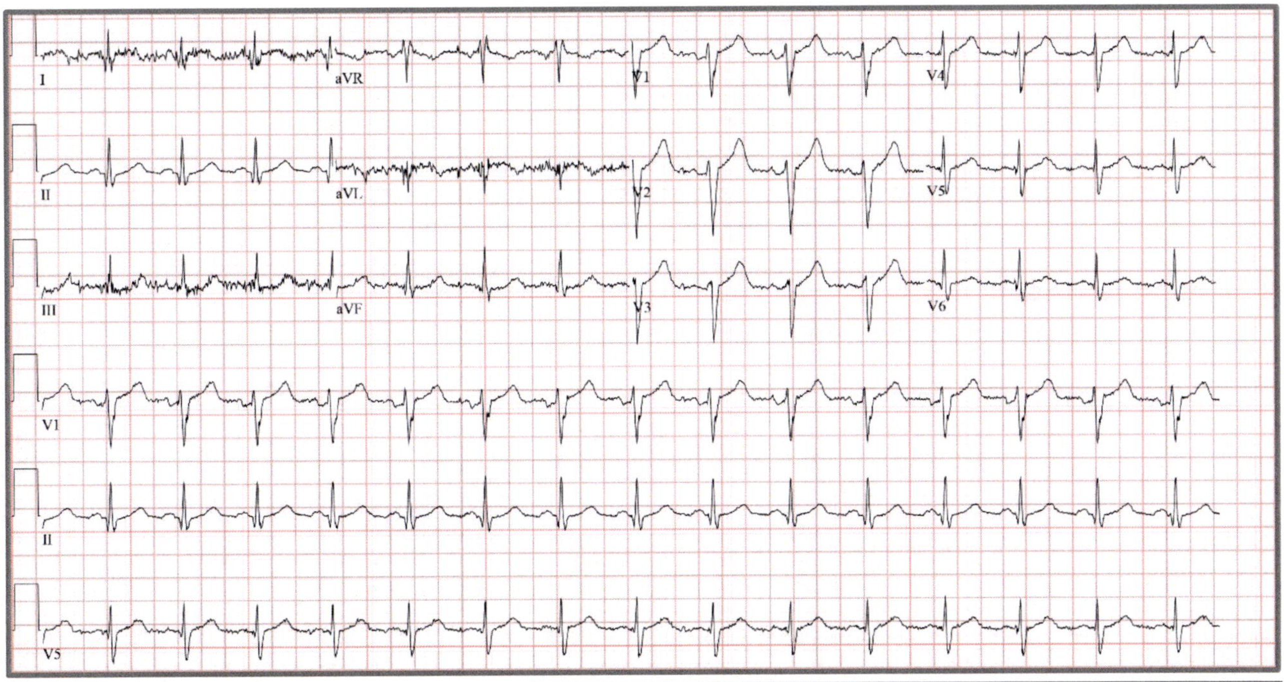

Rate: | **Rhythm:** | **Axis:** | **Intervals:** | **Ischemia:**

#138 – 72-year-old female presents with confusion

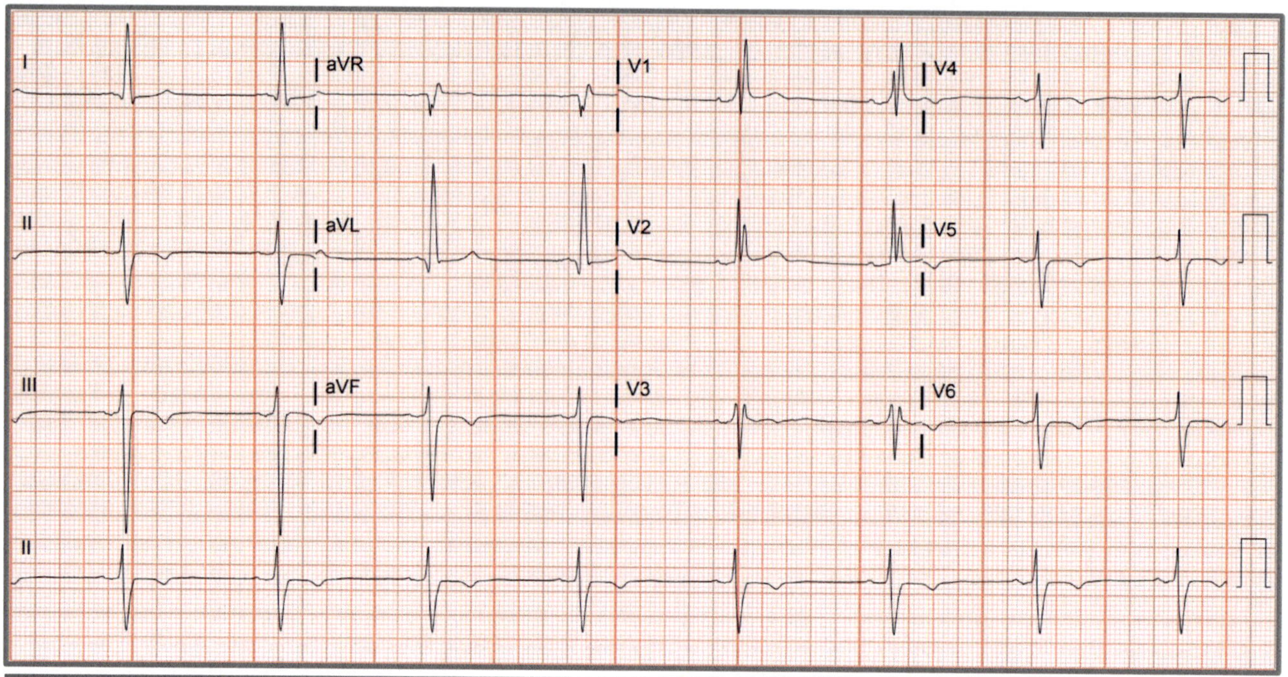

Rate: Rhythm: Axis: Intervals: Ischemia:

#139 – 16-year-old male presents with syncope

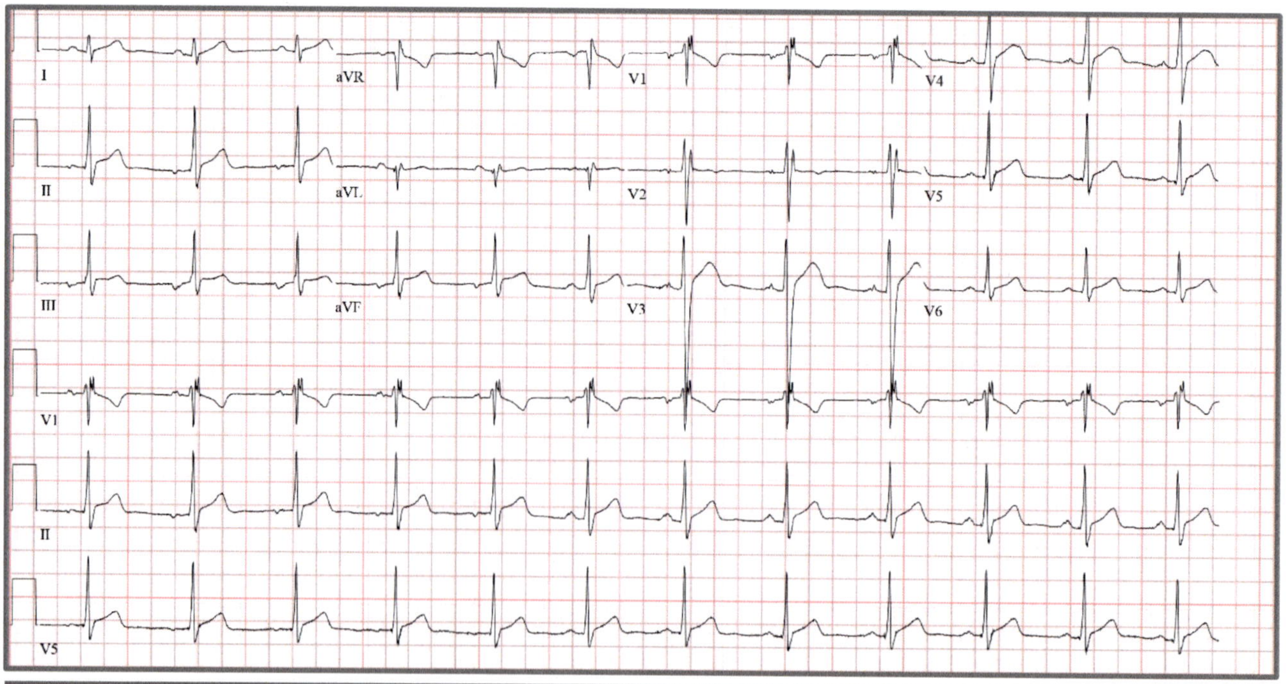

Rate: Rhythm: Axis: Intervals: Ischemia:

#140 – 86-year-old female presents with confusion

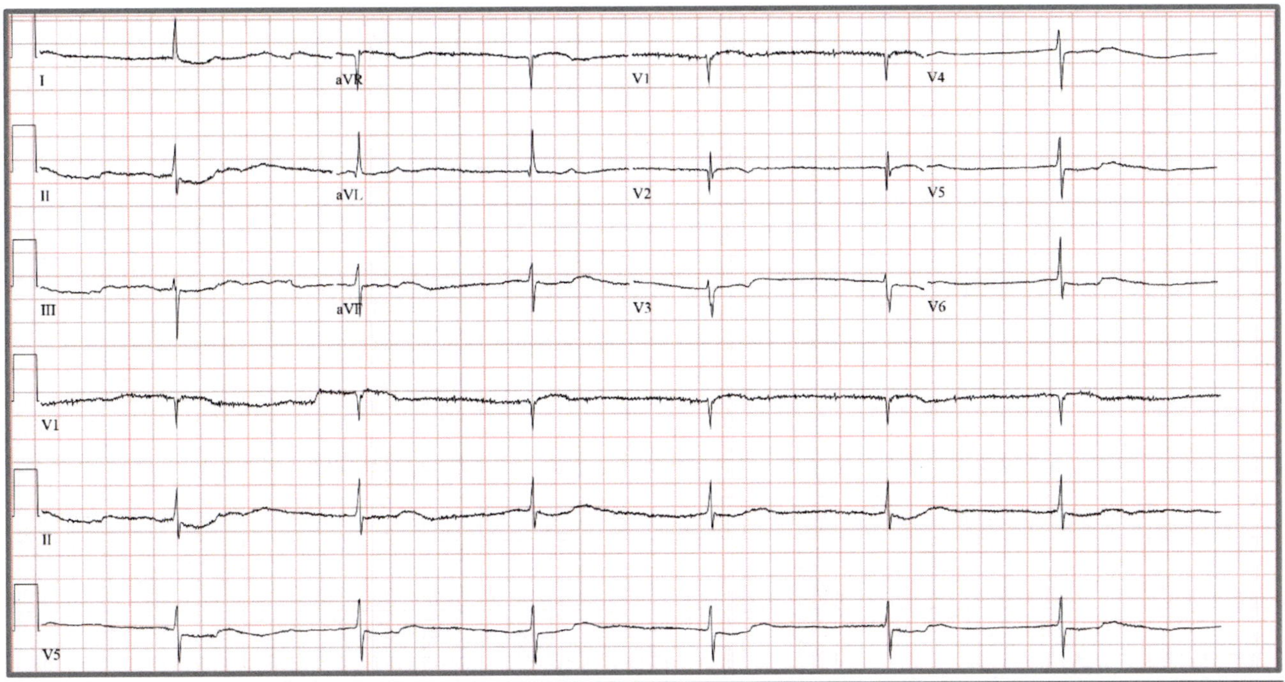

Rate:		Rhythm:		Axis:		Intervals:		Ischemia:	

#141 – 50-year-old male presents with dyspnea

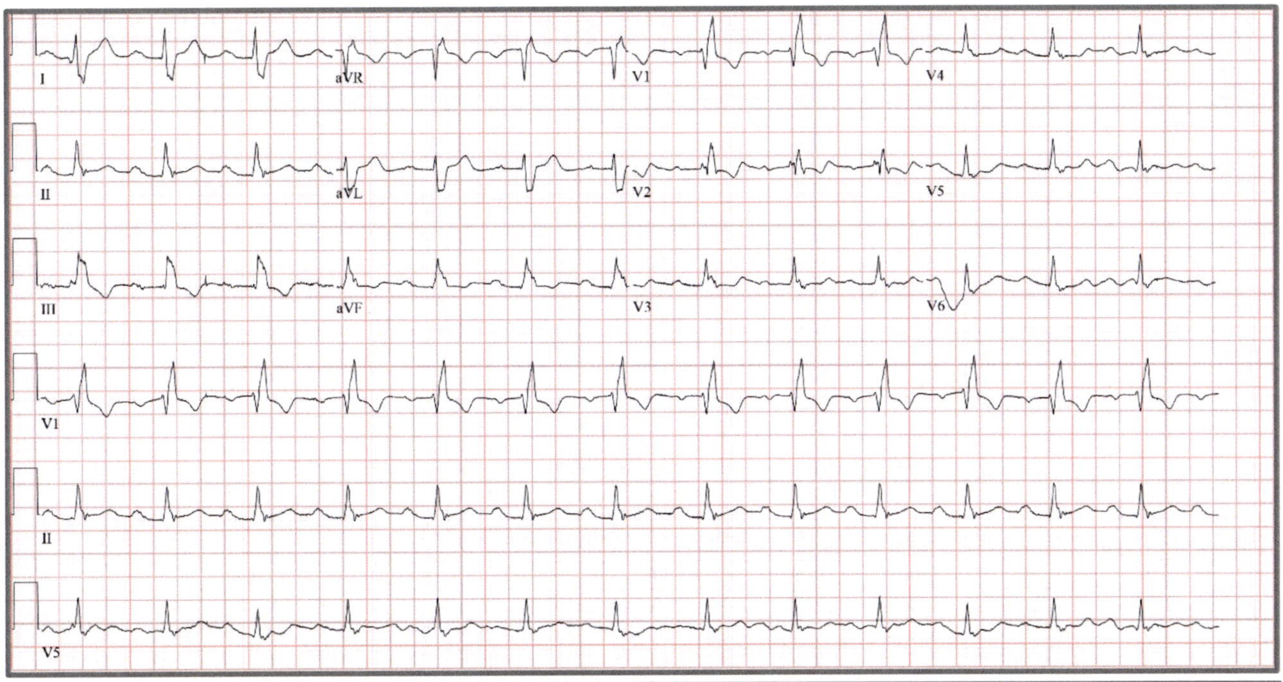

Rate:		Rhythm:		Axis:		Intervals:		Ischemia:	

#142 – 87-year-old female presents with cardiac arrest

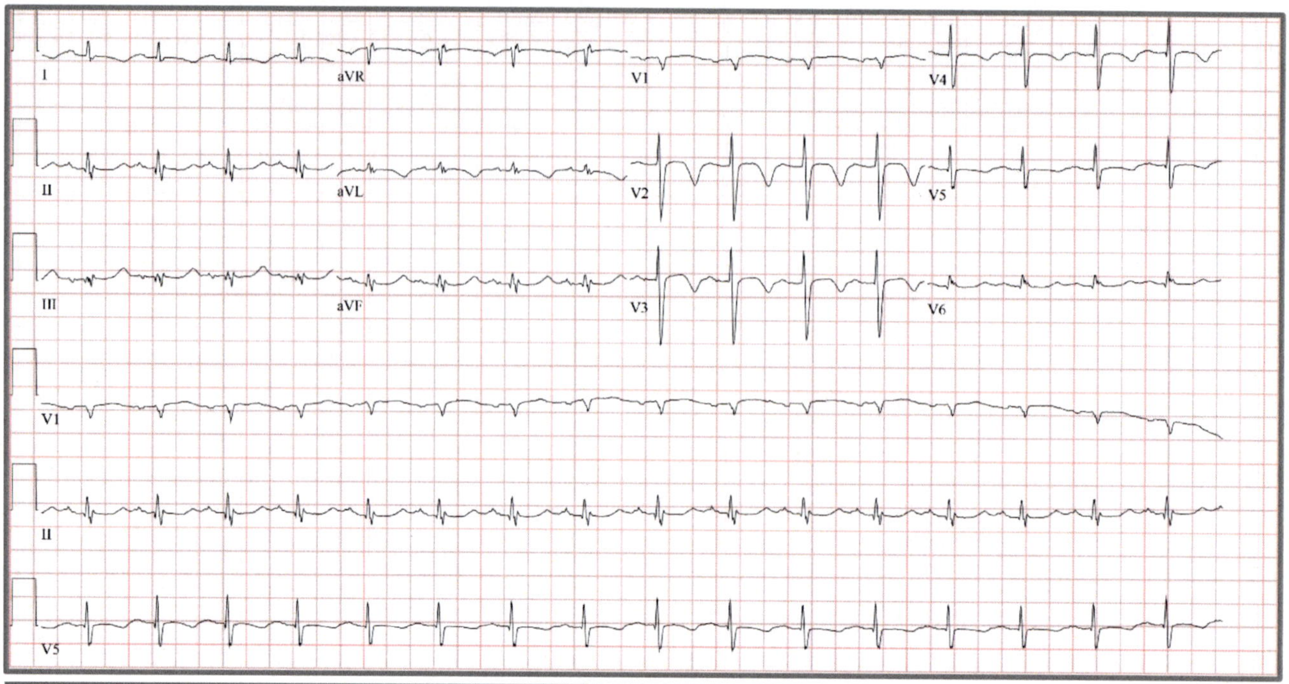

Rate:	Rhythm:	Axis:	Intervals:	Ischemia:

#143 – 35-year-old male presents with sickle cell pain crisis

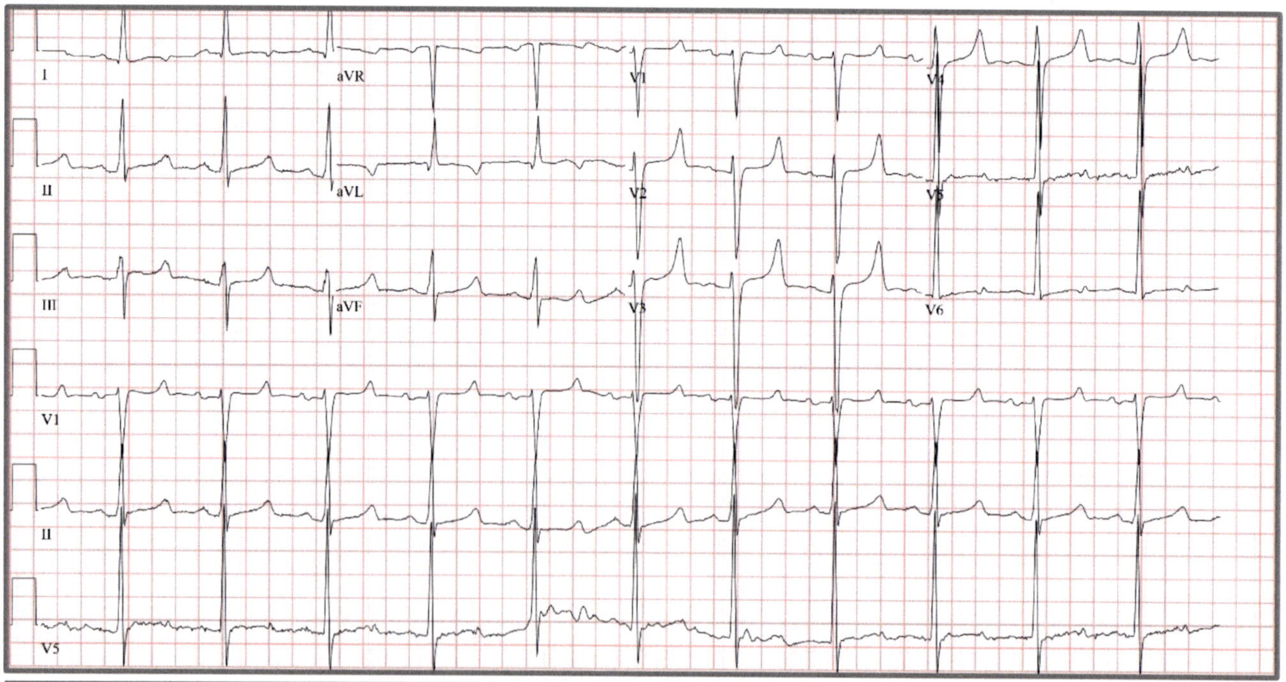

Rate:	Rhythm:	Axis:	Intervals:	Ischemia:

#144 – 42-year-old female presents status post assault

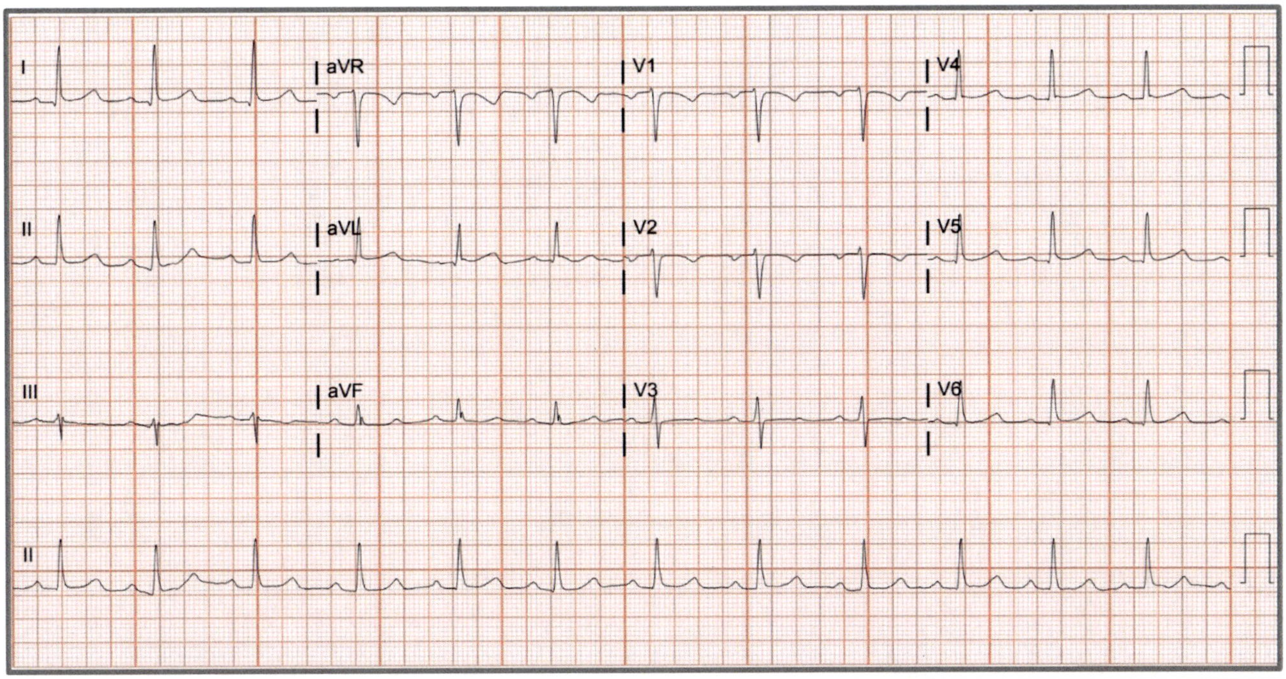

Rate:	Rhythm:	Axis:	Intervals:	Ischemia:

#145 – 58-year-old female presents with abdominal pain

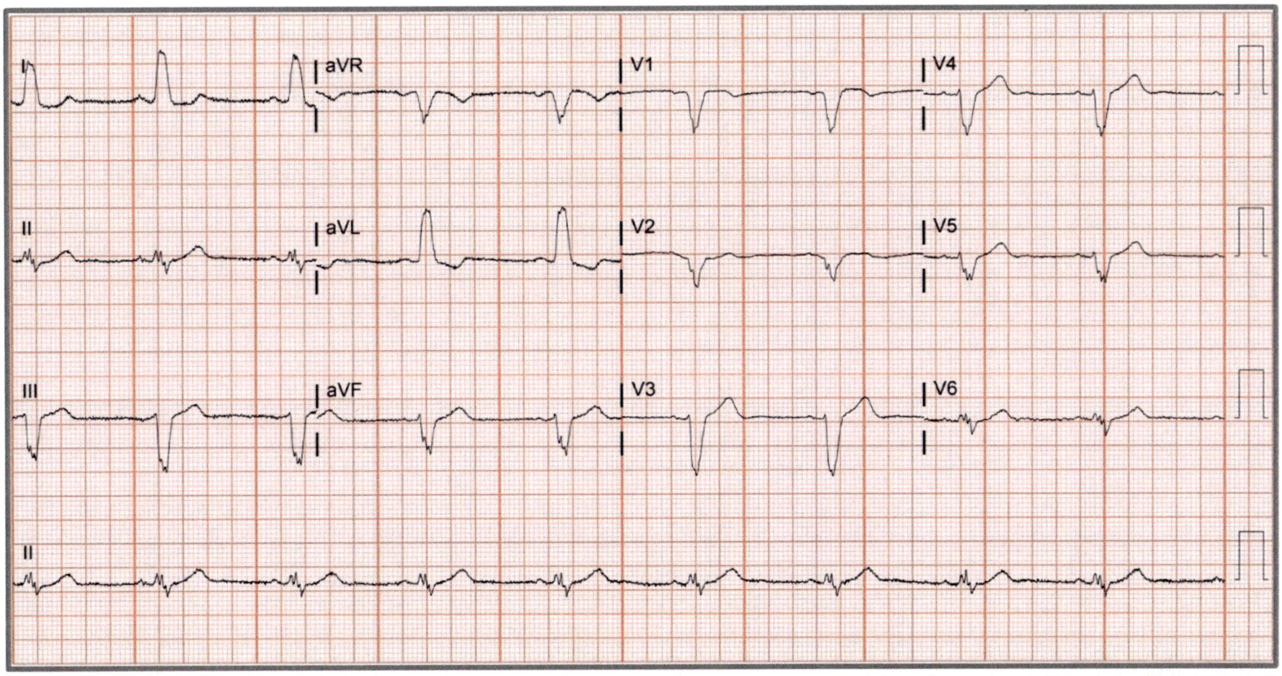

Rate:	Rhythm:	Axis:	Intervals:	Ischemia:

#146 – 64-year-old male presents with palpitations

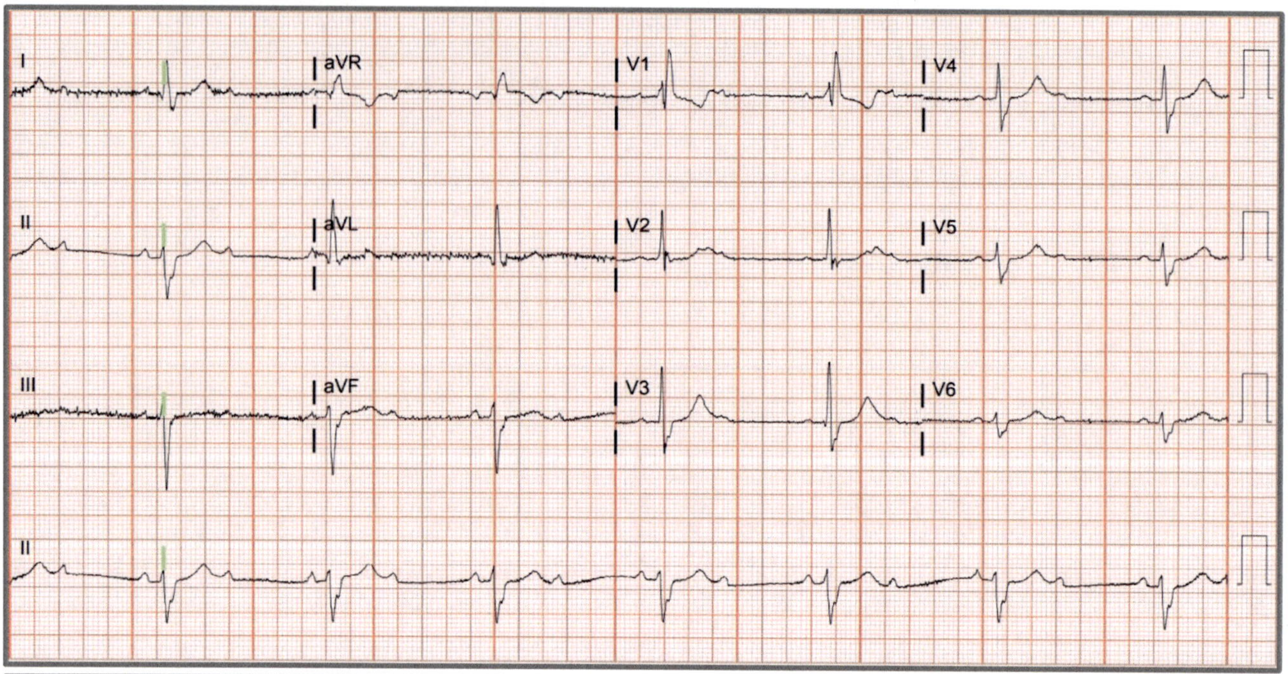

Rate:	Rhythm:	Axis:	Intervals:	Ischemia:

#147 – 64-year-old female presents with dyspnea

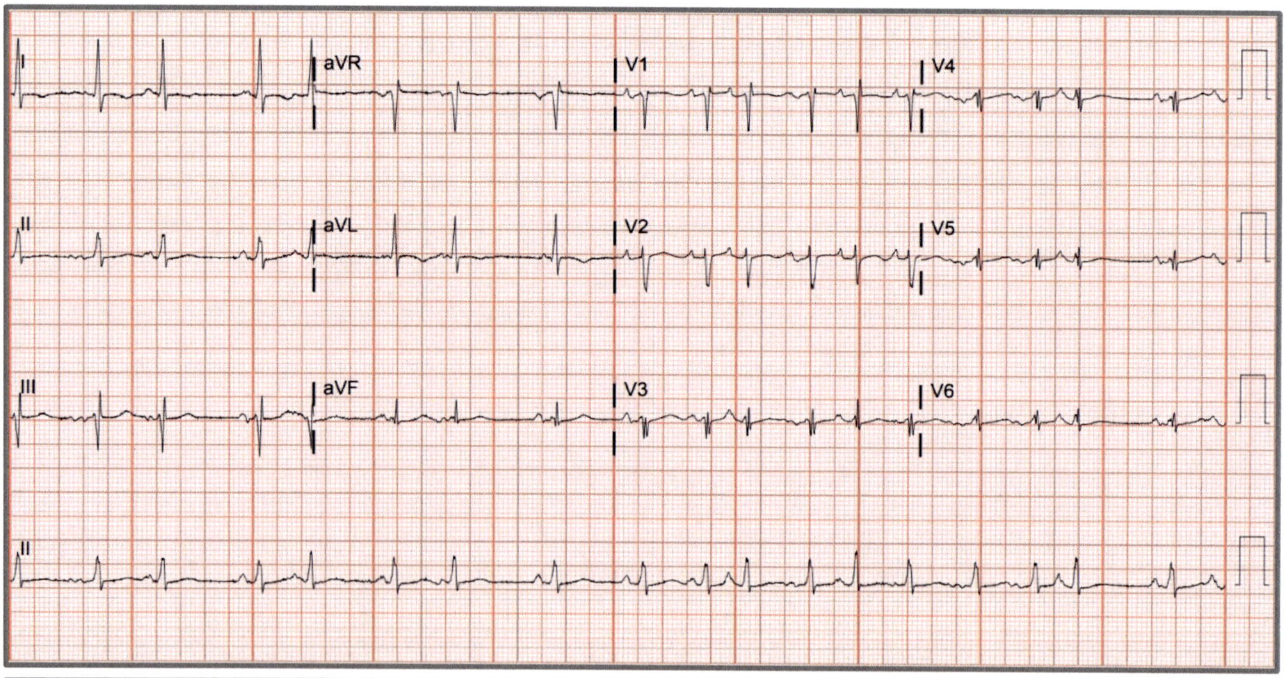

Rate:	Rhythm:	Axis:	Intervals:	Ischemia:

#148 – 50-year-old male presents with palpitations

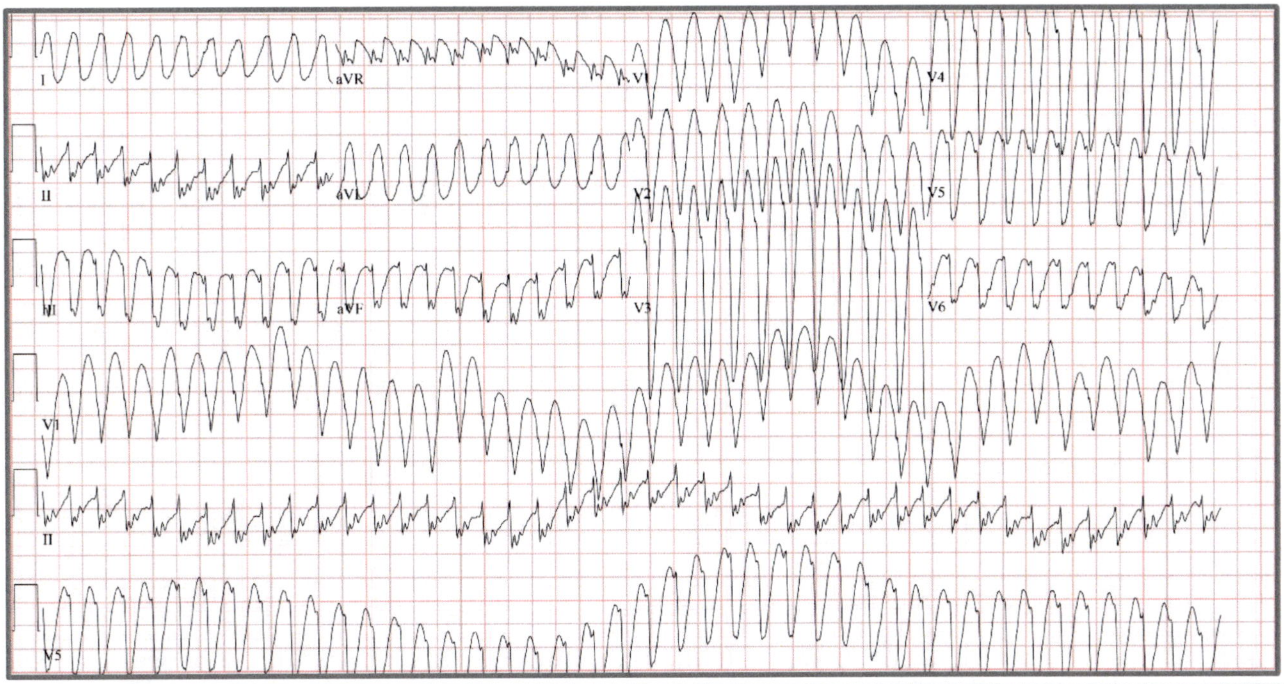

Rate: Rhythm: Axis: Intervals: Ischemia:

#149 – 54-year-old female presents with chest pain

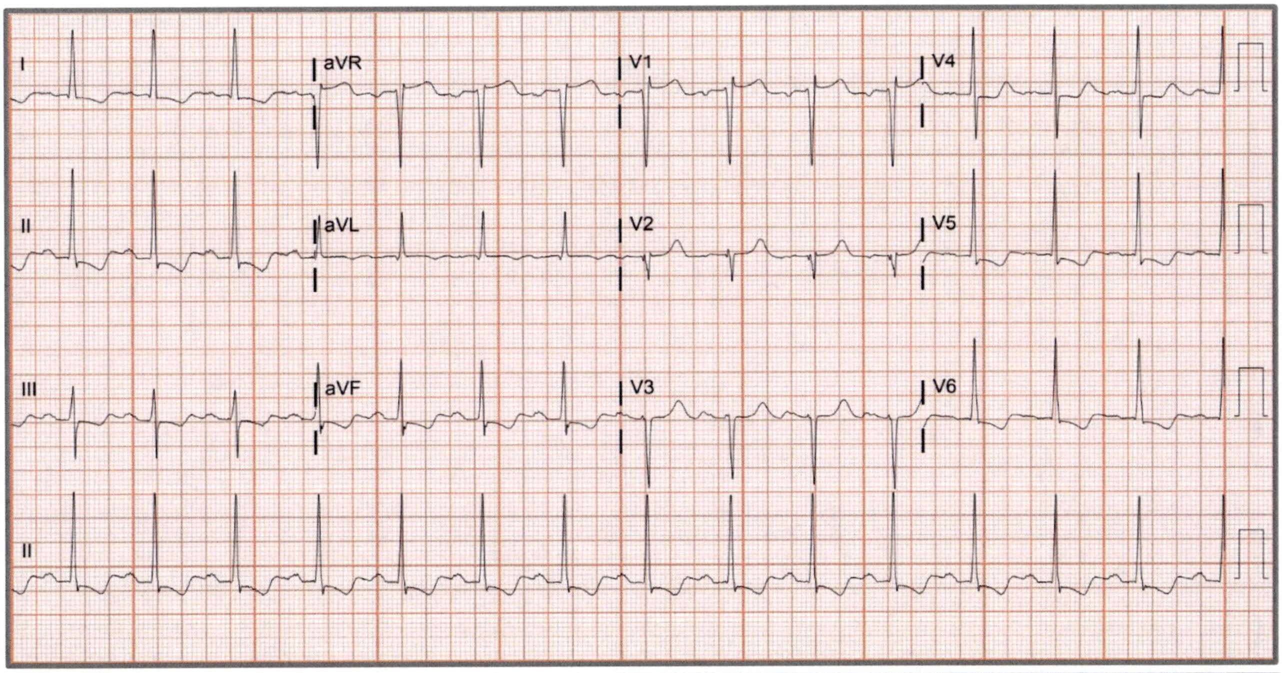

Rate: Rhythm: Axis: Intervals: Ischemia:

#150 – 52-year-old female presents with palpitations

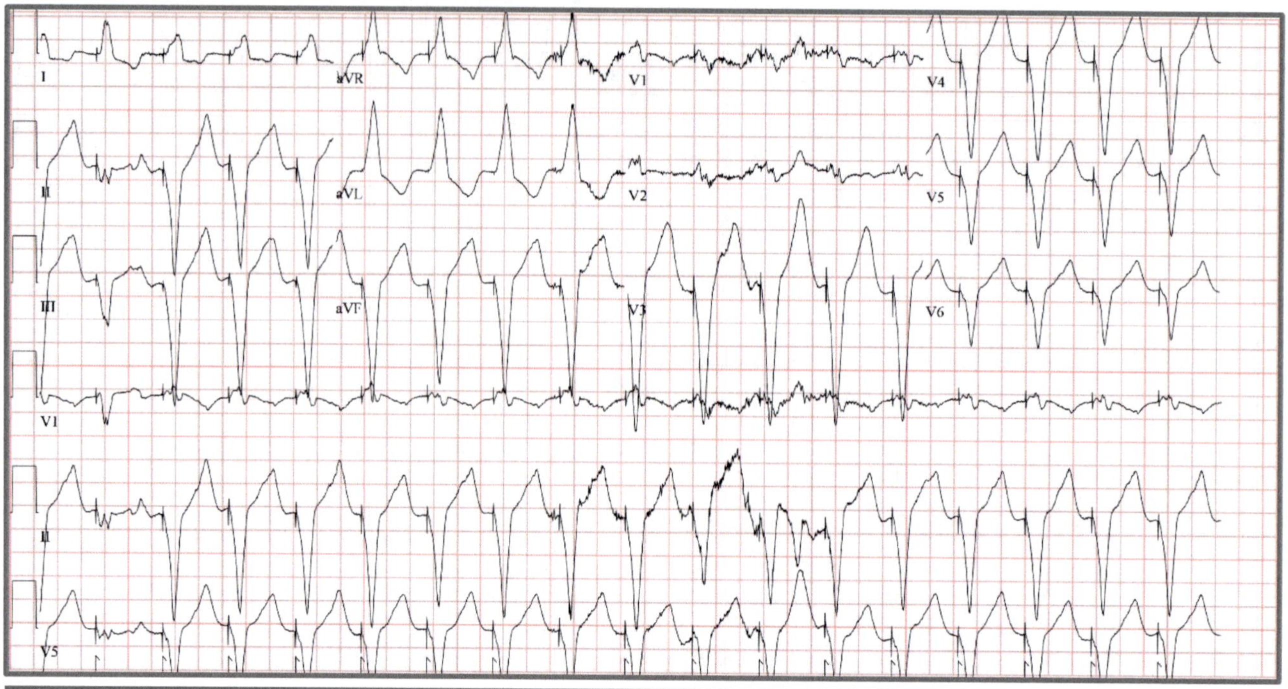

Rate: Rhythm: Axis: Intervals: Ischemia:

#151 – 55-year-old male presents with dyspnea

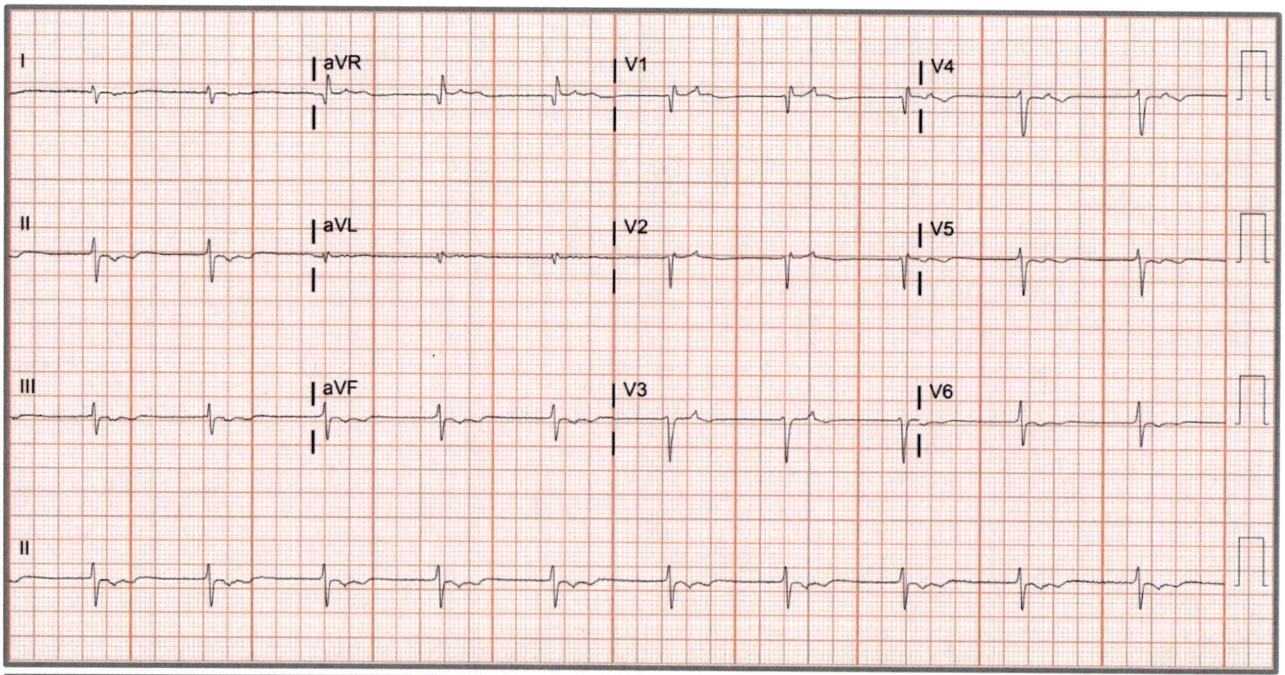

Rate: Rhythm: Axis: Intervals: Ischemia:

#152 – 66-year-old male presents with weakness

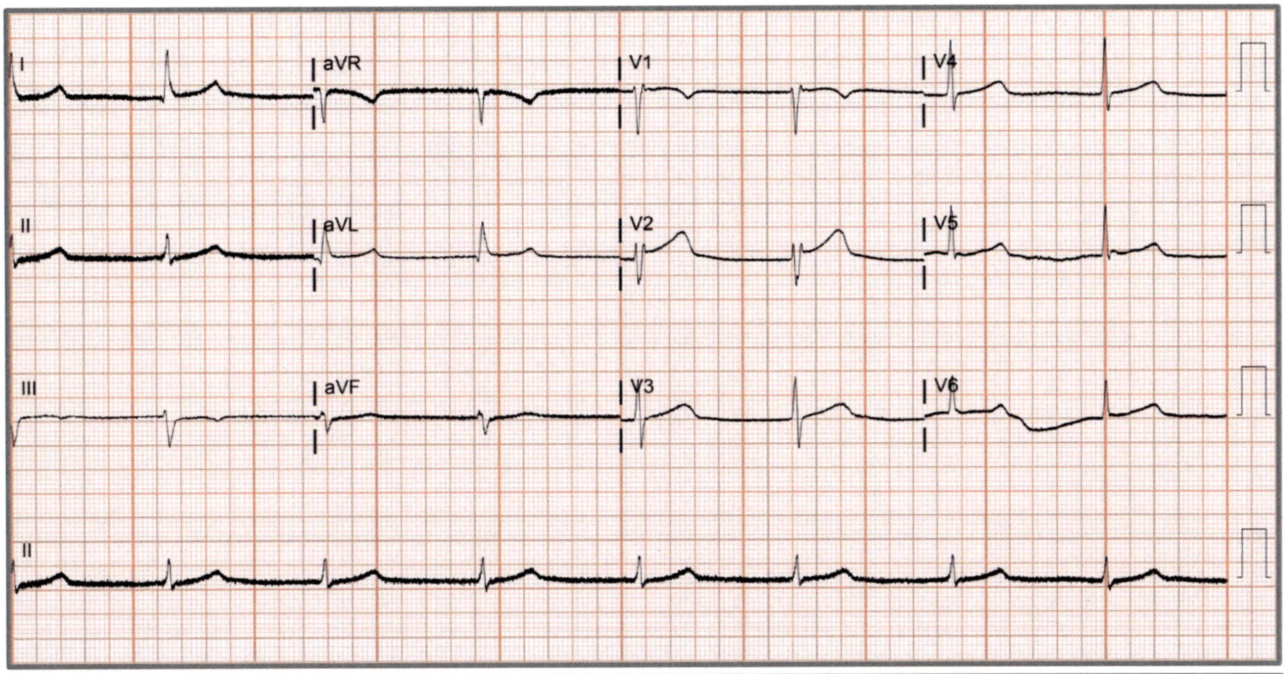

Rate: **Rhythm:**   **Axis:**   **Intervals:**   **Ischemia:**

#153 – 66-year-old male presents with weakness

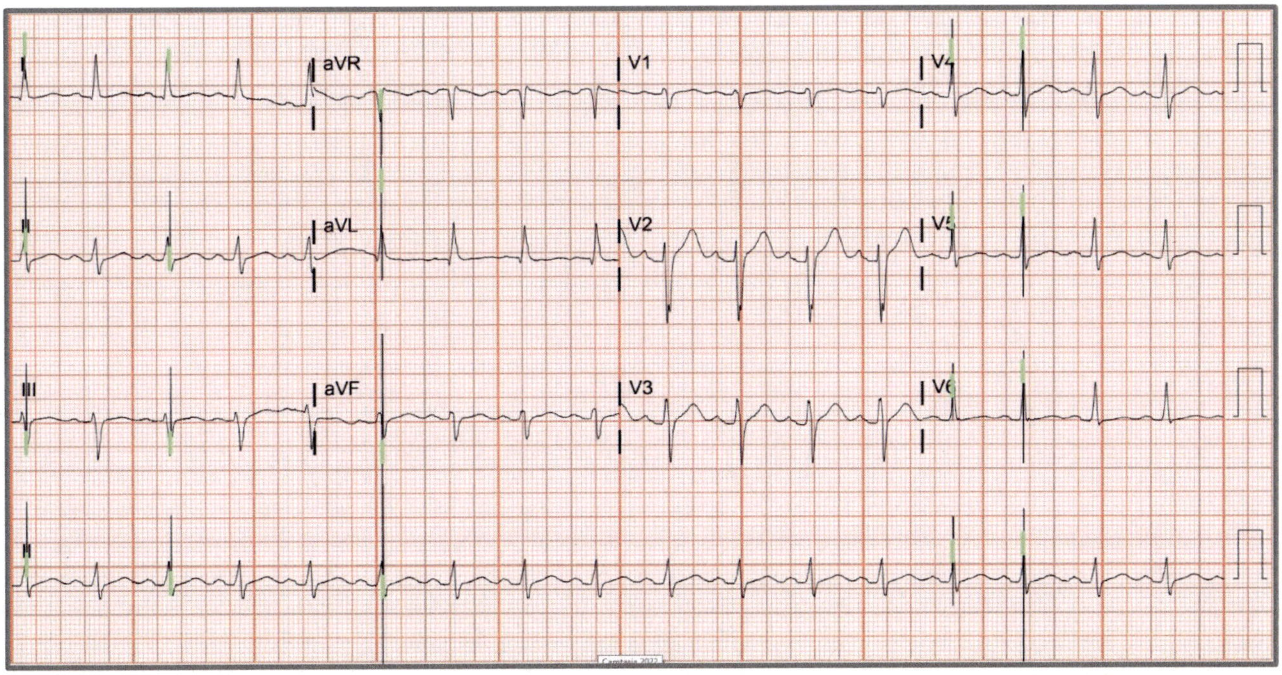

Rate: **Rhythm:**   **Axis:**   **Intervals:**   **Ischemia:**

#154 – 69-year-old male presents with chest pain

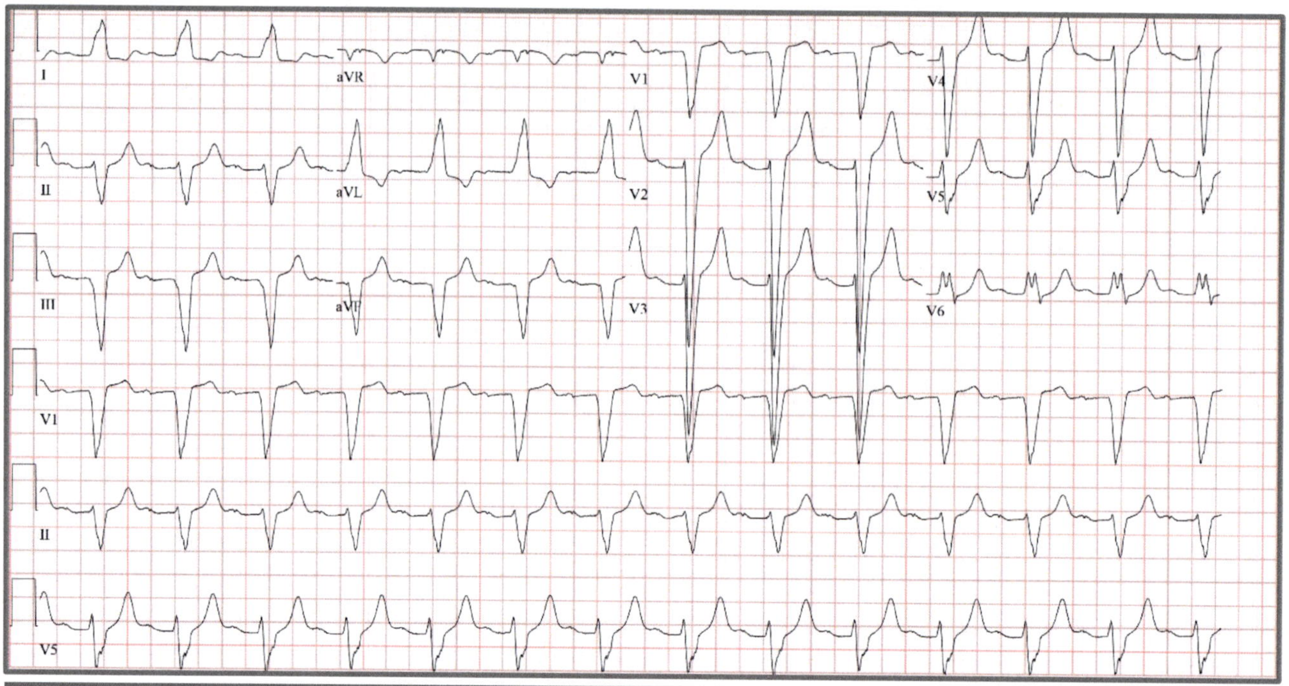

Rate: Rhythm: Axis: Intervals: Ischemia:

#155 – 26-year-old male presents with abdominal pain

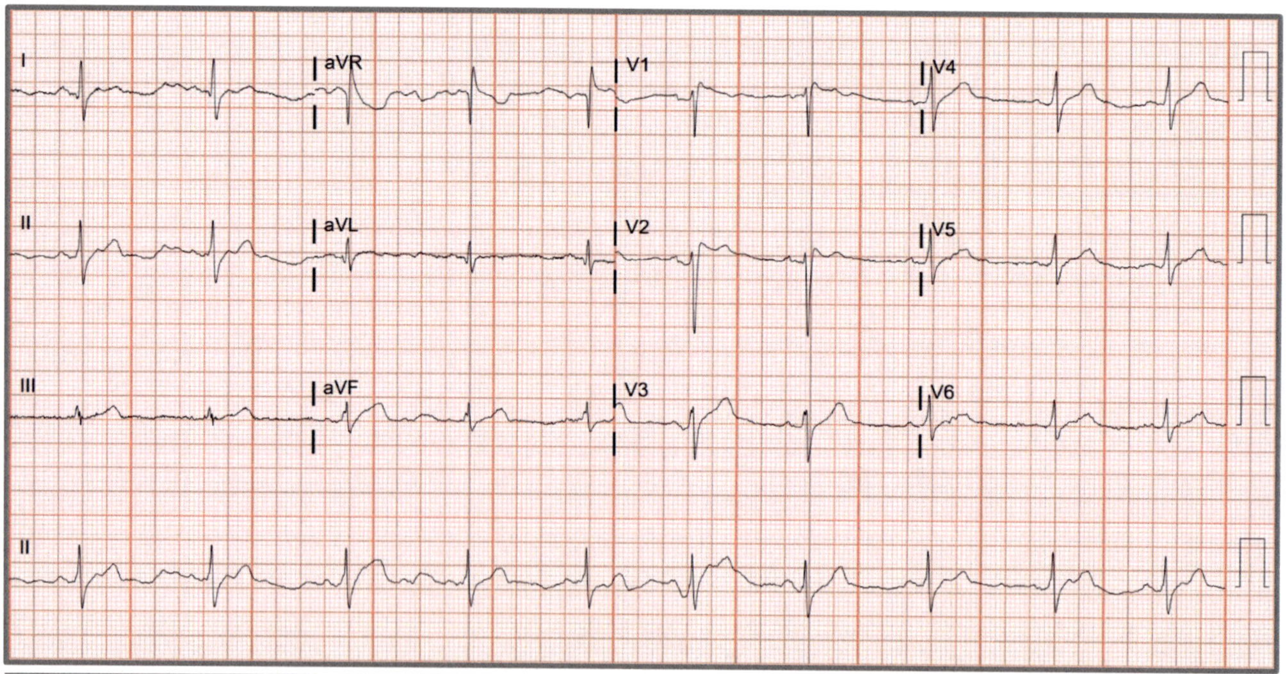

Rate: Rhythm: Axis: Intervals: Ischemia:

#156 – 56-year-old male presents with chest pain

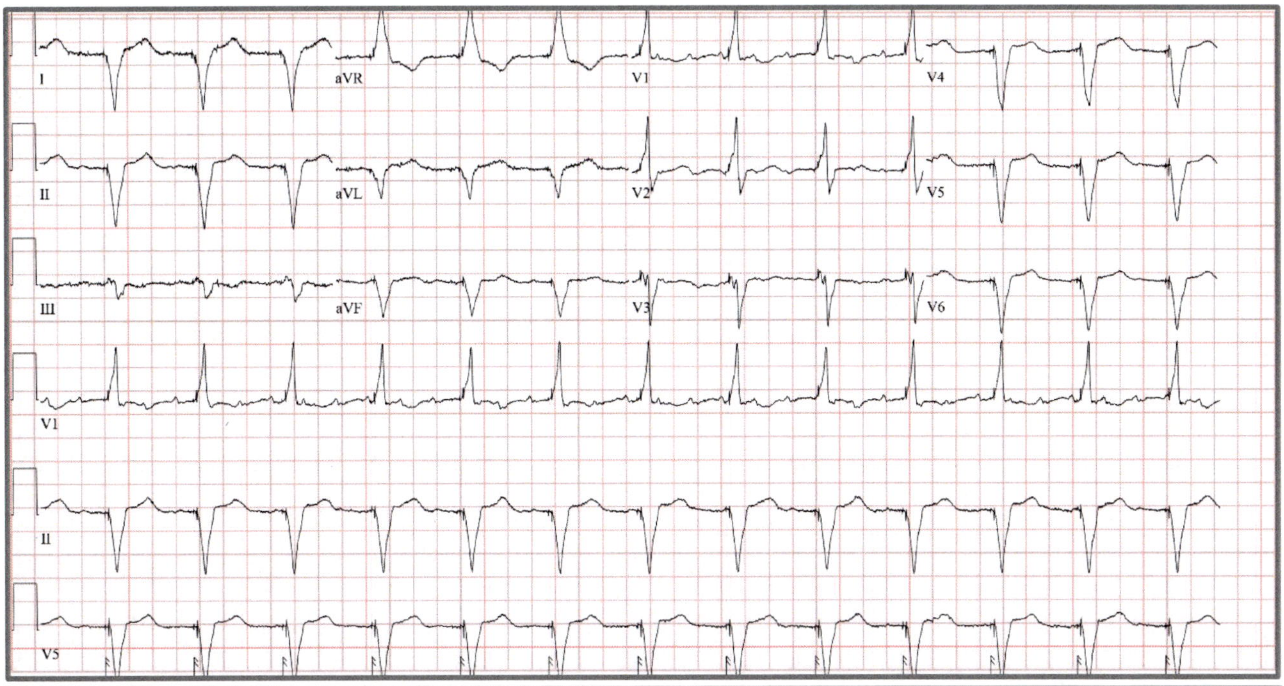

Rate: **Rhythm:** **Axis:** **Intervals:** **Ischemia:**

#157 – 67-year-old male presents with dyspnea and fever

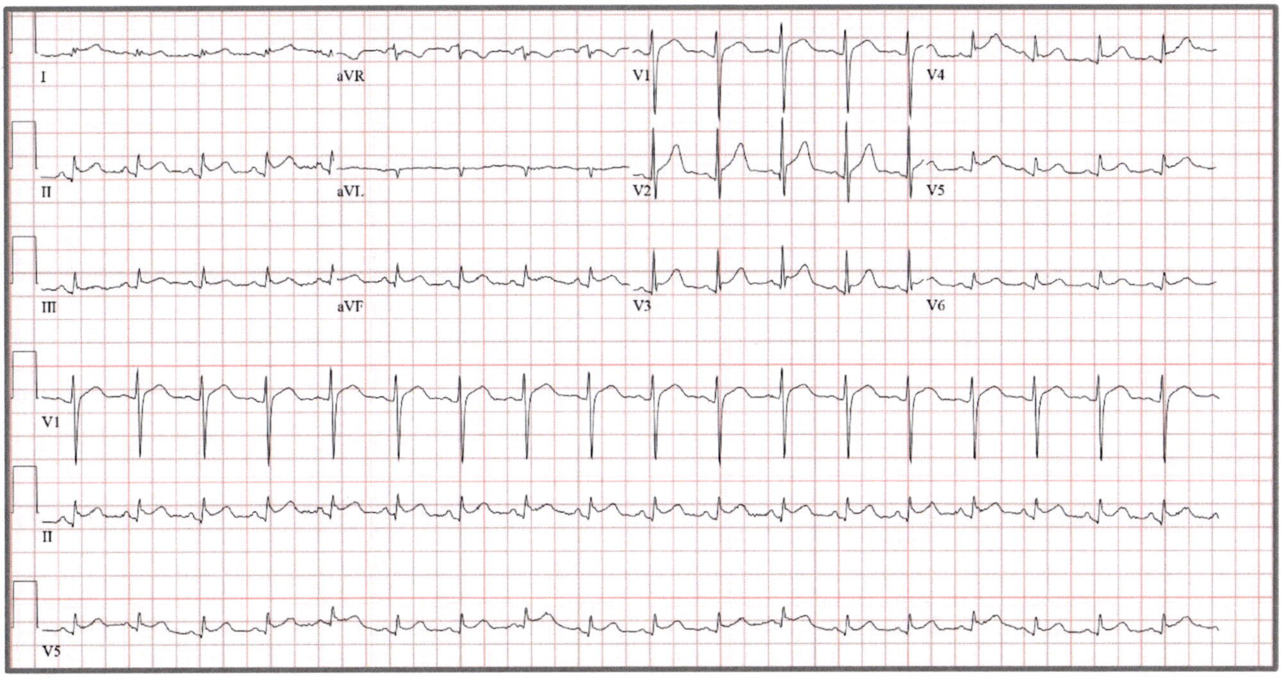

Rate: **Rhythm:** **Axis:** **Intervals:** **Ischemia:**

#158 – 8-year-old female presents with palpitations

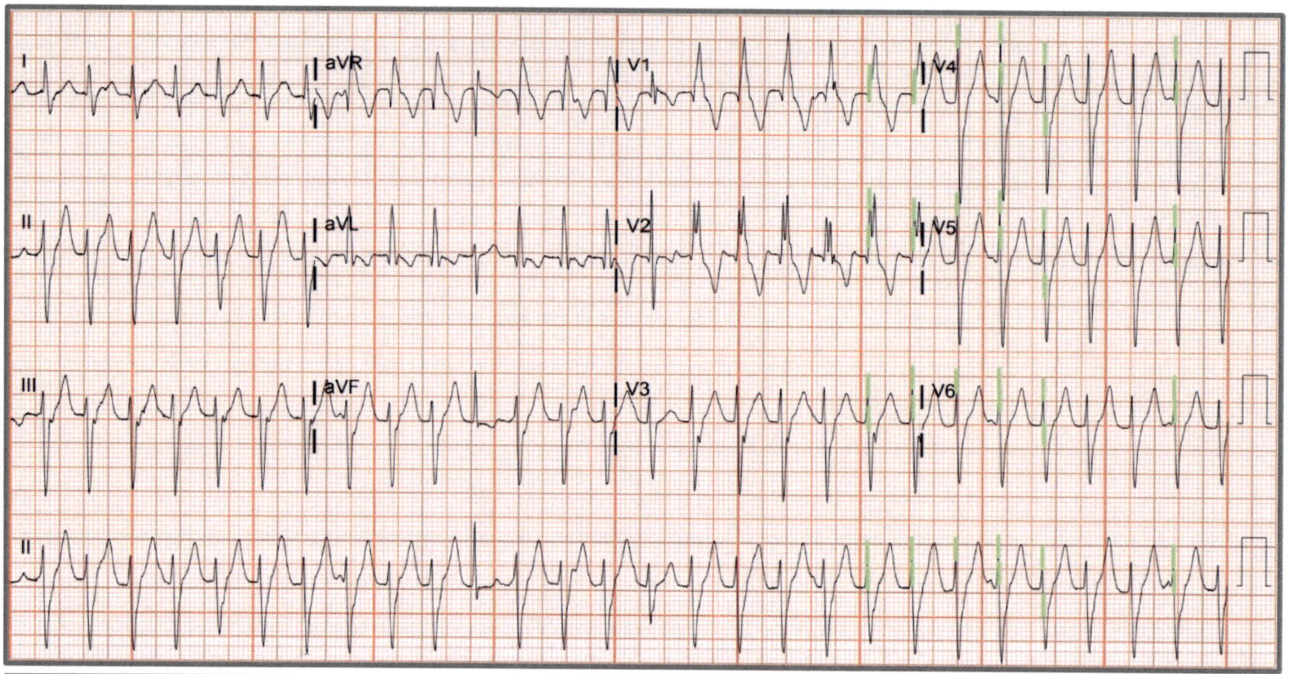

Rate: Rhythm: Axis: Intervals: Ischemia:

#159 – 32-year-old male presents with palpitations

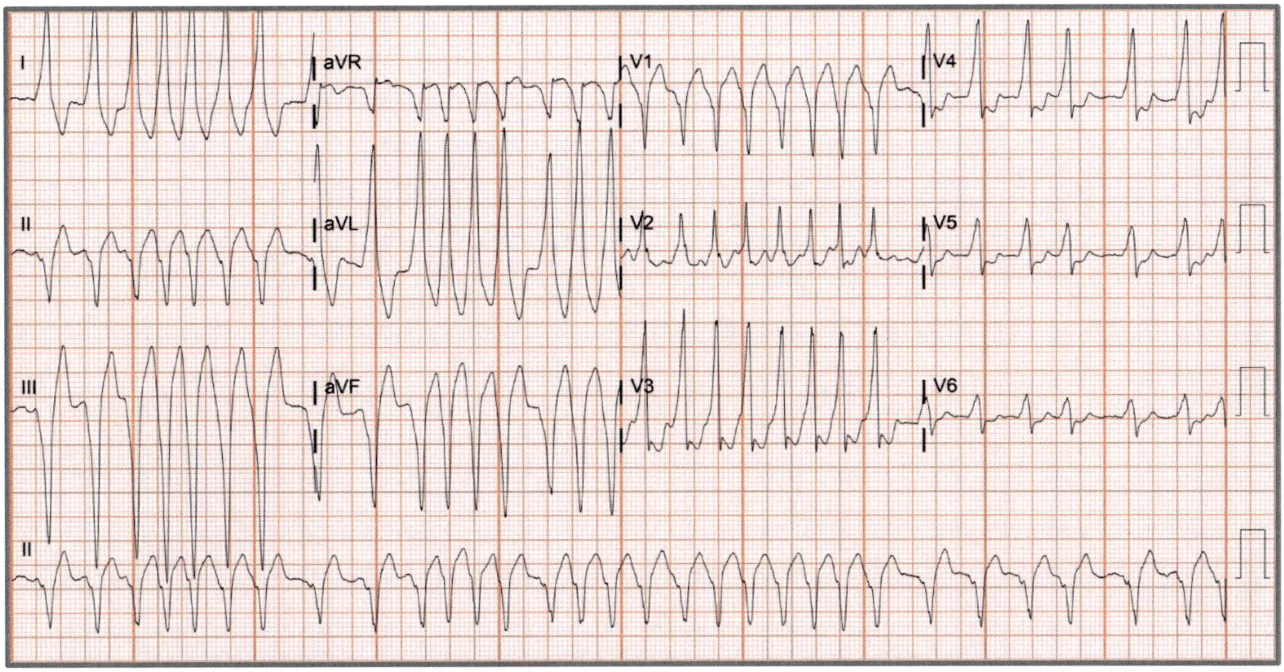

Rate:		Rhythm:		Axis:		Intervals:		Ischemia:	

⇩ Prior ECG ⇩

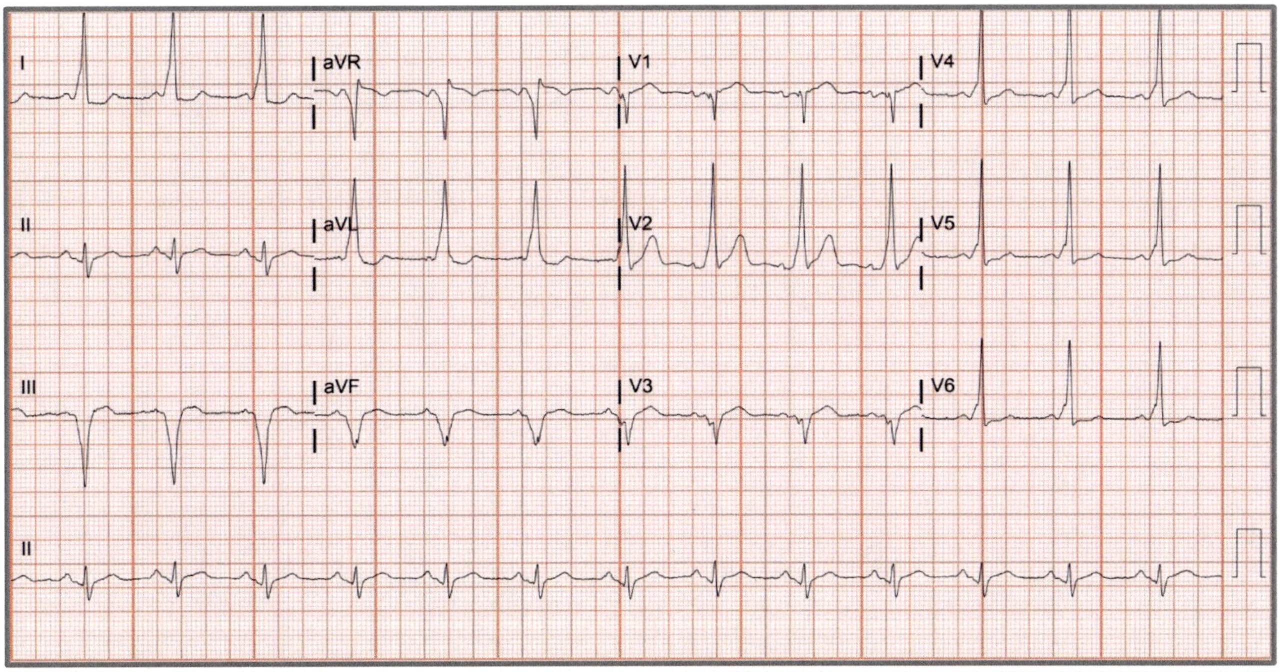

Rate:		Rhythm:		Axis:		Intervals:		Ischemia:	

#160 – 50-year-old female presents post cardiac arrest

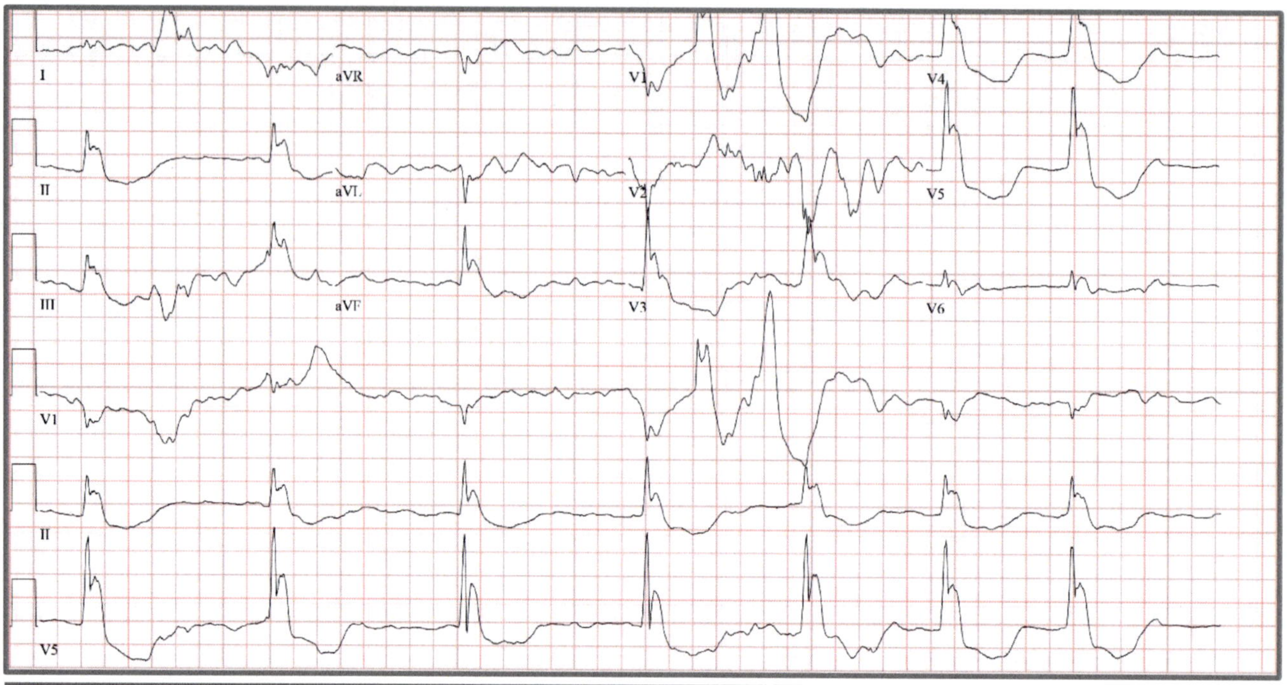

Rate:	Rhythm:	Axis:	Intervals:	Ischemia:

#161 – 50-year-old male presents with chest pain

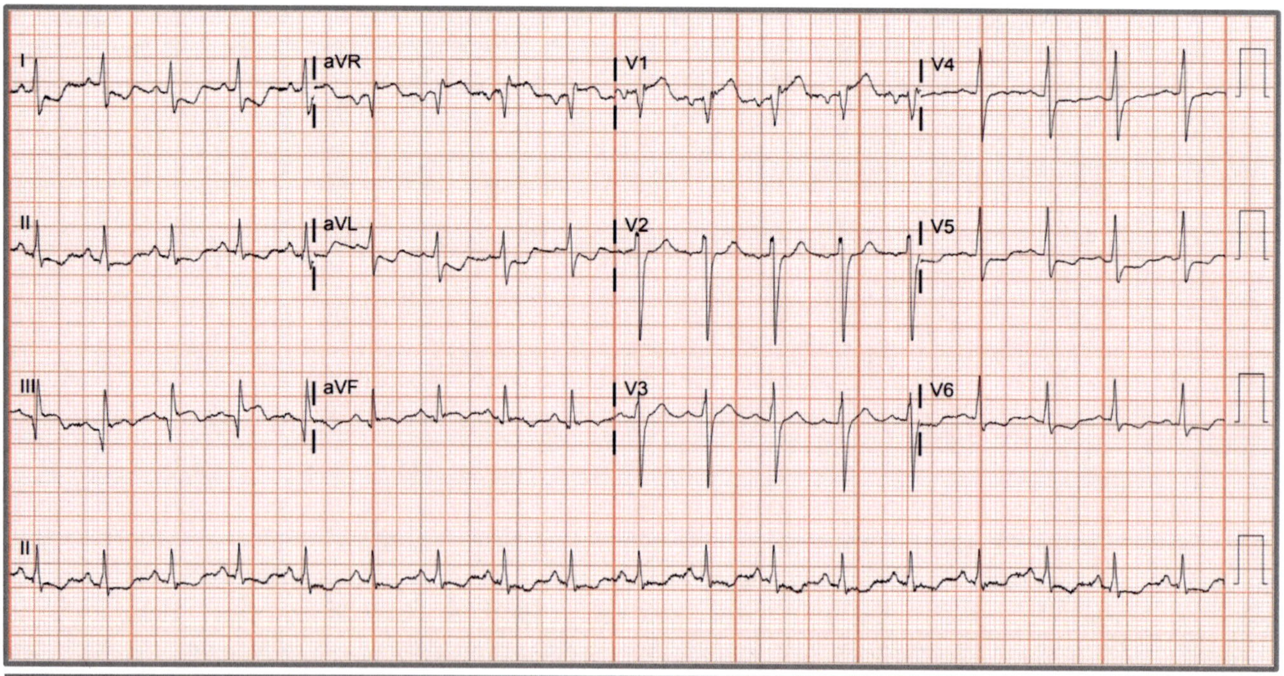

Rate:	Rhythm:	Axis:	Intervals:	Ischemia:

#162 – 64-year-old male presents with chest pain

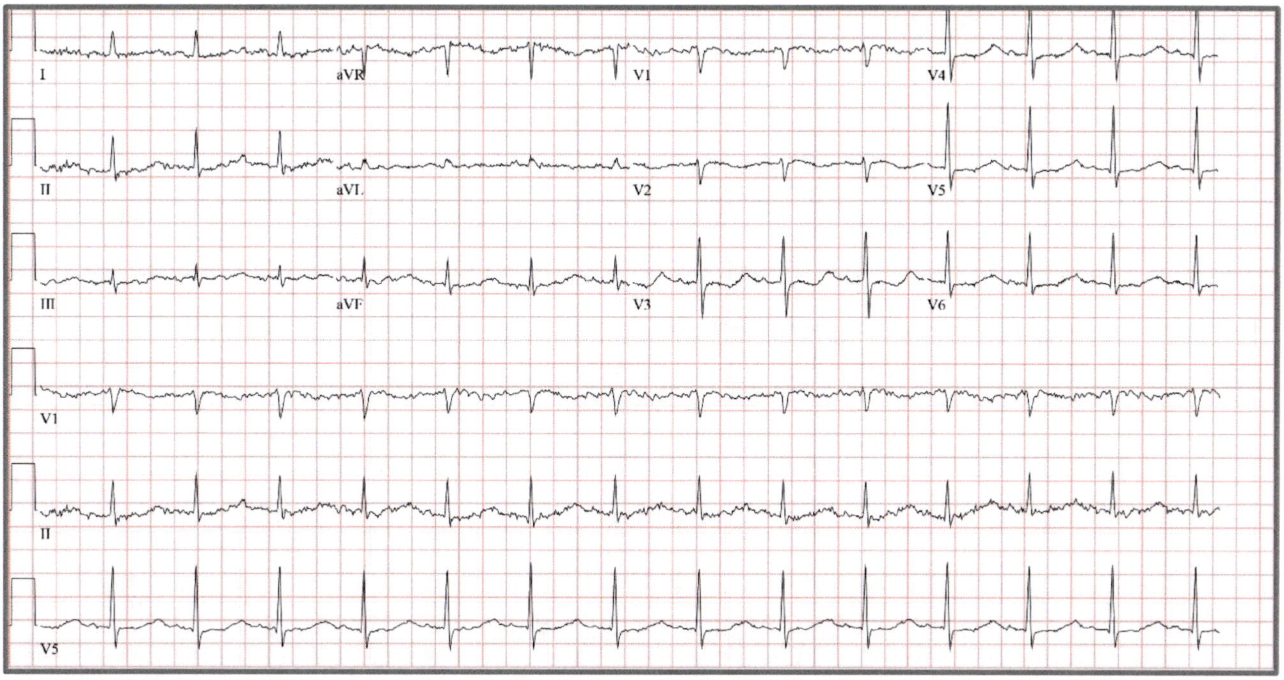

Rate: Rhythm: Axis: Intervals: Ischemia:

#163 – 64-year-old male presents with chest pain

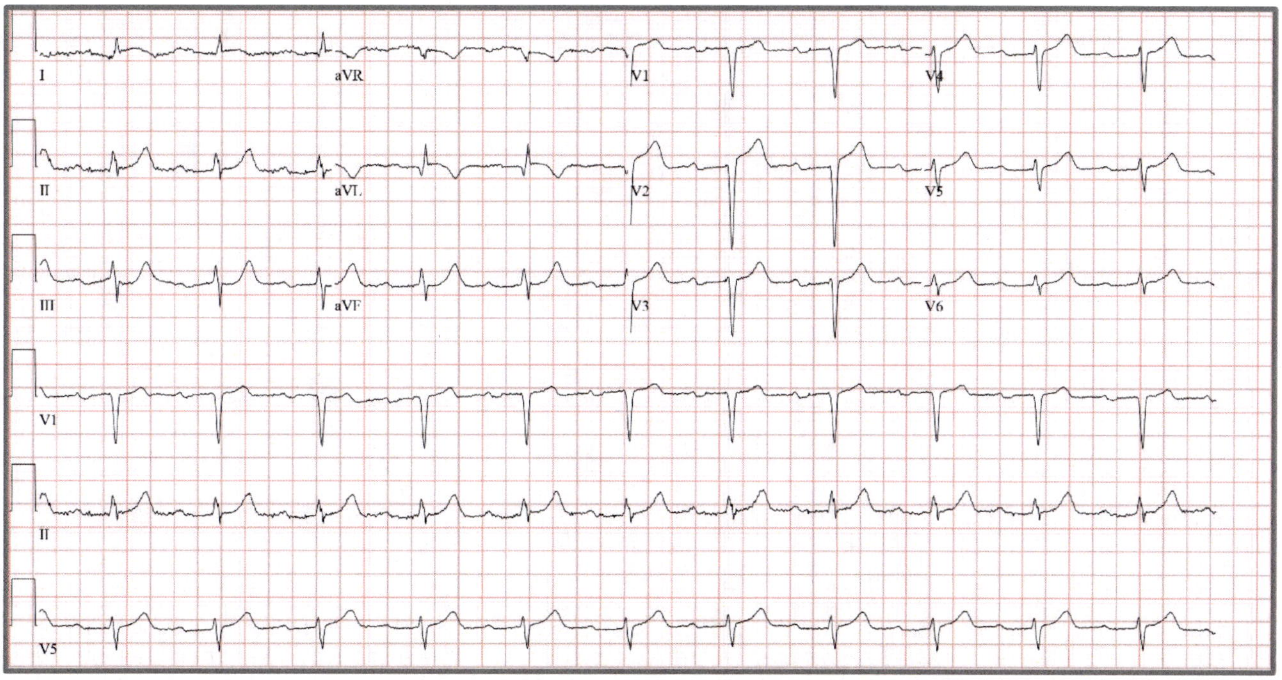

Rate: Rhythm: Axis: Intervals: Ischemia:

#164 – 65-year-old female presents with chest pain, dyspnea

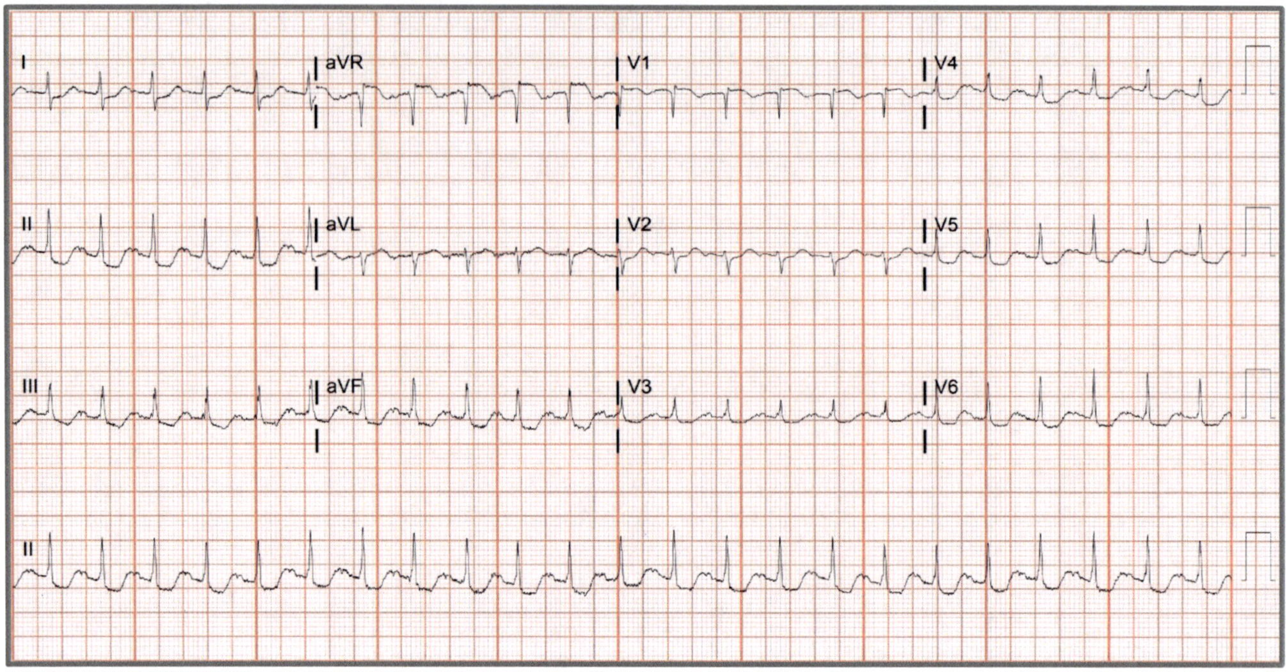

Rate: Rhythm: Axis: Intervals: Ischemia:

#165 – 62-year-old male presents with dyspnea

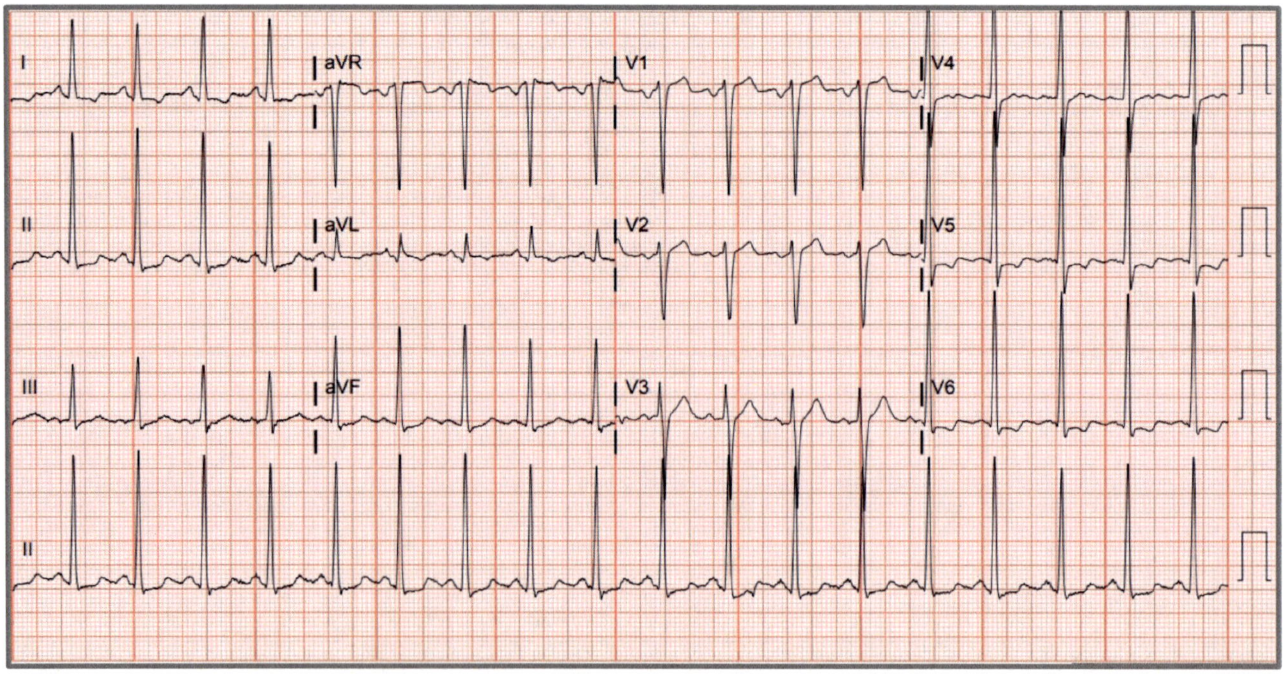

Rate: Rhythm: Axis: Intervals: Ischemia:

#166 – 87-year-old female presents with melena

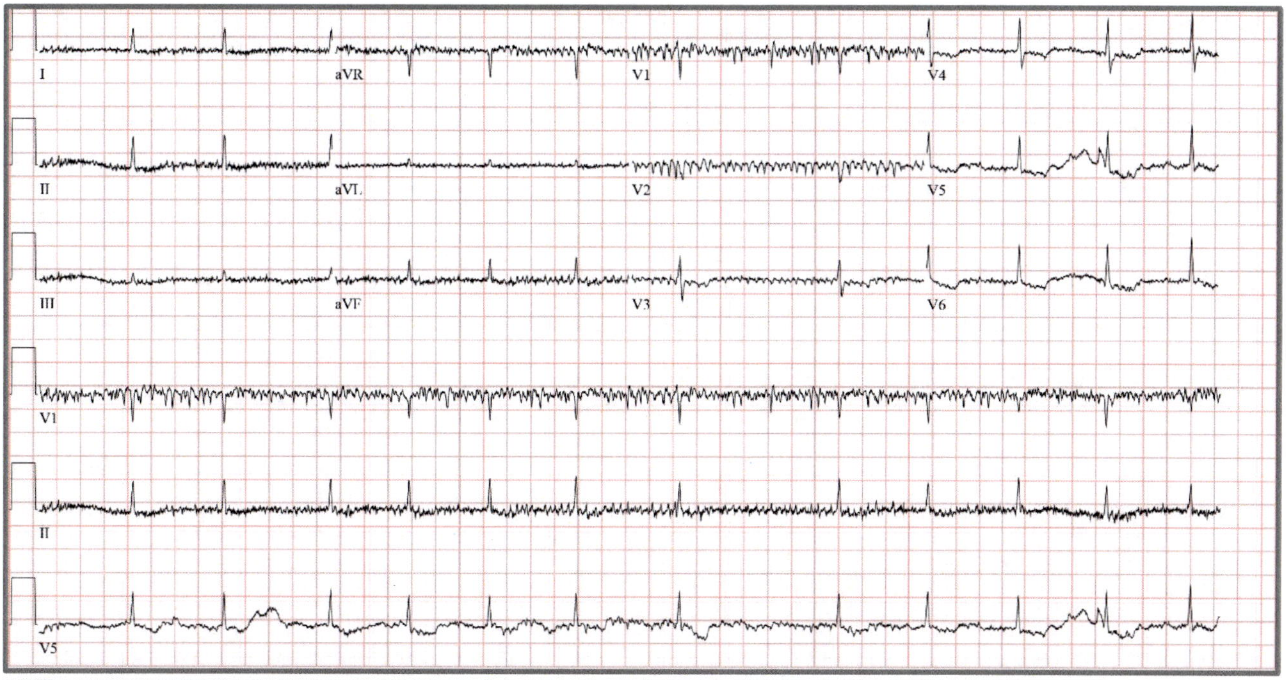

Rate:		Rhythm:		Axis:		Intervals:		Ischemia:	

#167 – 31-year-old male presents with dyspnea

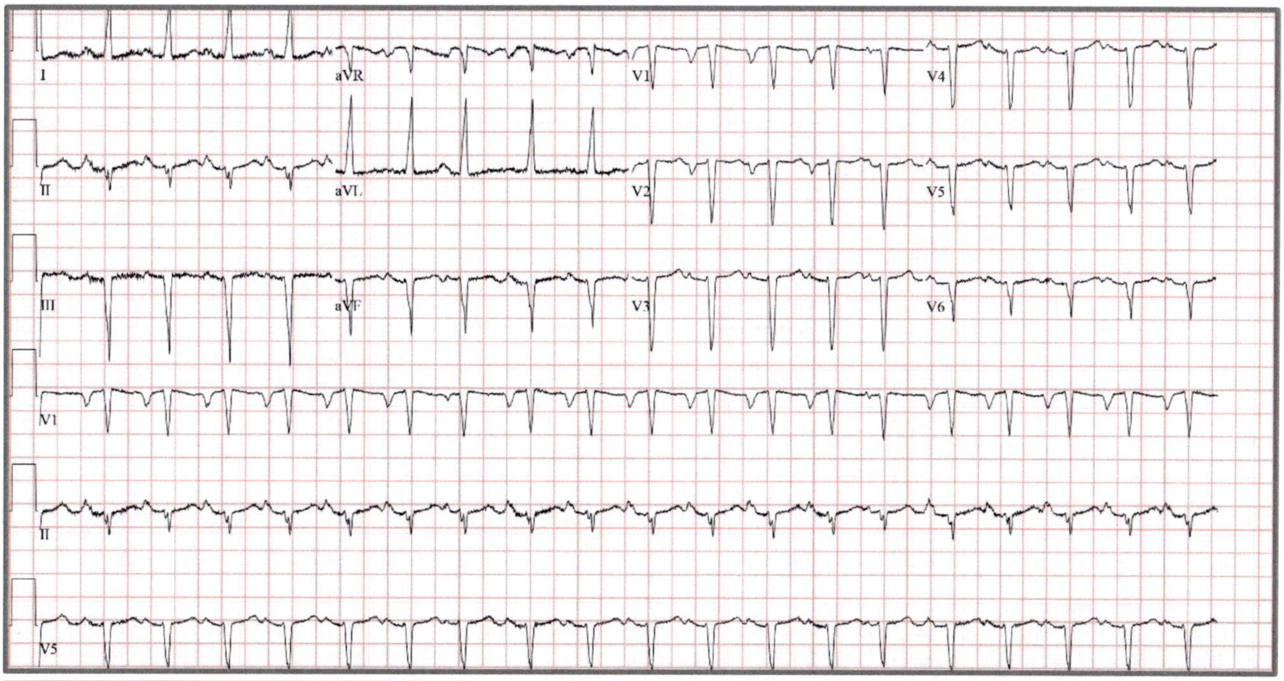

Rate:		Rhythm:		Axis:		Intervals:		Ischemia:	

#168 – 64-year-old female presents with vomiting

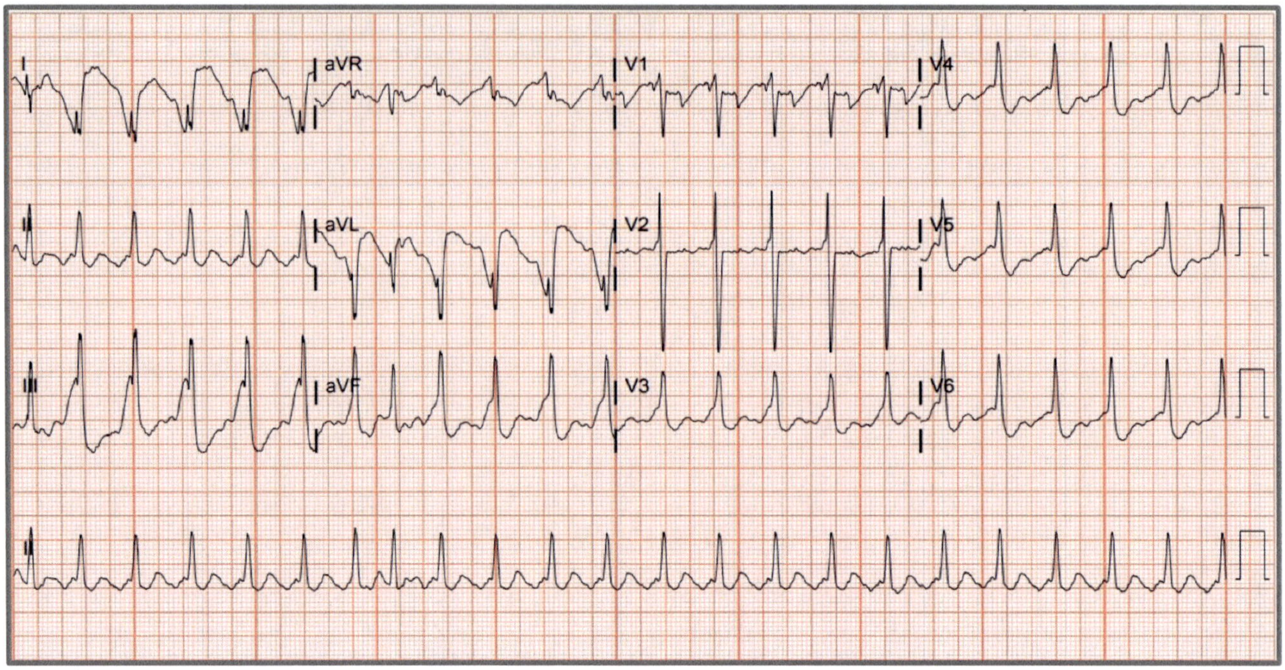

Rate: **Rhythm:** **Axis:** **Intervals:** **Ischemia:**

#169 – 54-year-old male presents with chest pain

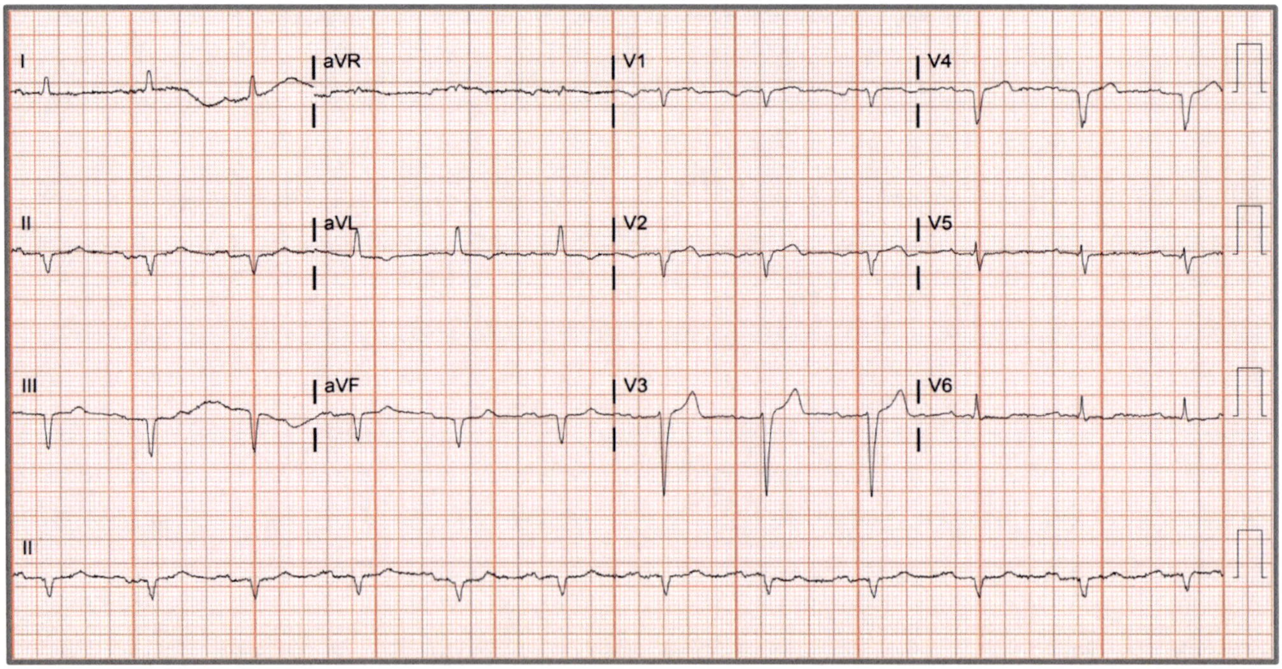

Rate: **Rhythm:** **Axis:** **Intervals:** **Ischemia:**

#170 – 76-year-old female presents with dyspnea

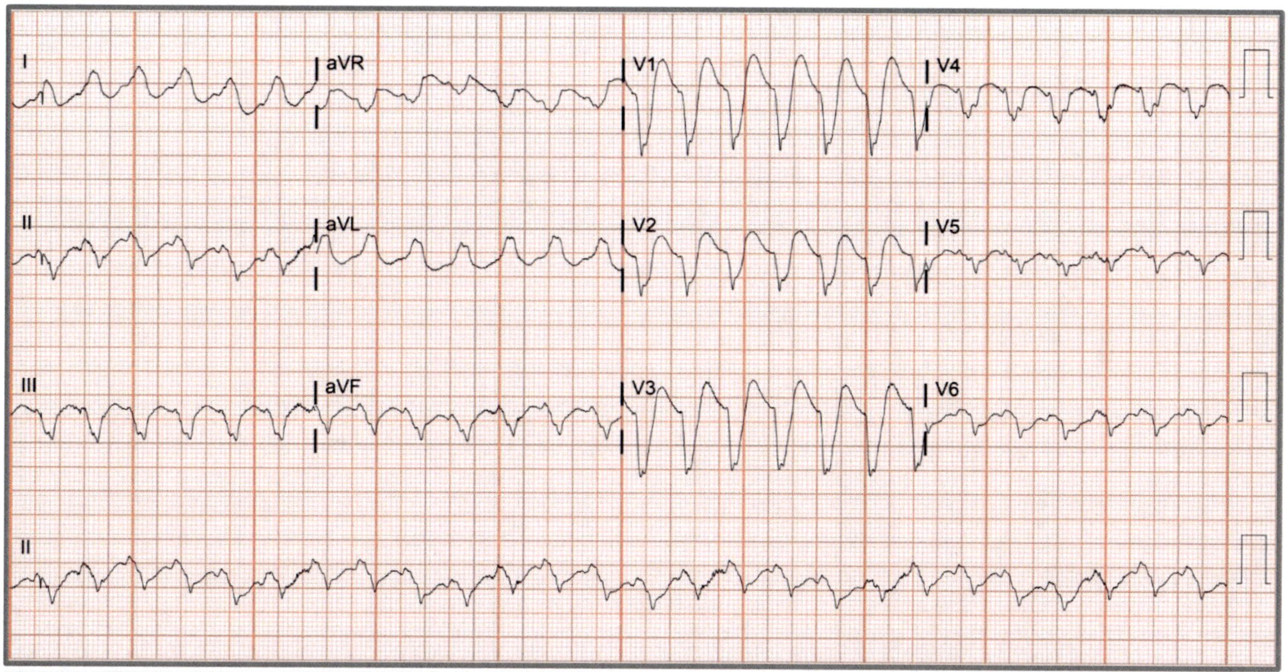

Rate: Rhythm: Axis: Intervals: Ischemia:

#171 – 61-year-old male presents with dyspnea

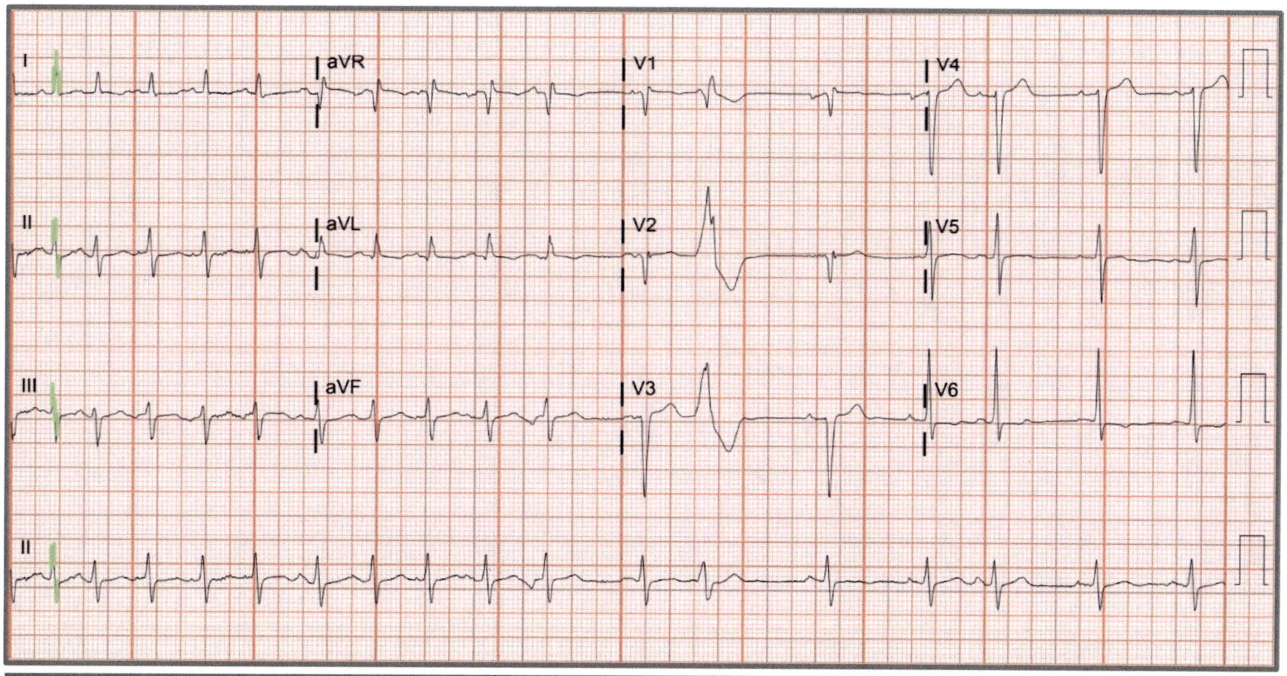

Rate: Rhythm: Axis: Intervals: Ischemia:

#172 – 41-year-old female presents with presyncope

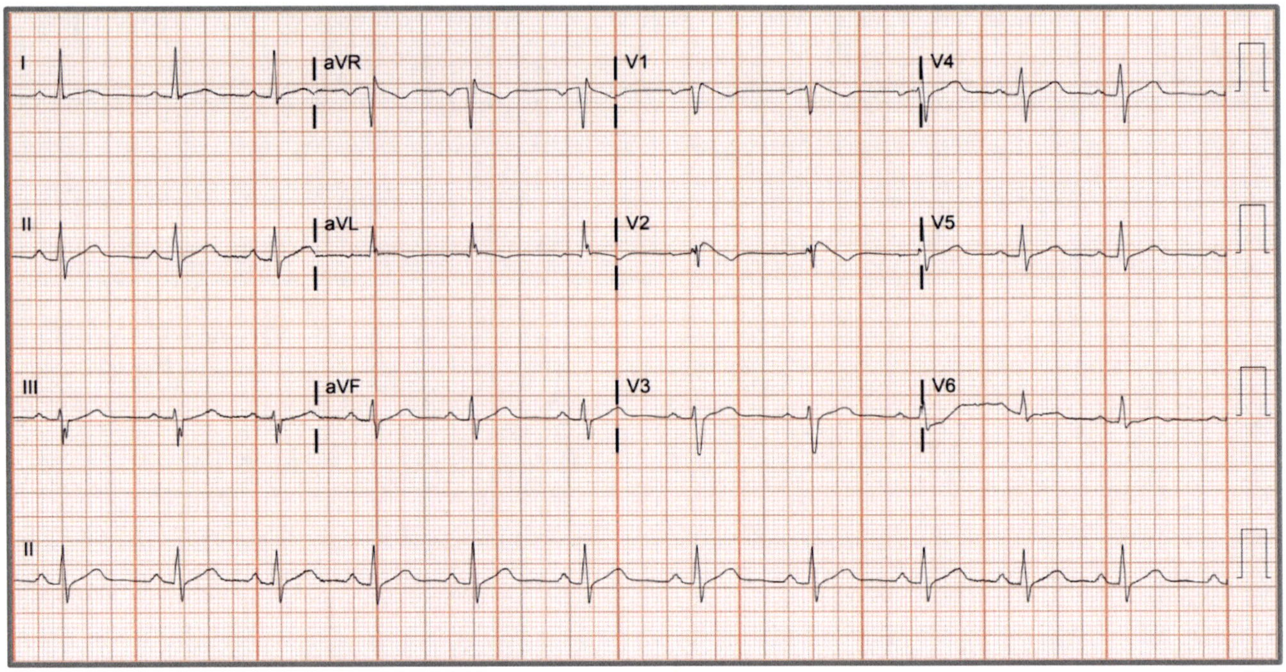

Rate:	Rhythm:	Axis:	Intervals:	Ischemia:

#173 – 29-year-old male presents with weakness

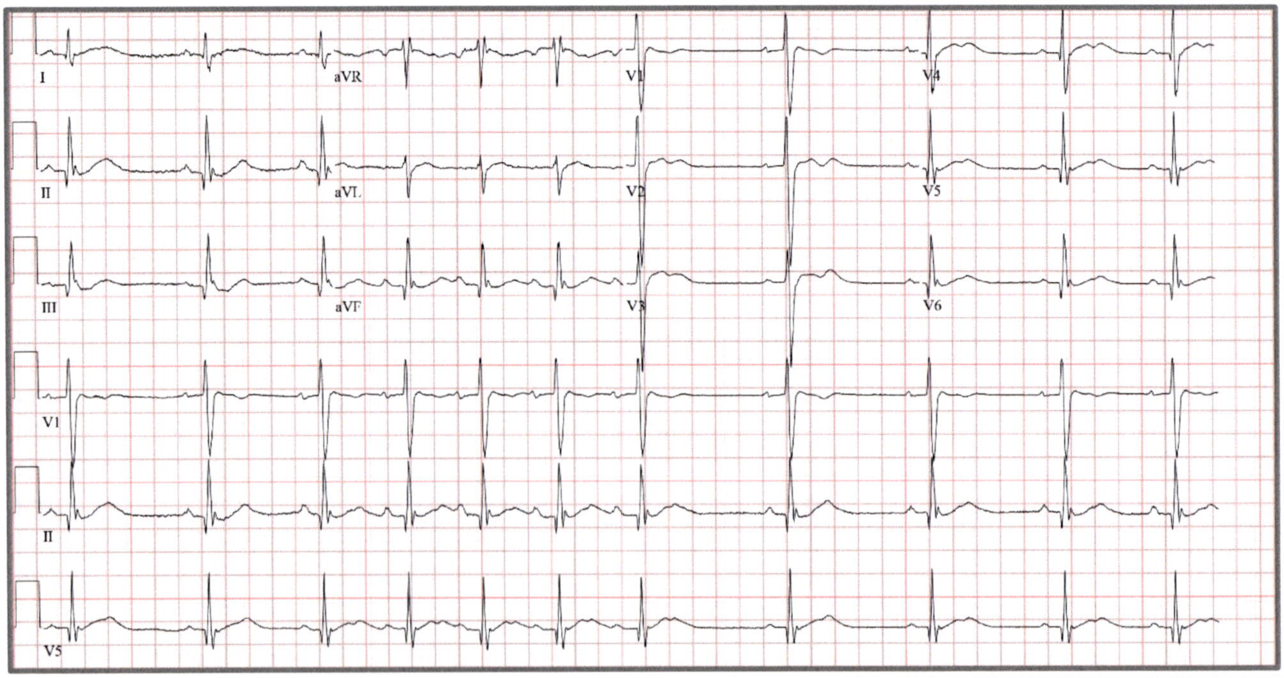

Rate:	Rhythm:	Axis:	Intervals:	Ischemia:

#174 – 87-year-old female presents with fall

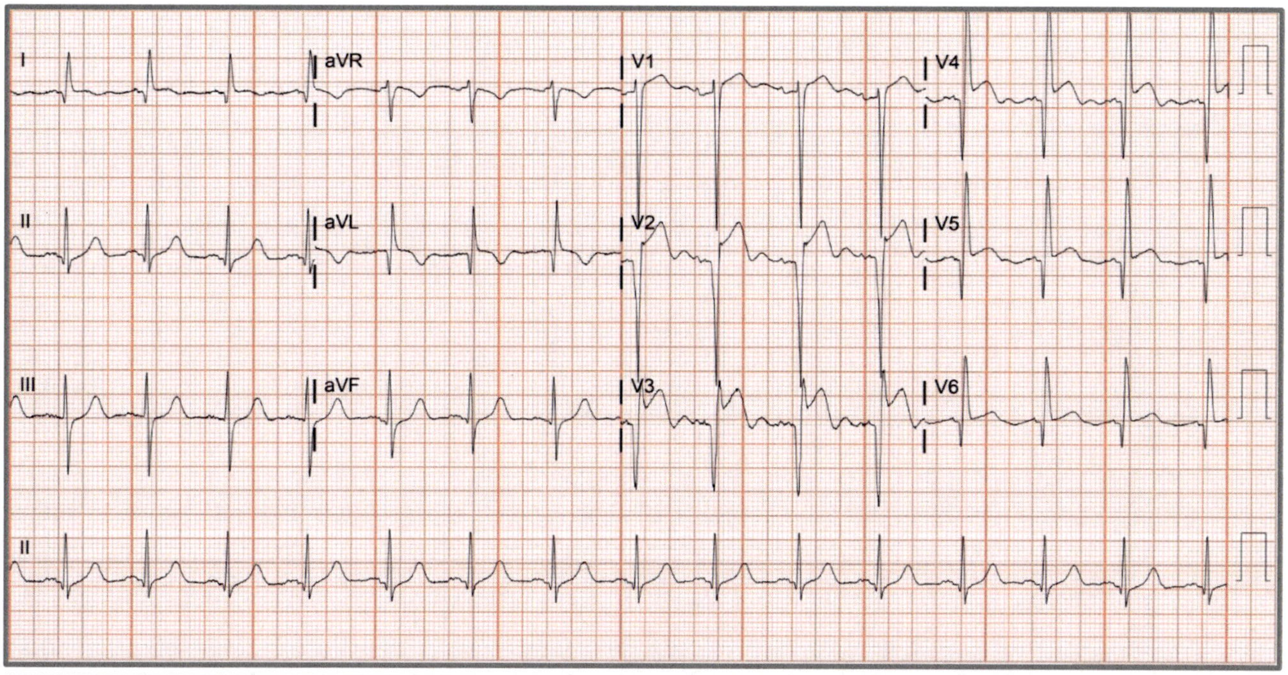

Rate: **Rhythm:** **Axis:** **Intervals:** **Ischemia:**

#175 – 45-year-old male presents with dyspnea

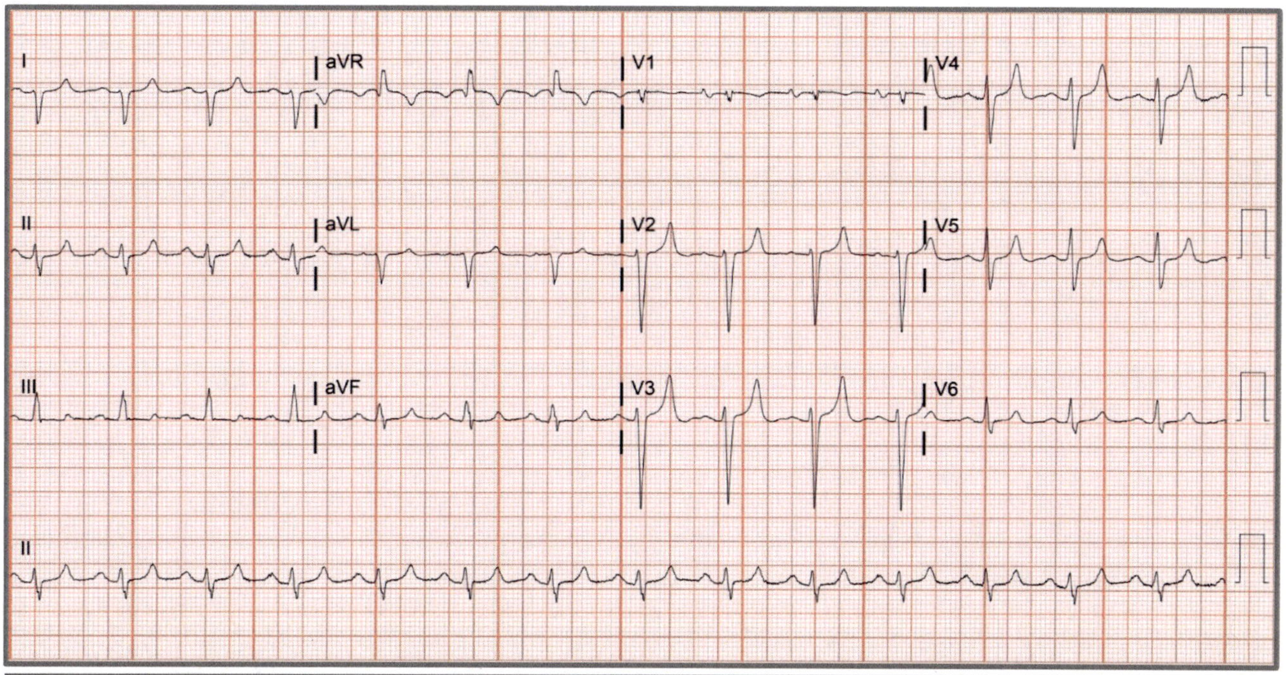

Rate: **Rhythm:** **Axis:** **Intervals:** **Ischemia:**

#176 – 33-year-old male presents with gunshot wound

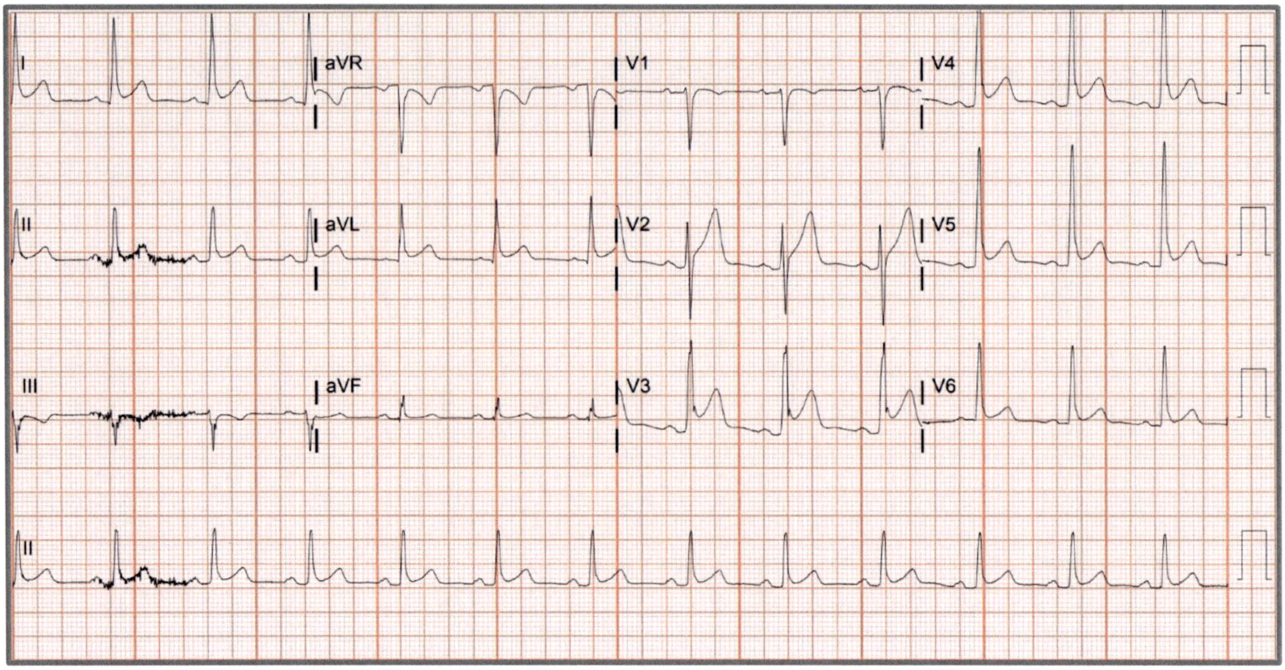

Rate:	**Rhythm:**	**Axis:**	**Intervals:**	**Ischemia:**

#177 – 40-year-old female presents with chest pain

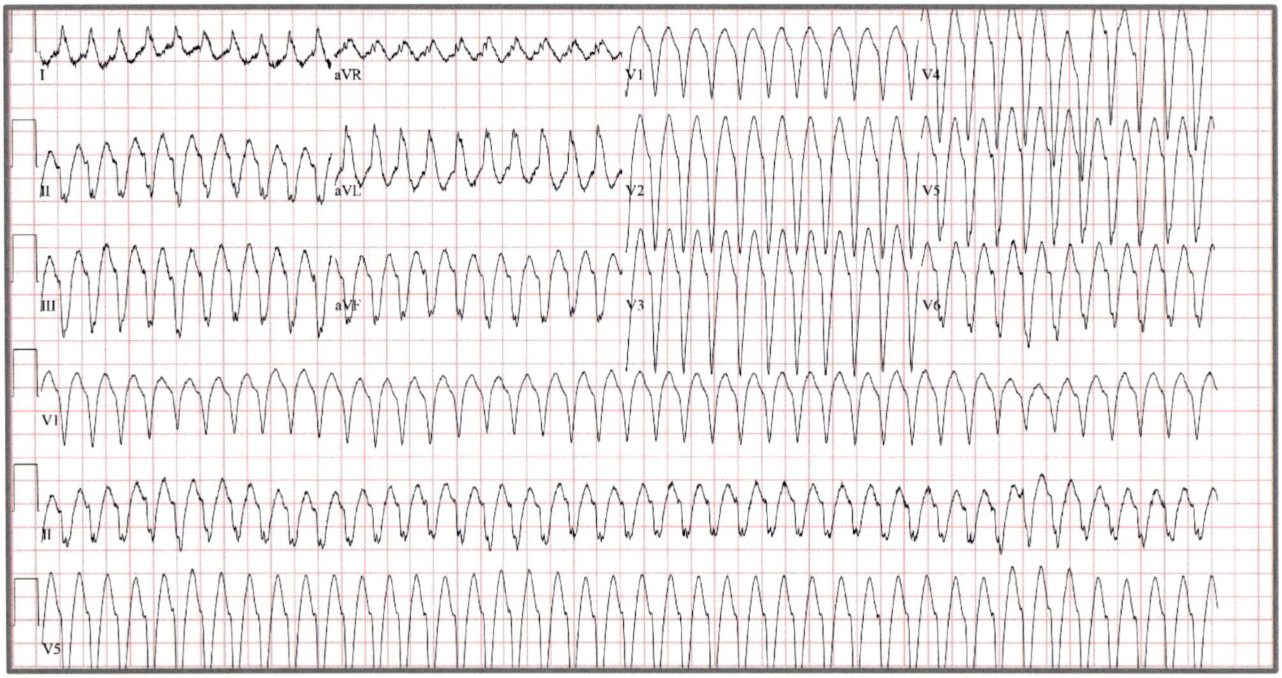

Rate:	**Rhythm:**	**Axis:**	**Intervals:**	**Ischemia:**

#178 – 61-year-old male presents with exertional chest pain

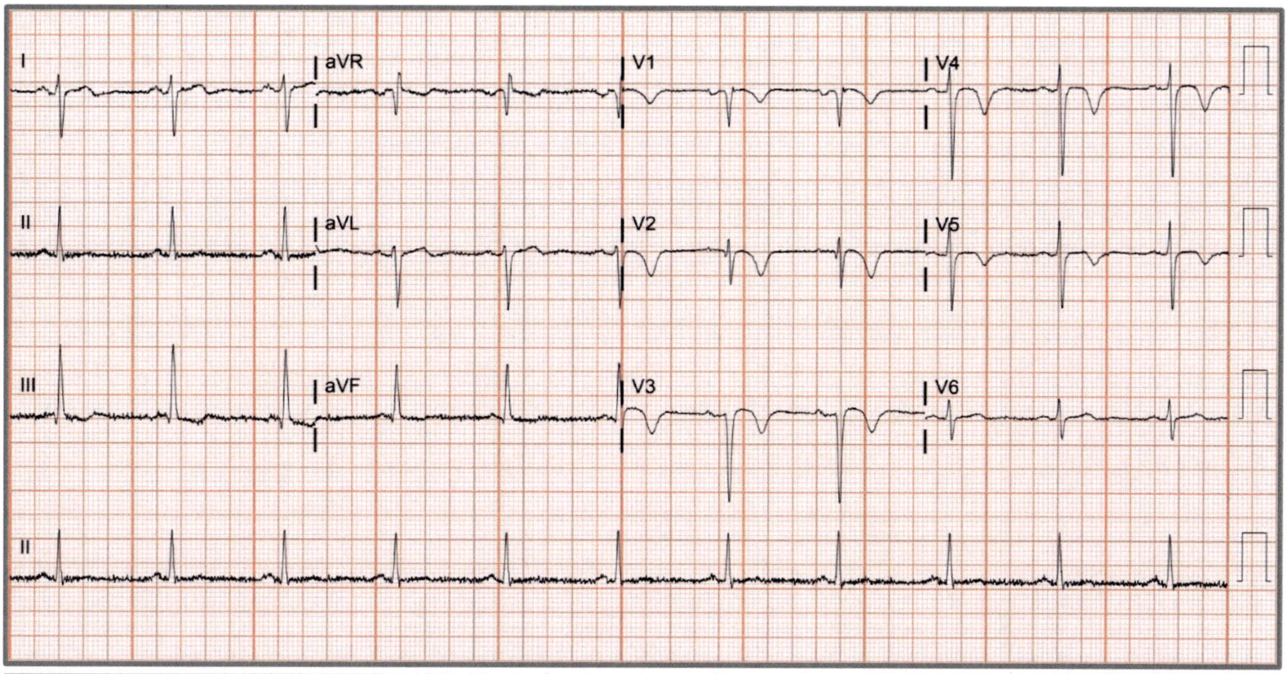

Rate:	Rhythm:	Axis:	Intervals:	Ischemia:

#179 – 62-year-old male presents with altered mental status

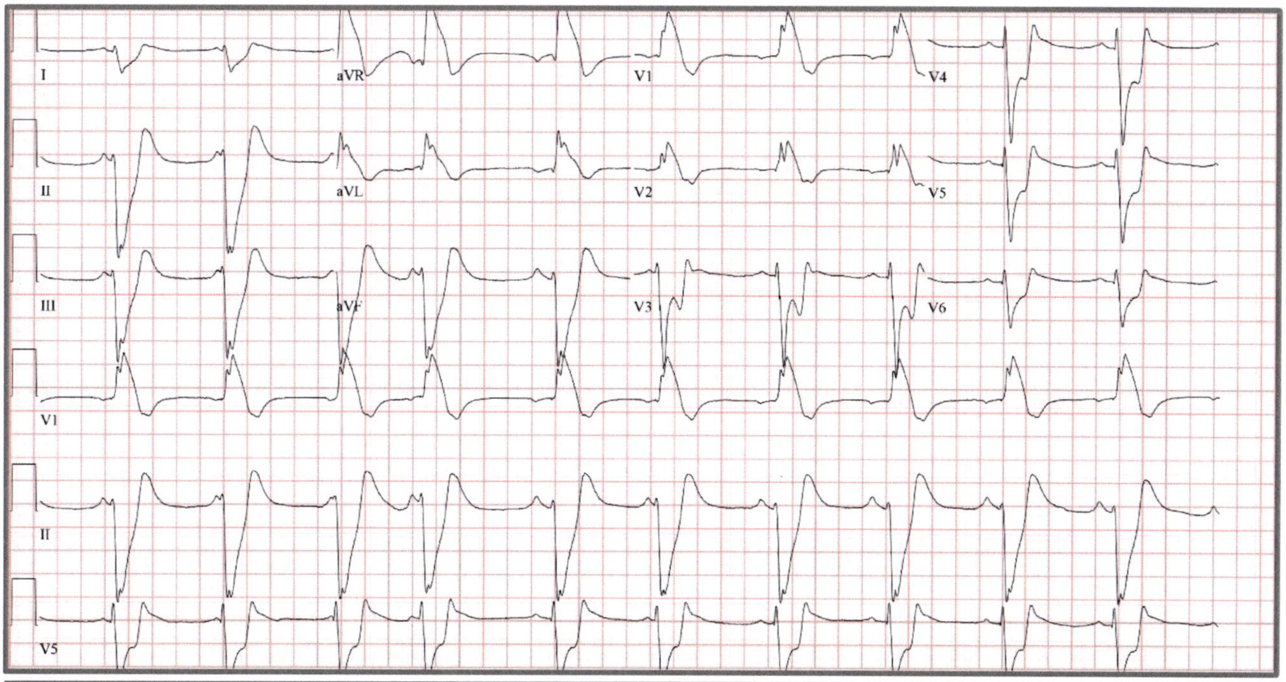

Rate:	Rhythm:	Axis:	Intervals:	Ischemia:

#180 – 61-year-old male presents with syncope

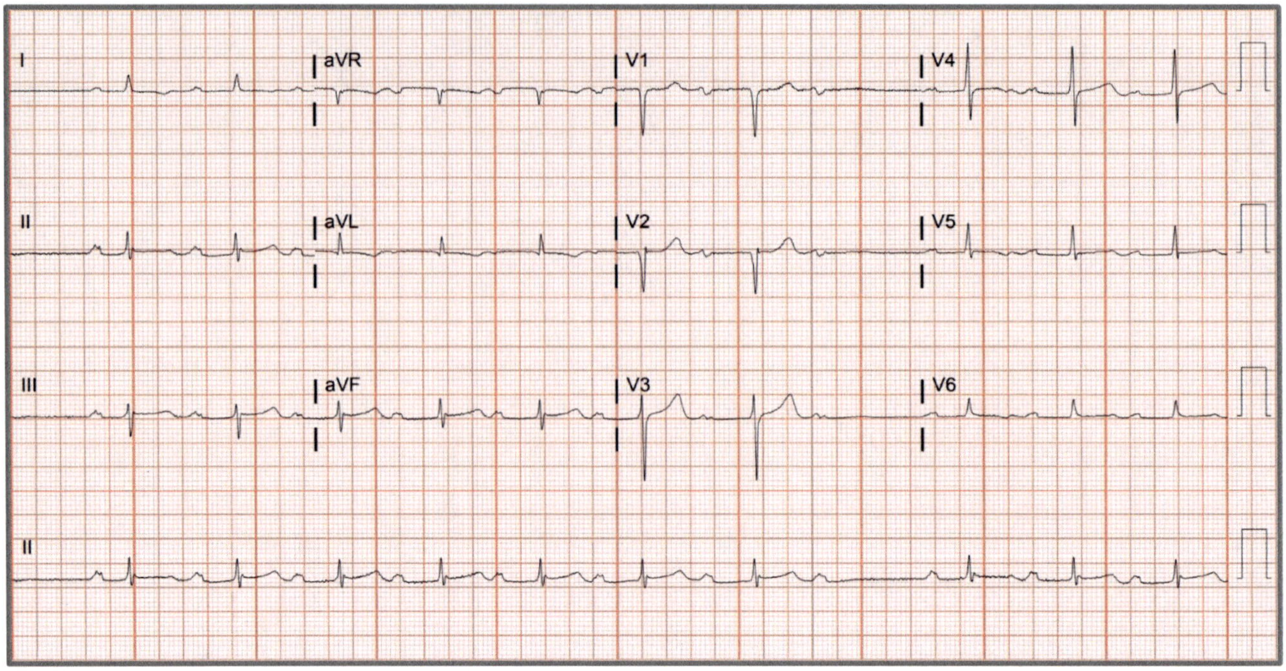

Rate:		Rhythm:		Axis:		Intervals:		Ischemia:	

#181 – 57-year-old male presents with dyspnea

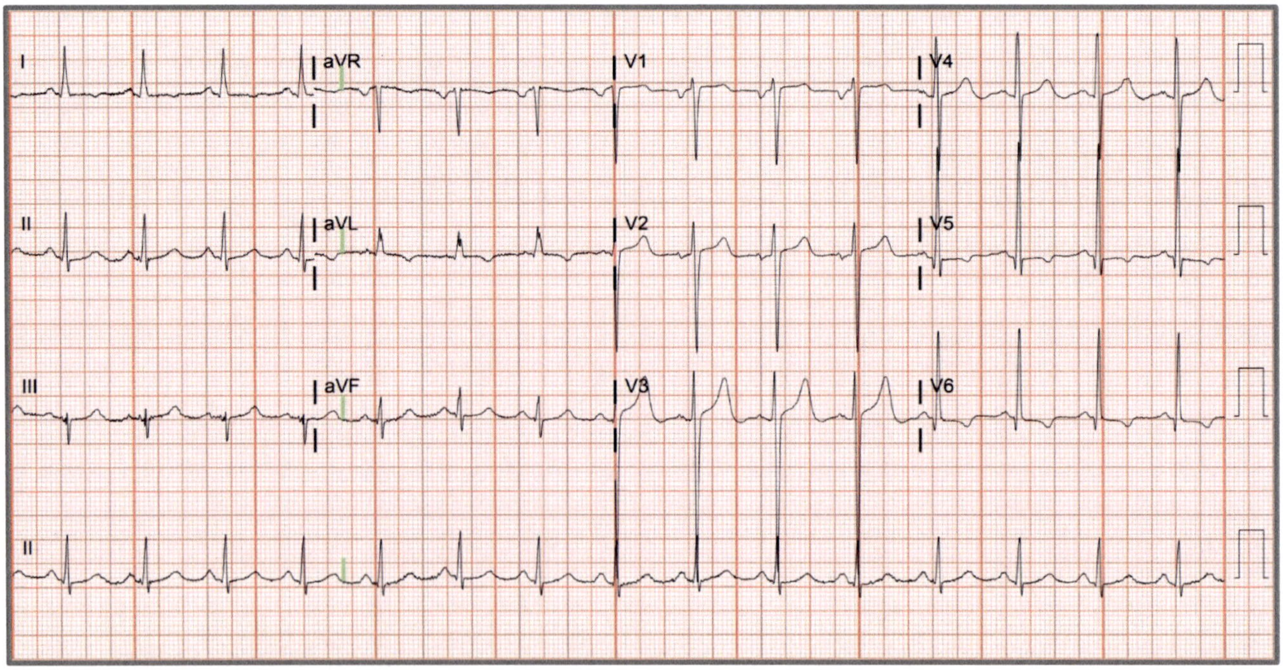

Rate:		Rhythm:		Axis:		Intervals:		Ischemia:	

#182 – 42-year-old female presents with fatigue and syncope

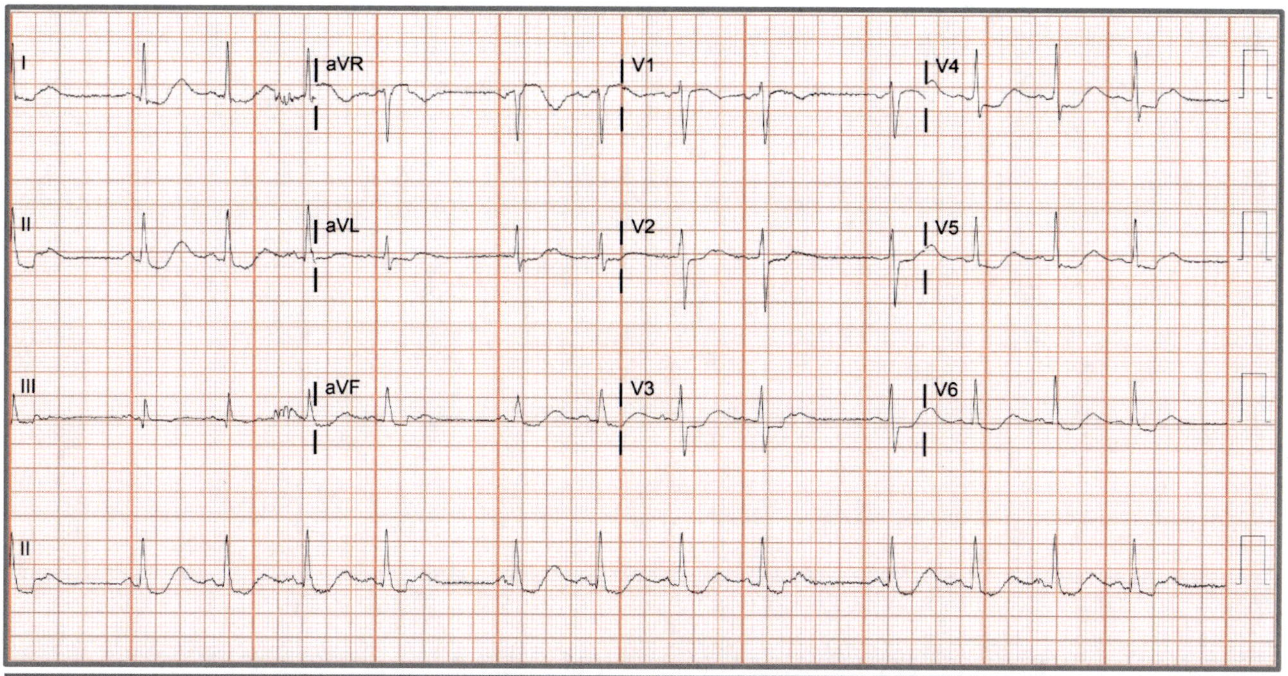

Rate: Rhythm: Axis: Intervals: Ischemia:

#183 – 62-year-old male presents with dyspnea

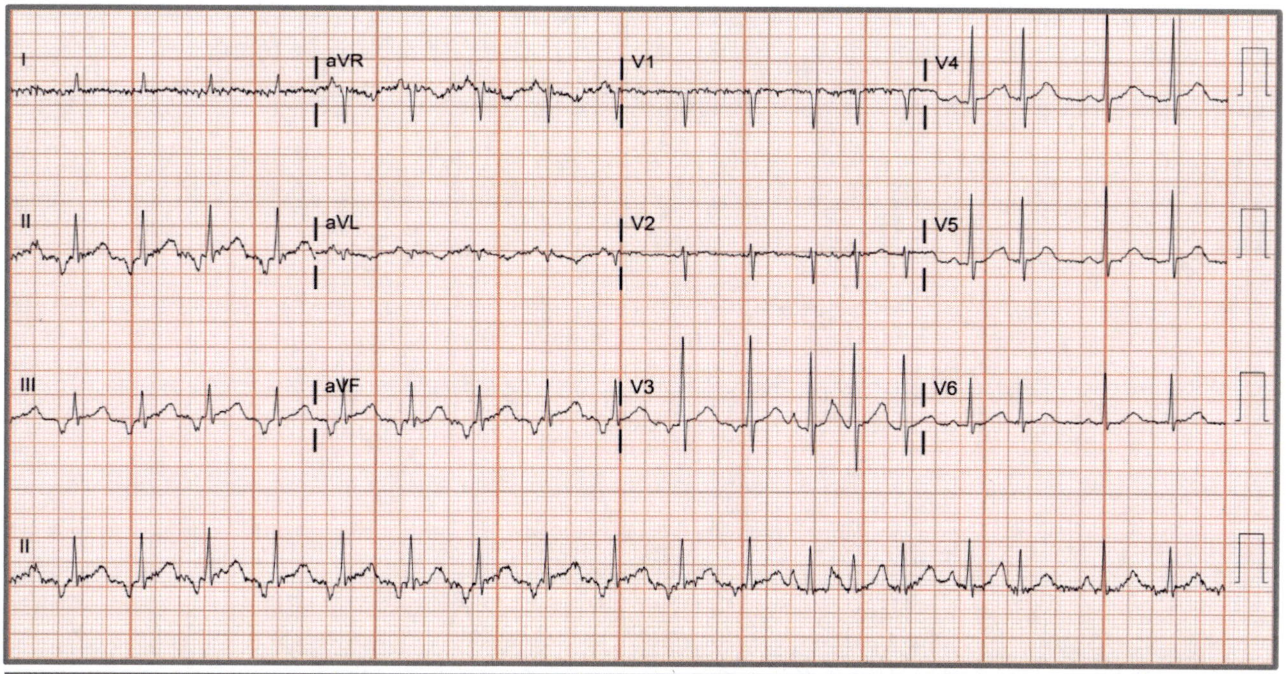

Rate: Rhythm: Axis: Intervals: Ischemia:

#184 – 44-year-old male presents with palpitations

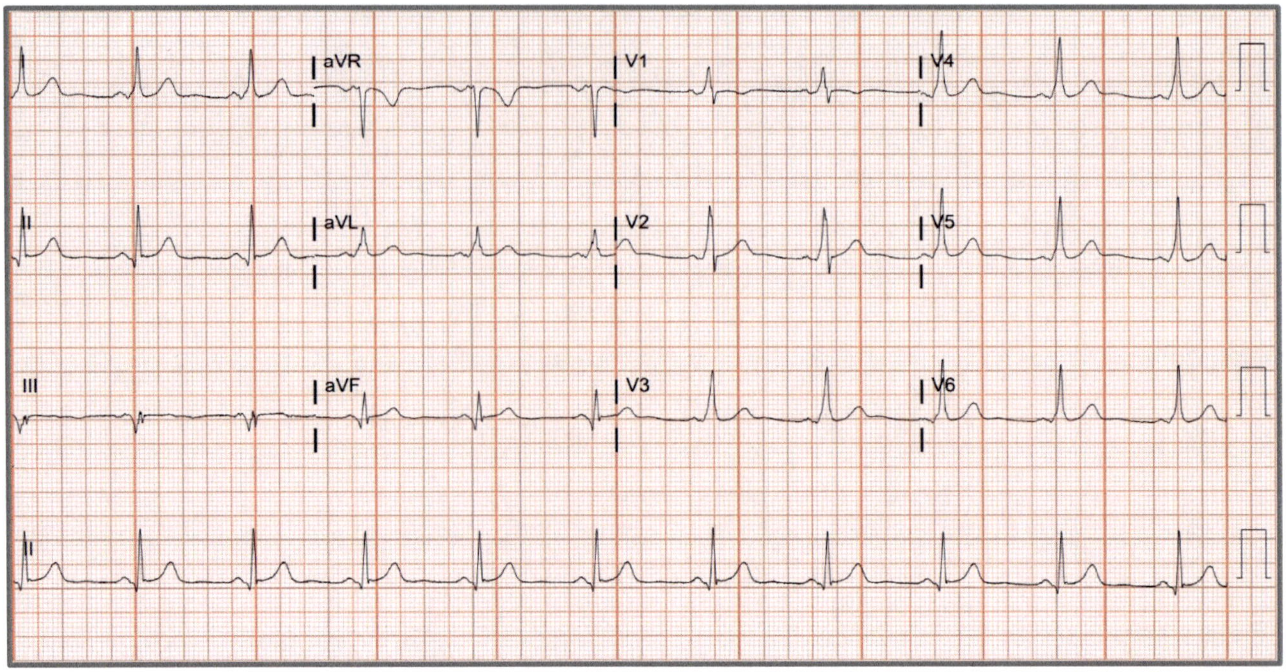

Rate: **Rhythm:** **Axis:** **Intervals:** **Ischemia:**

#185 – 62-year-old male presents with chest pain x 1 week

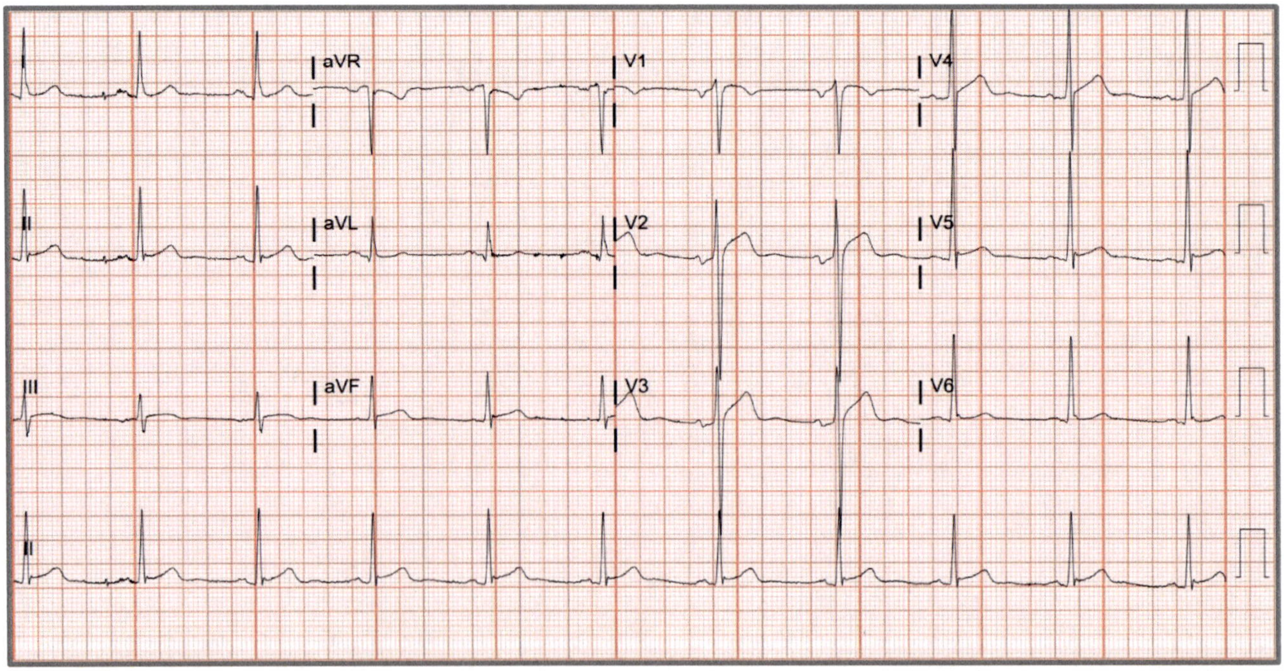

Rate: **Rhythm:** **Axis:** **Intervals:** **Ischemia:**

#186 – 71-year-old male presents with chest pain

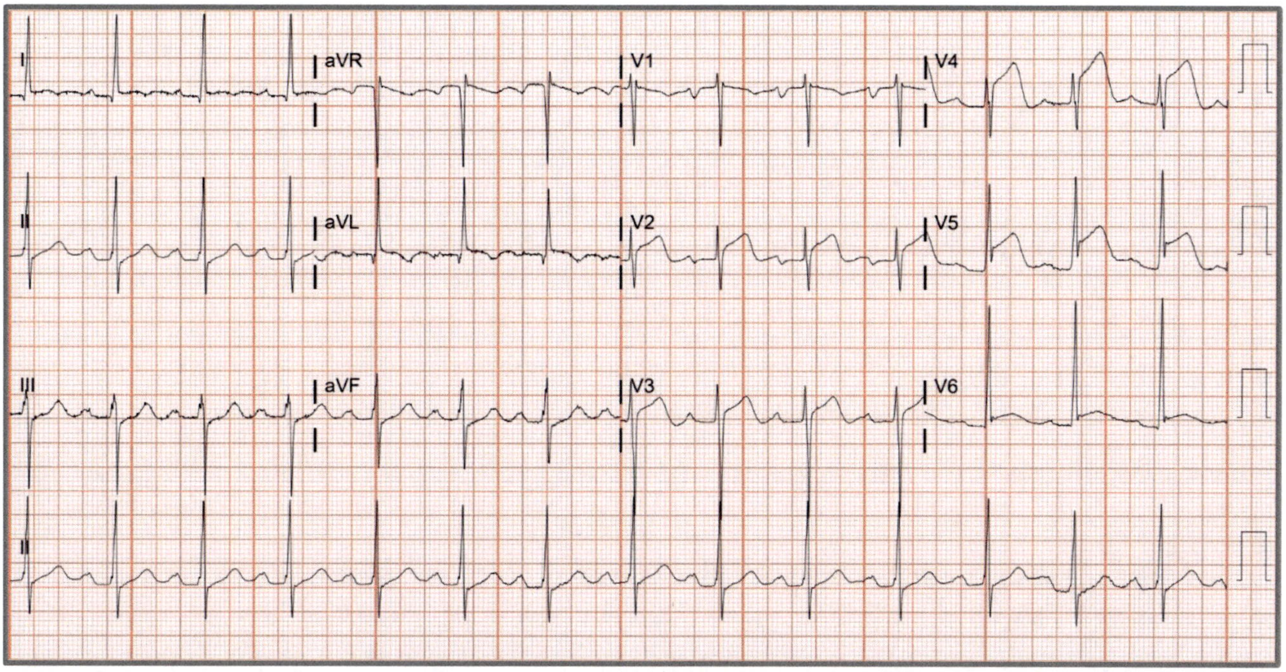

Rate:	Rhythm:	Axis:	Intervals:	Ischemia:

#187 – 60-year-old male presents with chest pain

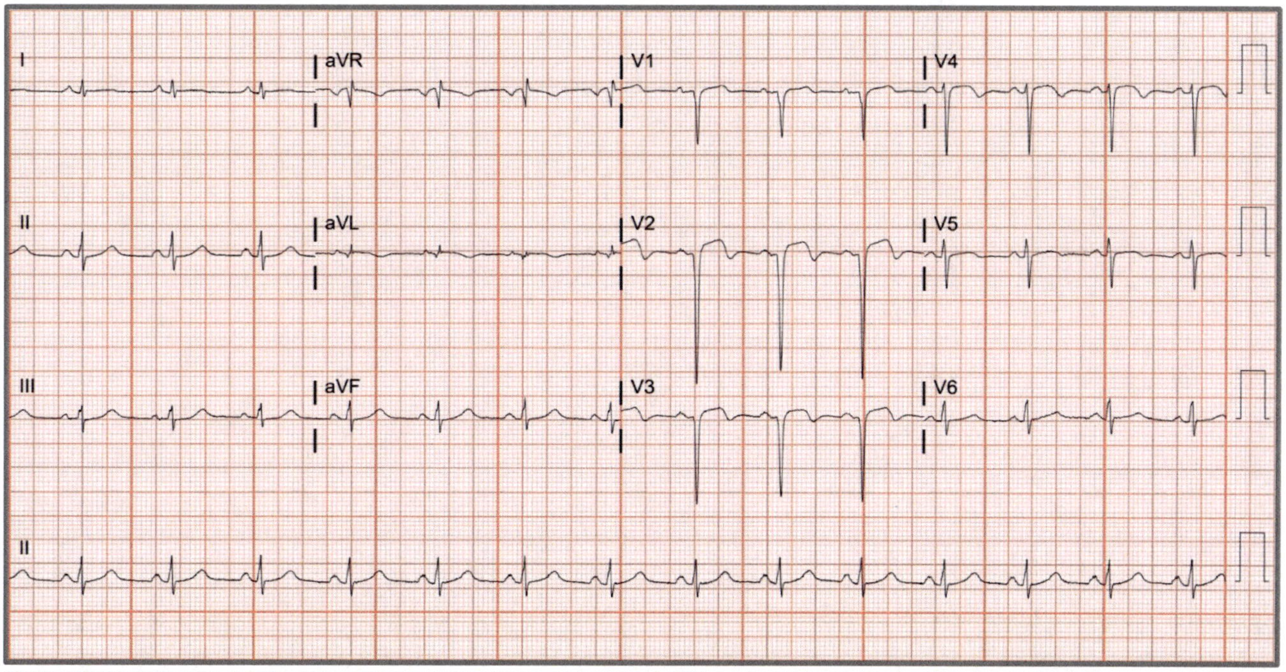

Rate:	Rhythm:	Axis:	Intervals:	Ischemia:

#188 – 47-year-old male presents with chest pain

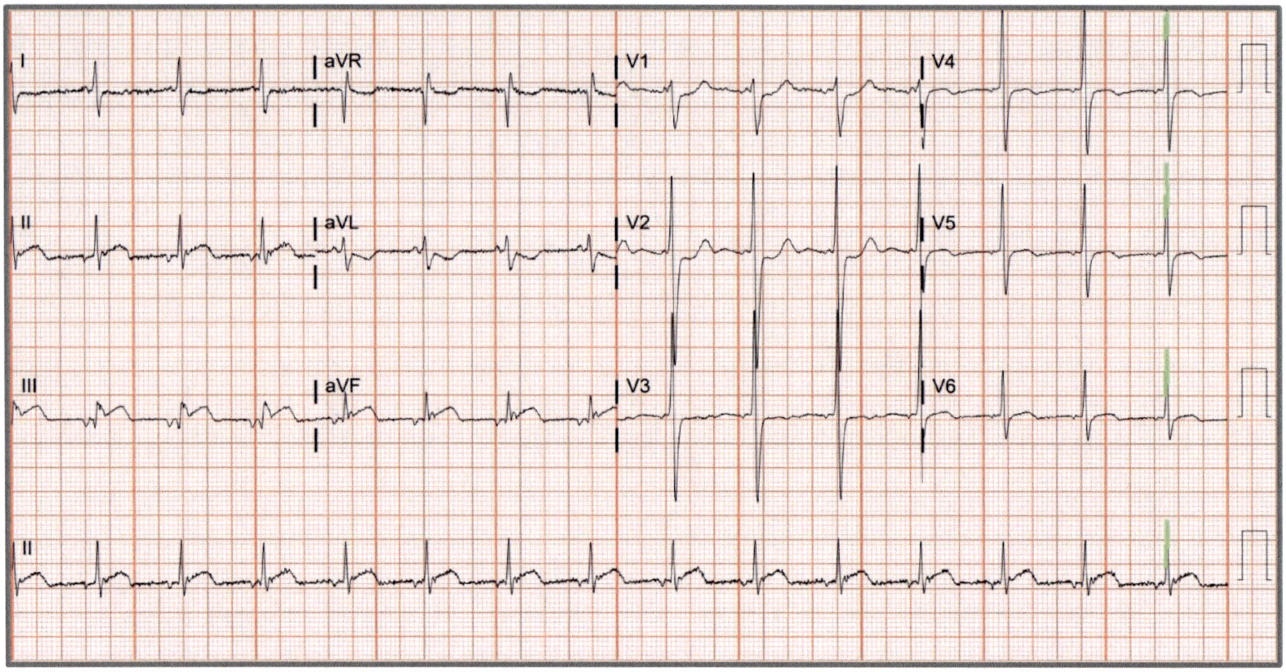

Rate: Rhythm: Axis: Intervals: Ischemia:

#189 – 73-year-old male presents with chest pain

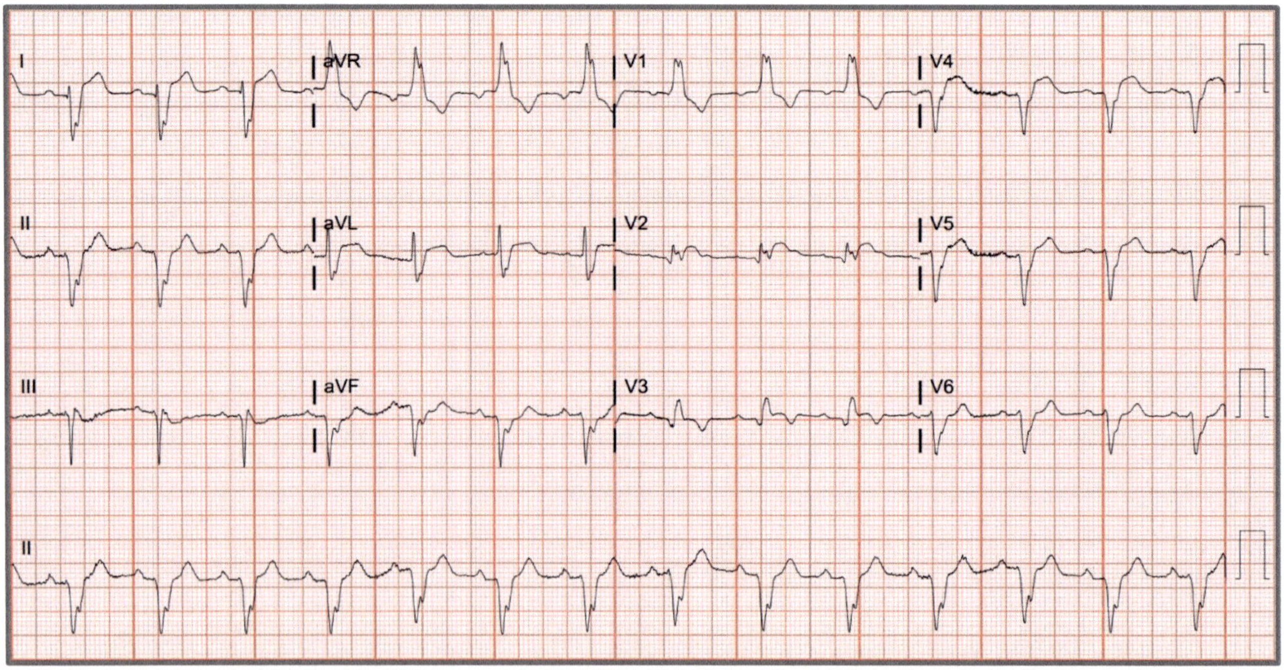

Rate: Rhythm: Axis: Intervals: Ischemia:

#190 – 67-year-old male presents with fatigue

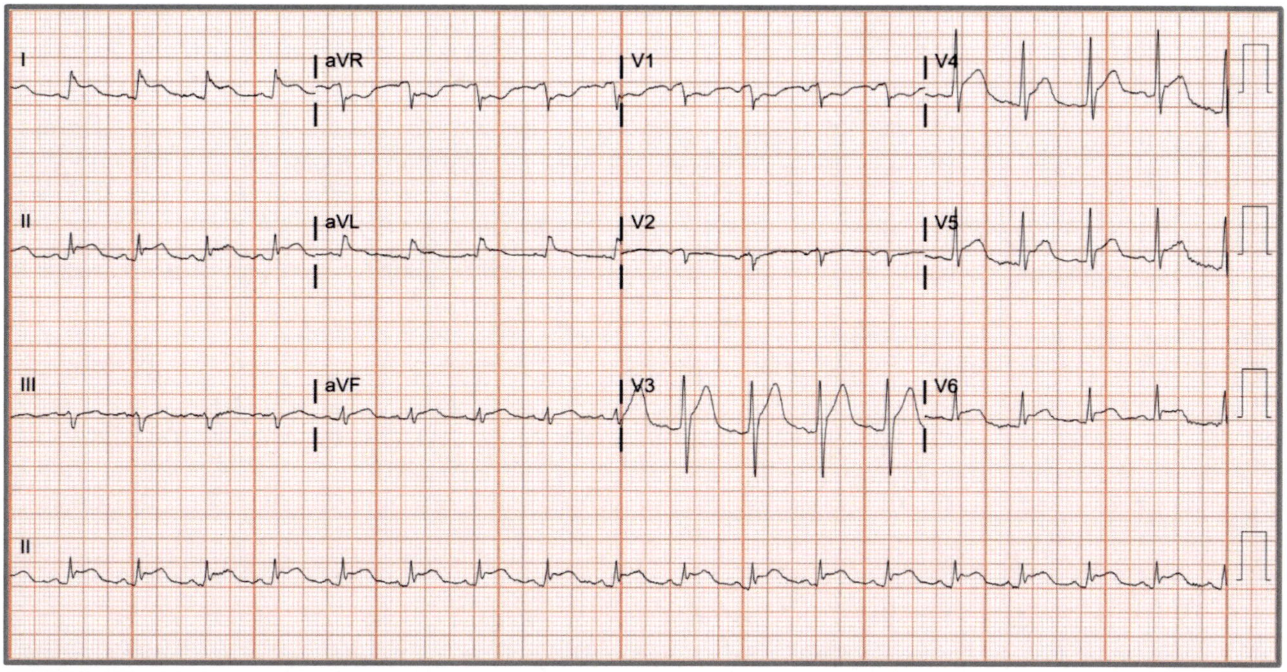

Rate:	Rhythm:	Axis:	Intervals:	Ischemia:

#191 – 64-year-old female presents with epistaxis

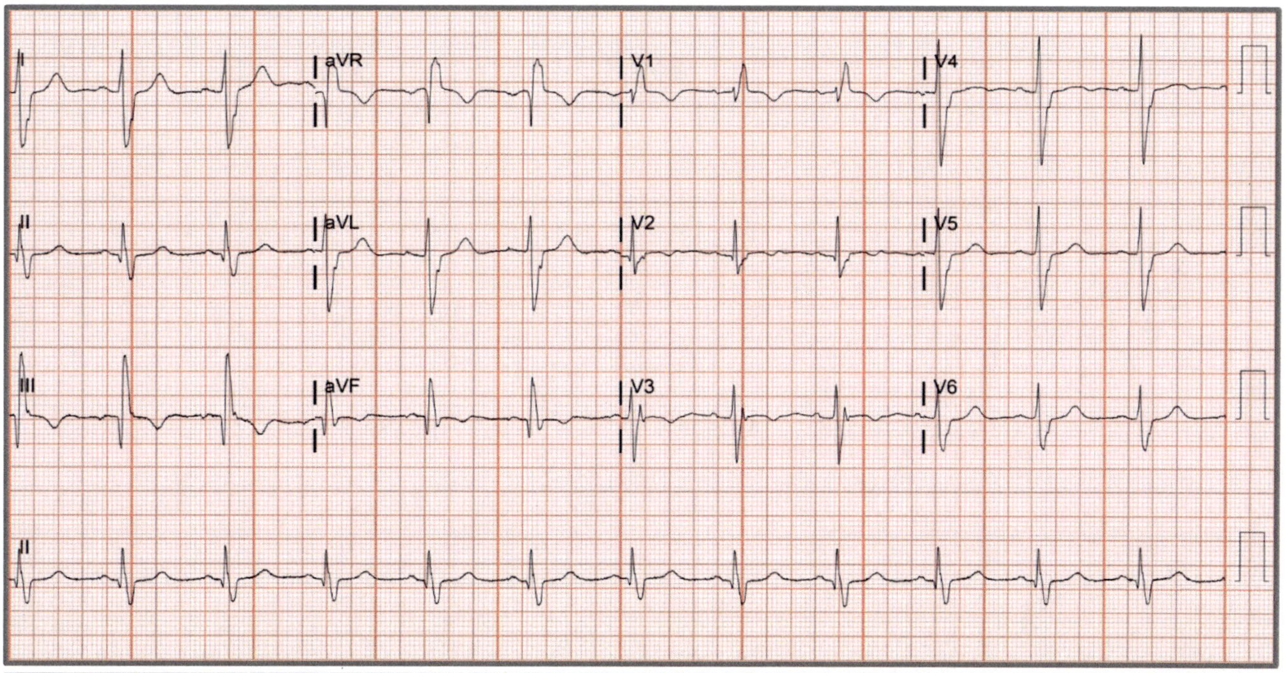

Rate:	Rhythm:	Axis:	Intervals:	Ischemia:

#192 – 68-year-old male presents with dyspnea

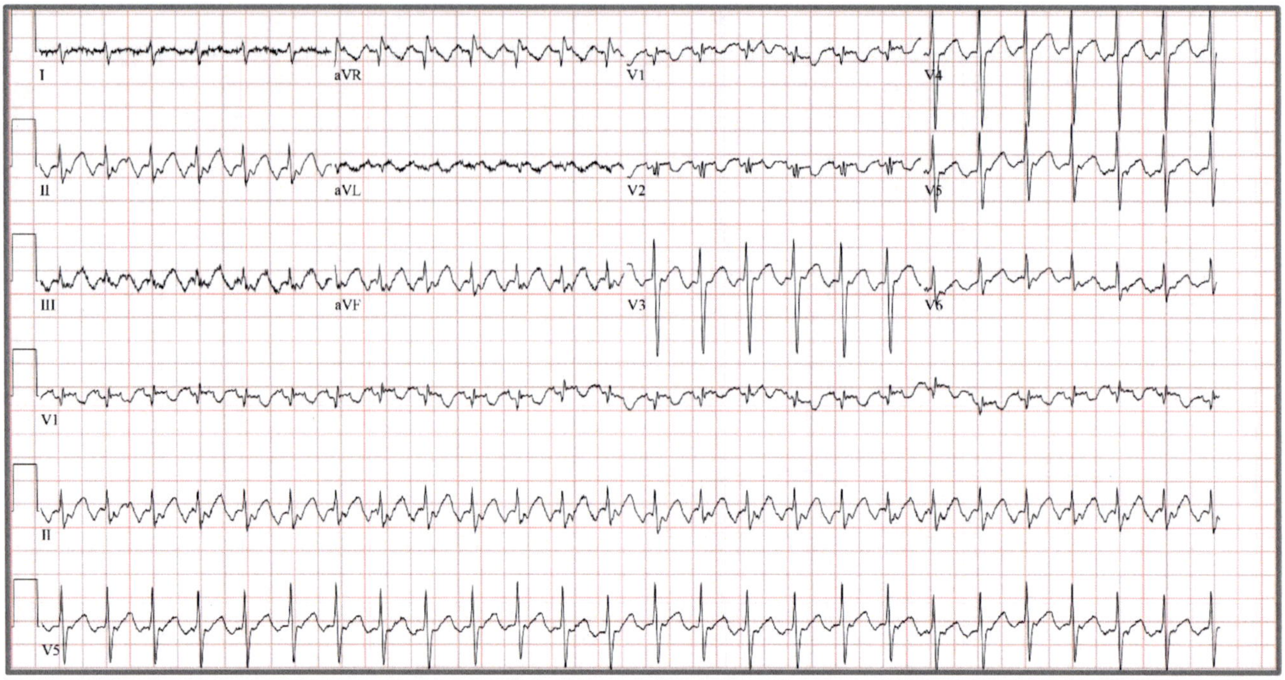

Rate: Rhythm: Axis: Intervals: Ischemia:

#193 – 59-year-old male presents with dizziness

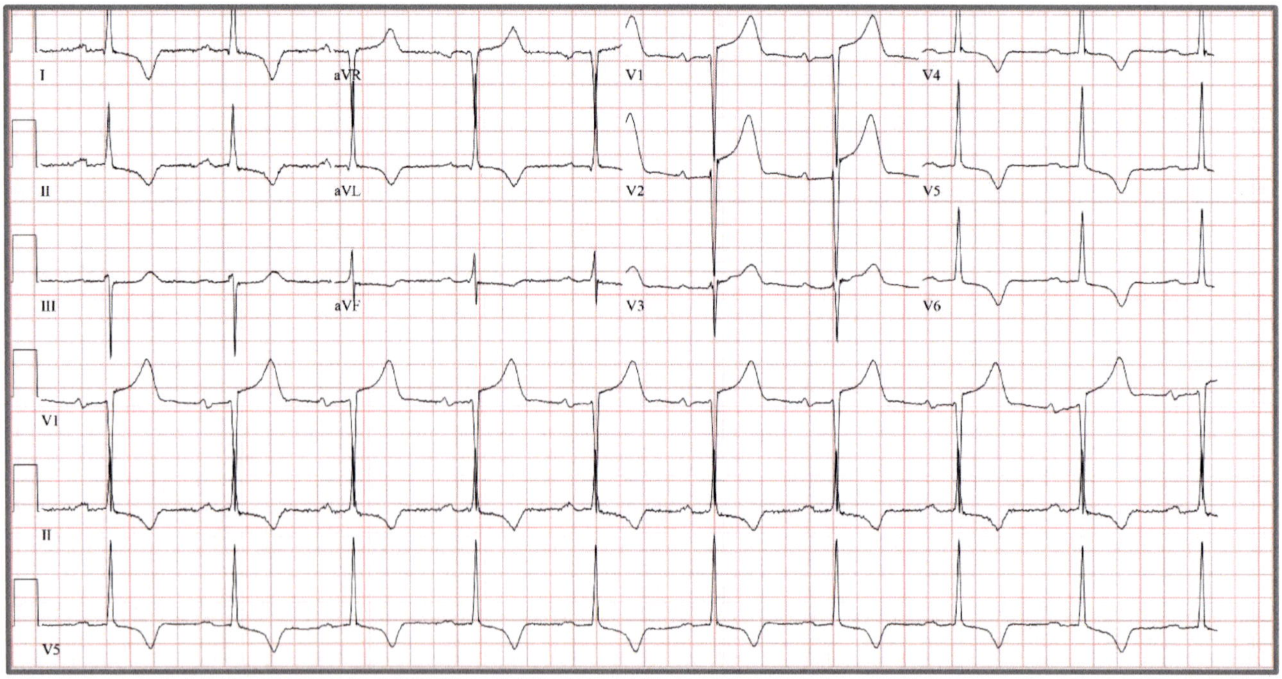

Rate: Rhythm: Axis: Intervals: Ischemia:

#194 – 59-year-old male presents with dyspnea

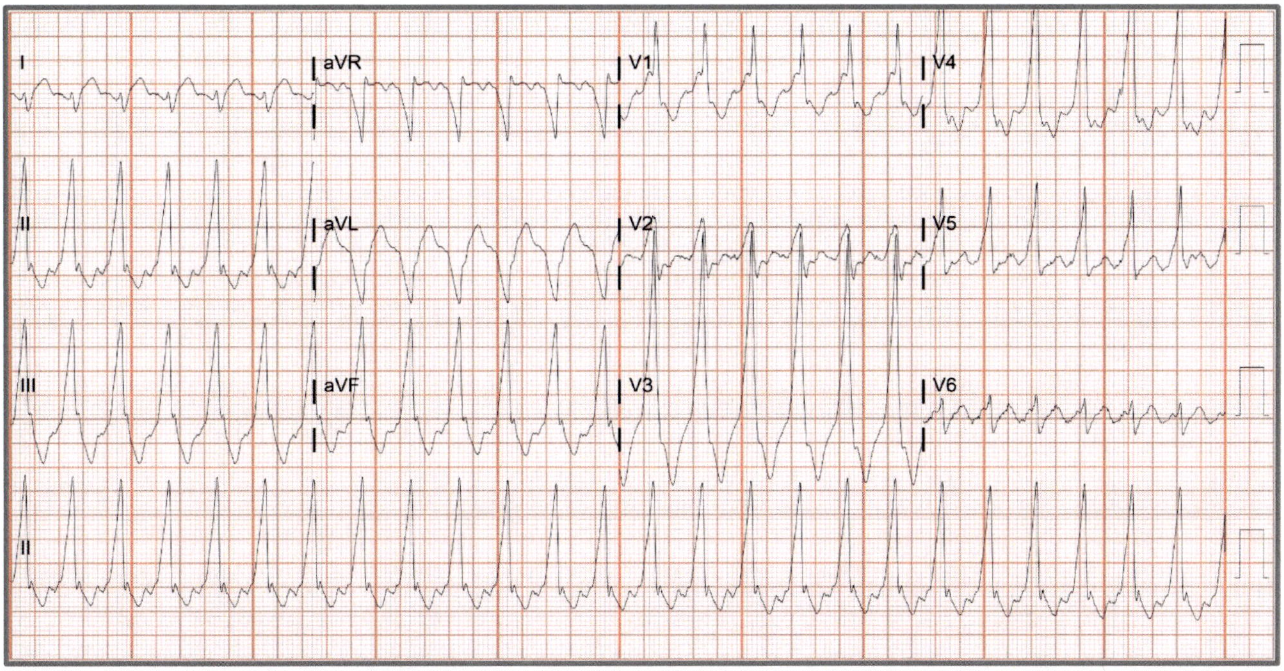

Rate:	Rhythm:	Axis:	Intervals:	Ischemia:

⇩ Post-conversion ECG ⇩

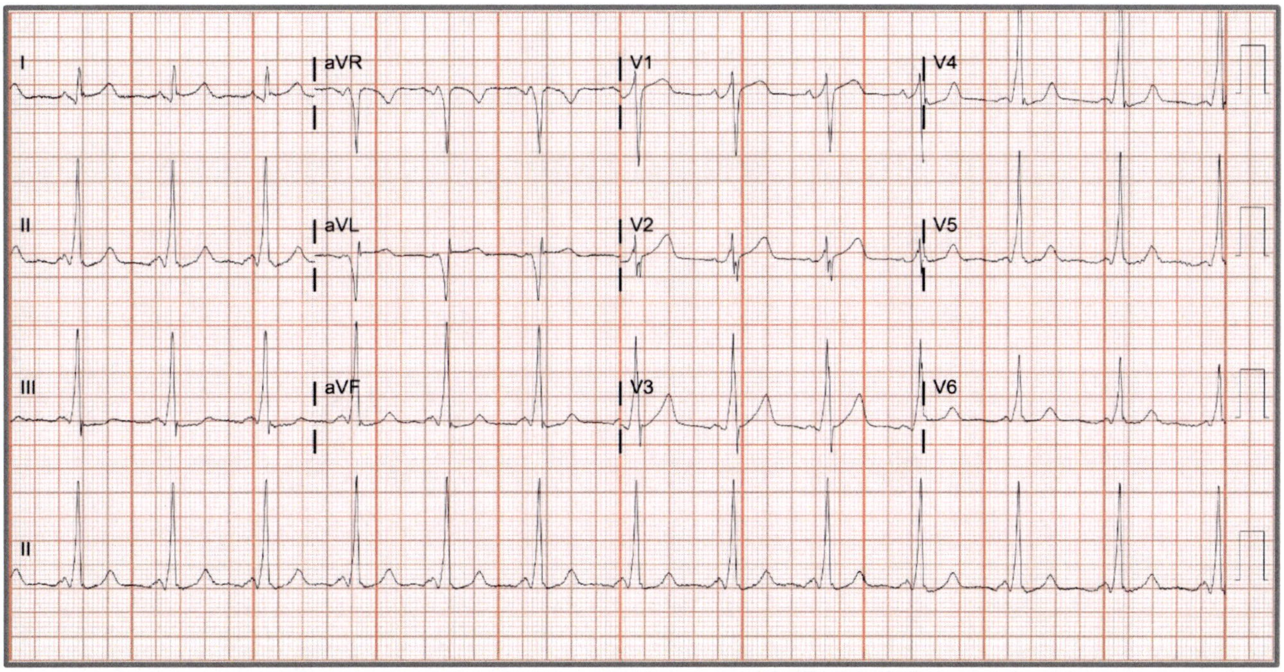

Rate:	Rhythm:	Axis:	Intervals:	Ischemia:

#195 – 57-year-old male presents with altered mental status

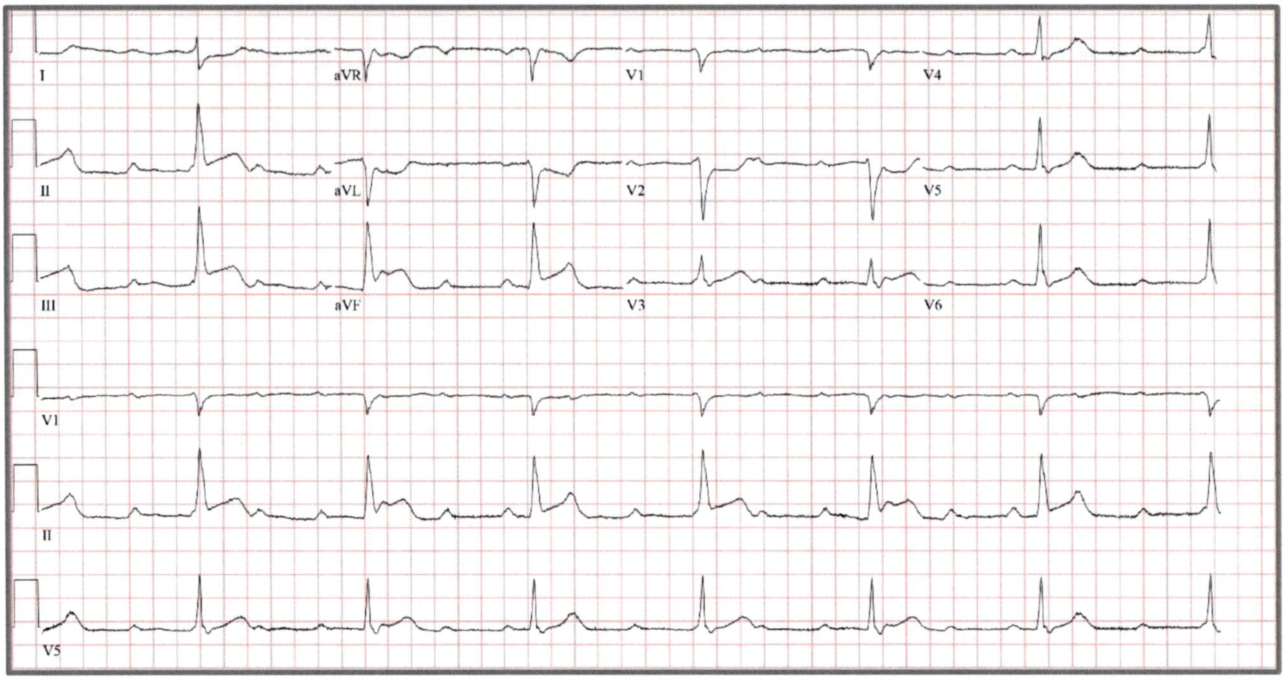

Rate: Rhythm: Axis: Intervals: Ischemia:

#196 – 69-year-old female presents with chest pain

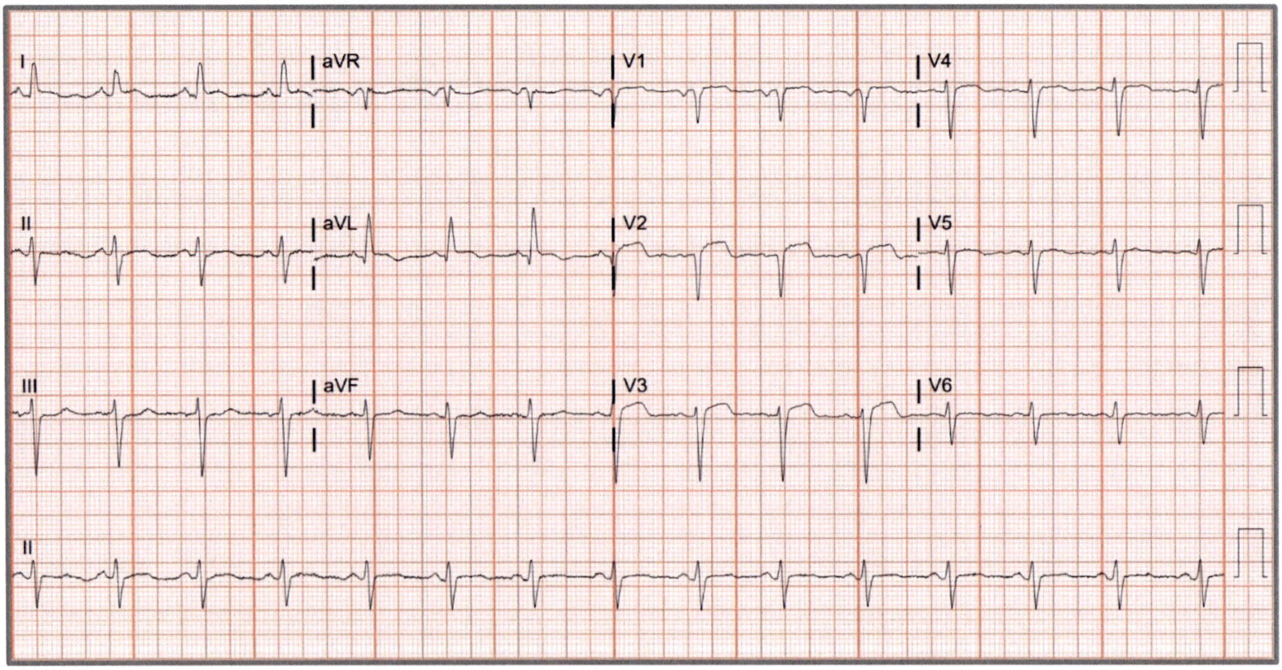

Rate: Rhythm: Axis: Intervals: Ischemia:

#197 – 38-year-old male presents with dyspnea

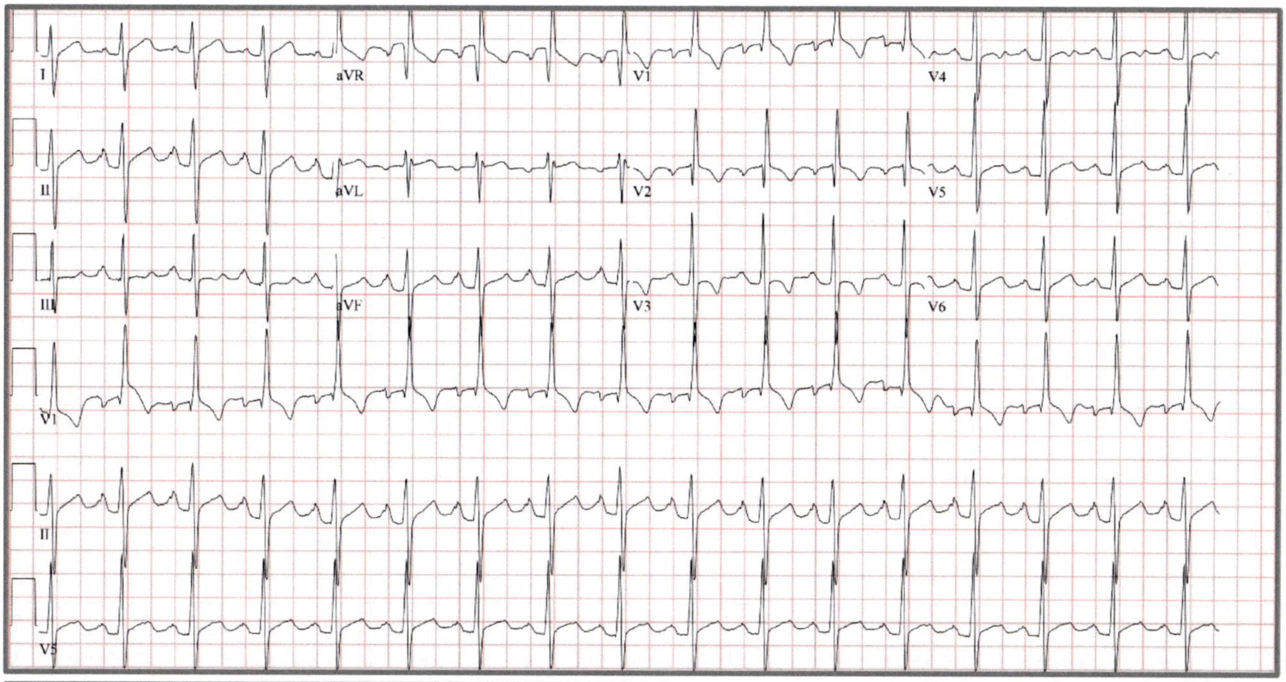

Rate:		Rhythm:		Axis:		Intervals:		Ischemia:	

#198 – 80-year-old male presents with chest pain

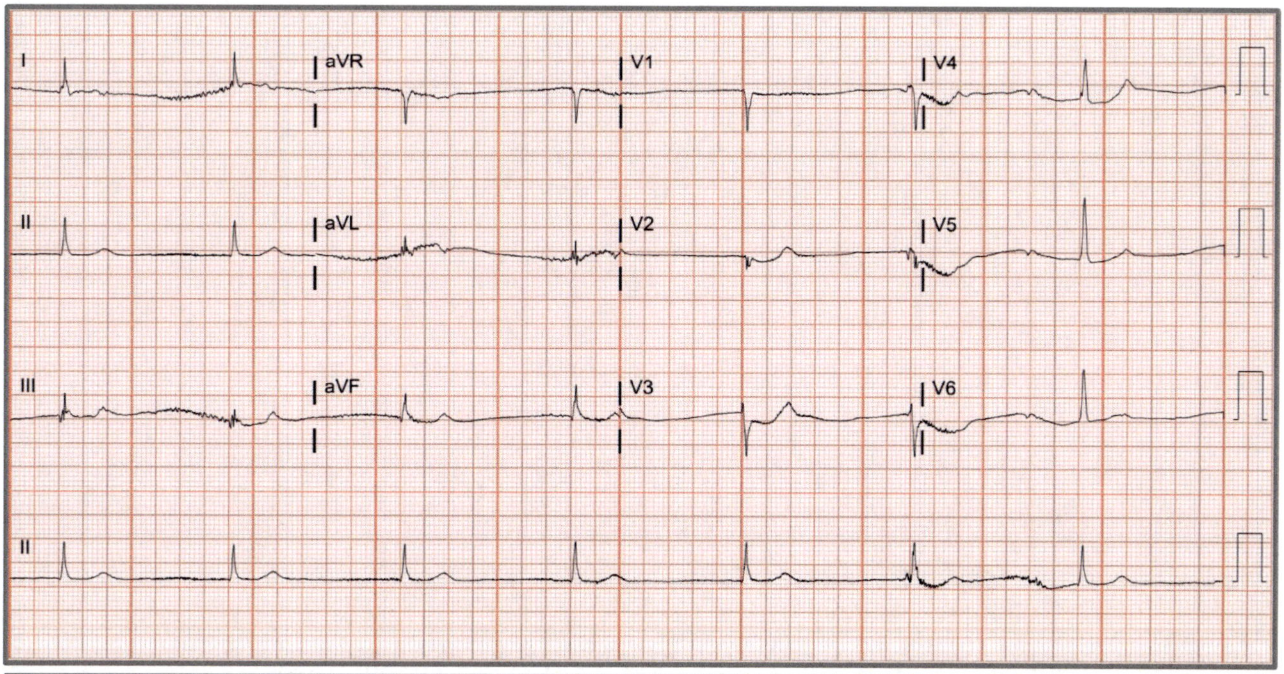

Rate:		Rhythm:		Axis:		Intervals:		Ischemia:	

#199 – 52-year-old male presents with epigastric pain

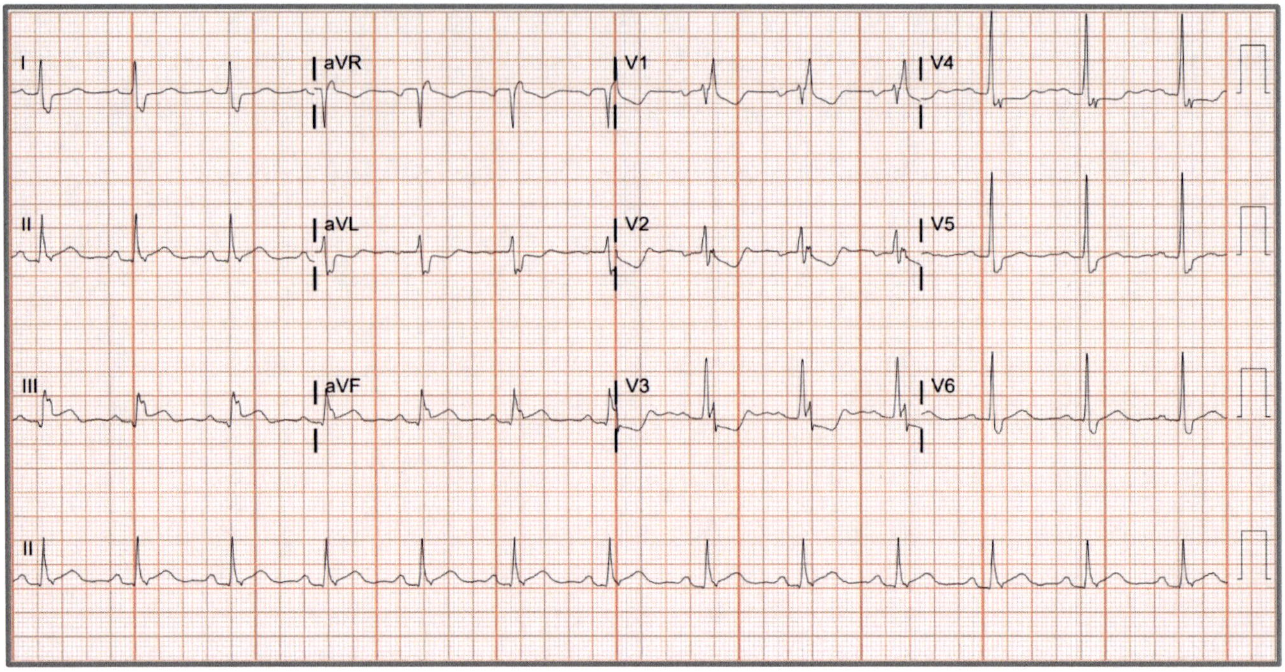

Rate: Rhythm: Axis: Intervals: Ischemia:

#200 – 63-year-old male presents with dyspnea

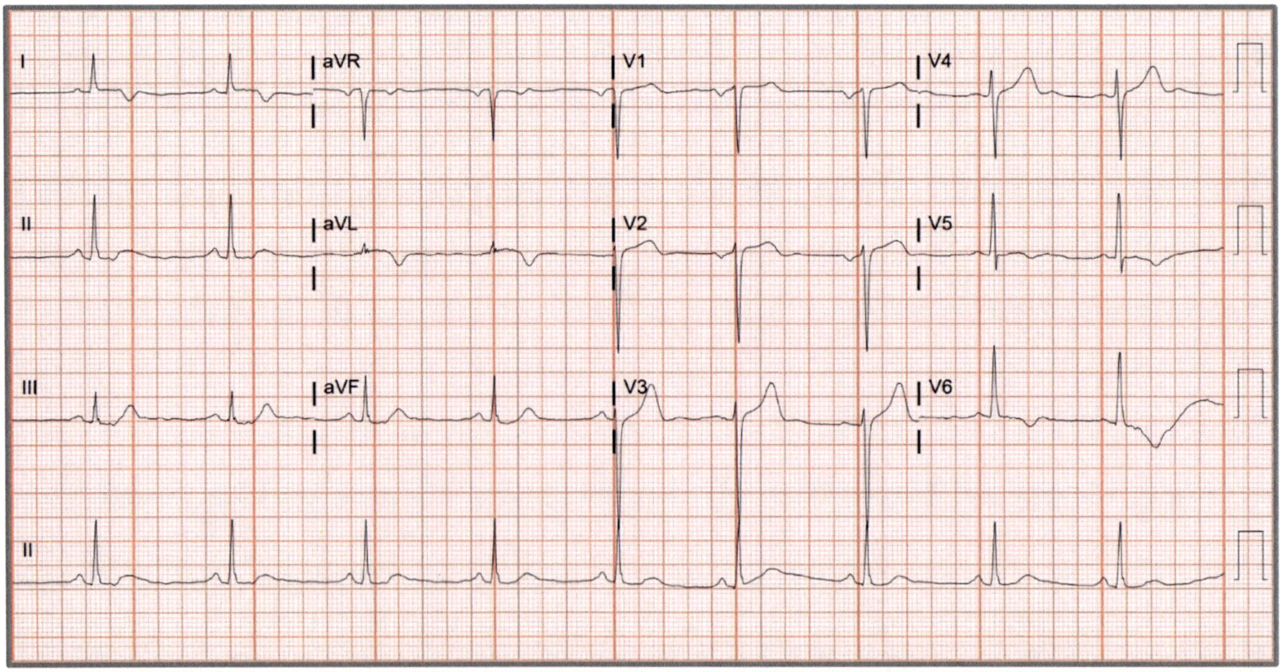

Rate: Rhythm: Axis: Intervals: Ischemia:

The Explanations

1. **Third Degree Atrioventricular Block with Ventricular Escape**. There is atrioventricular dissociation and a severely bradycardic ventricular escape rhythm. The term atrioventricular dissociation refers to the independent contraction of the atria and ventricles and suggests a disturbance in the normal conduction pathway;[1] in this case, third degree (i.e., complete) atrioventricular block. The conduction system contains a series of intrinsic pacemaker cells, all suppressed by the most superior one (i.e., the sinus node under normal circumstances). When signals fail to transmit distally, pacemaker cells can "escape" their suppression. The more distal the escape rhythm, the slower and less reliable it is. Junctional escape rhythms tend to be narrow complex (<120 ms) with rates between 40 and 60 beats per minute. Here, the wide (>120 ms), and slow (<40 beats per minute) QRS complexes suggest a ventricular escape rhythm (Figure 1).[2]

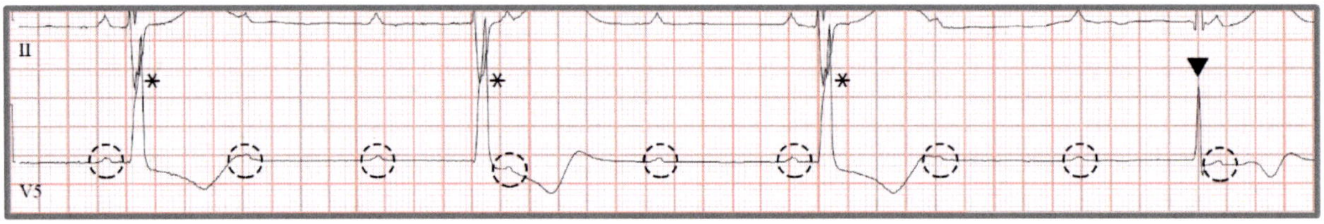

Figure 1. The atrial rate is 60 beats per minute (dashed circles), and the ventricular escape rate is 24 beats per minute (asterisks). There is a single junctional escape complex (arrowhead).

2. **Inferior ST-elevation Myocardial Infarction**. Inferior ST-segment elevation with reciprocal changes in aVL. Reciprocal changes refer to ST-segment depression in leads opposing the infarct region and are strong predictors of occlusion. Left heart catheterization revealed proximal right coronary artery occlusion and percutaneous coronary intervention was performed.

3. **Trifascicular Disease, Right Bundle Branch Block, Left Anterior Fascicular Block.** The wide QRS, rSR' in the anterior precordial leads (V1, V2), and deep S-waves in the lateral leads (I, V6) indicate the presence of a right bundle branch block (Figure 2).

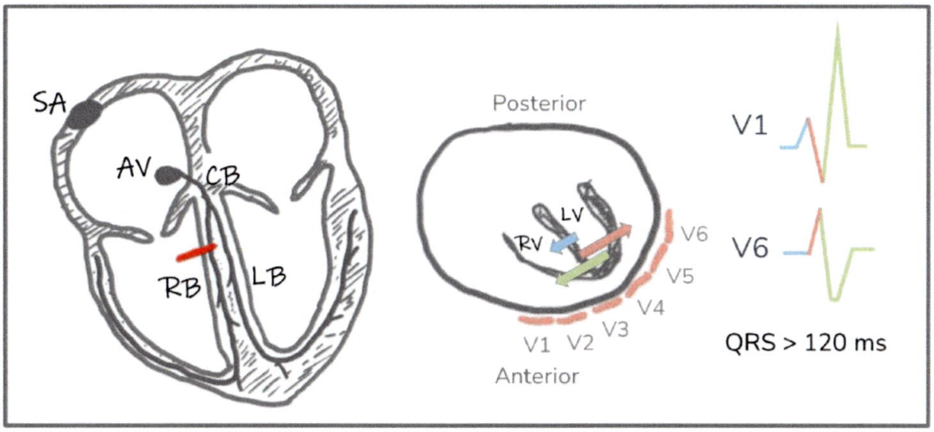

Figure 2. Direction of depolarization in right bundle branch block. The septum first depolarizes from left to right (blue arrow), followed by left ventricular depolarization (pink arrow), and, finally, right ventricular depolarization (green arrow). The result is an rSR' pattern in V1, and a wide S wave in the lateral leads (I, aVL, V5, V6). SA, sinoatrial node; AV, atrioventricular node; RB, right bundle; LB, left bundle; CB, common bundle; RV, right ventricle; LV, left ventricle; red dash represents a block of the right bundle.

The criteria for right bundle branch block are:

1. QRS greater than 120 ms
2. rSR' pattern in V1-3 ('M-shaped')
3. Wide/slurred S wave in the lateral leads (I, aVL, V5-6)

The right bundle branch block, however, does not explain the left axis deviation. Causes of left axis deviation are:

1. Left bundle branch block or paced rhythm,
2. Prior inferior myocardial infarction (inferior Q waves),
3. Left ventricular hypertrophy,
4. Ventricular preexcitation, and, finally,
5. Left anterior fascicular block.

When the left anterior fascicle is disrupted, current passes along the posterior fascicle and the left ventricle is depolarized in a leftward/upward direction - producing an extreme left axis deviation (i.e., more than 45 degrees, Figure 3).

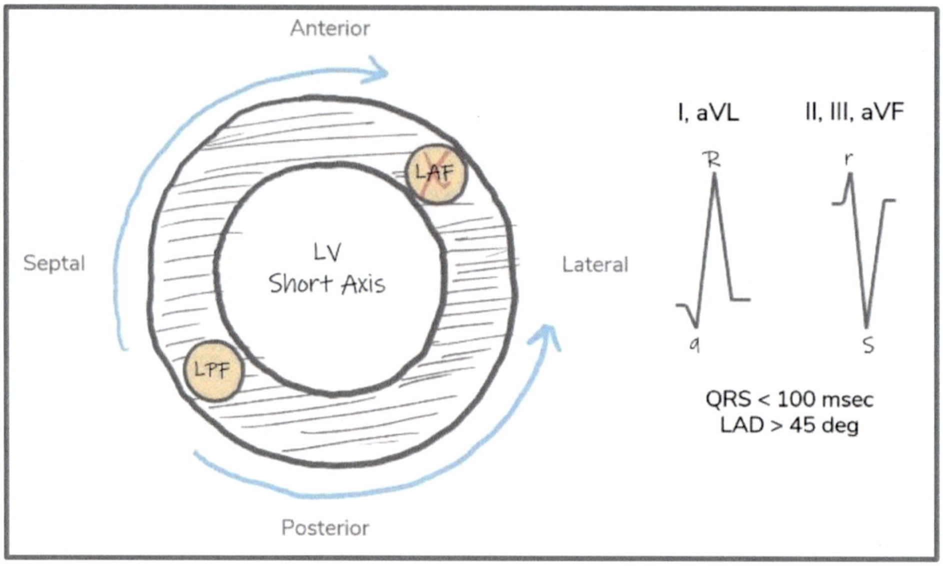

Figure 3. Relative locations of the anterior and posterior fascicles within the left ventricle. The blue arrows demonstrate the direction of depolarization. LV, left ventricle; LPF, left posterior fascicle; LAF, left anterior fascicle; LAD, left axis deviation.

This ECG demonstrates failure of two fascicles, the right bundle, and the left anterior fascicle, but there is also an associated first-degree atrioventricular block (i.e., prolonged PR interval). In the setting of severe conduction disease, first-degree atrioventricular block is likely to represent delayed conduction through a diseased third fascicle (i.e., trifascicular disease).[2–4] During sinus tachycardia, trifascicular disease can mimic ventricular tachycardia, but at slower rates, sinus conduction is confirmed. The prior ECG demonstrates atrial activity that can be more clearly seen in leads I and III (Figure 4).

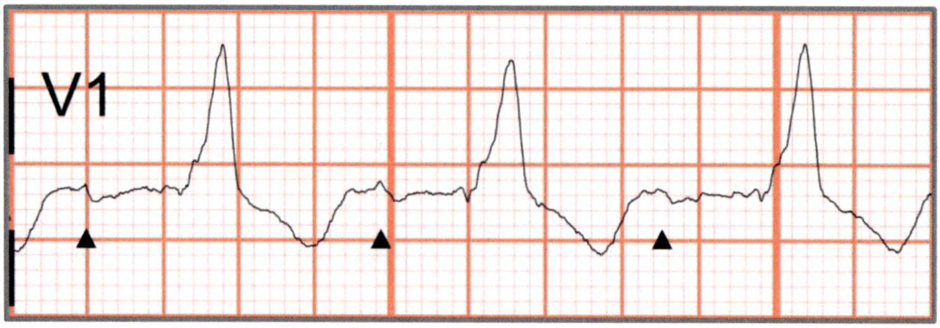

Figure 4. Right bundle branch block pattern in V1 with a prolonged PR interval. P waves are designated with arrowheads.

4. **Third Degree Atrioventricular Block, Atrial Fibrillation.** This patient had known atrial fibrillation yet has a regular rhythm (aside from the final premature complex). Atrial fibrillation with complete heart block will characteristically have a fibrillatory baseline and absent P waves but a regular escape rhythm.[5] When impulses from a superior pacemaker fail to transmit distally, an inferior one will "escape" it's usual suppression, leading to an "escape" rhythm. It is difficult to discern, but this patient

also had known right bundle branch and left anterior fascicular blocks whose morphologies exactly match the complexes in this ECG, making the junction the most plausible site for the escape rhythm.

5. **Global Subendocardial Ischemia**. This pattern of multilead ST-segment depressions and ST-segment elevation in aVR has been recognized as a predictor of triple vessel and/or left main disease;[6] however, this pattern can be seen with any pathology that causes a supply/demand mismatch. Differential considerations include acute pulmonary embolism, hypoxic respiratory failure, sepsis, severe anemia, hypokalemia, and left ventricular hypertrophy.[7–10] This patient presented with cardiac chest pain and was discovered to have diffuse disease on left heart catheterization. The patient underwent coronary artery bypass grafting.

6. **Atrial Fibrillation with Rapid Ventricular Response**. The differential for an irregularly irregular rhythm includes atrial fibrillation, atrial flutter with variable conduction, and multifocal atrial tachycardia. The apparent atrial activity in V1, at first glance, appears to represent flutter waves, but flutter waves are regular in appearance and cause ventricular activation (R-R intervals) at intervals that are multiples of atrial activation (P-P interval) - not the case here. Therefore, the apparent atrial activity in V1 is just baseline artifact and this is atrial fibrillation.

7. **Right Bundle Branch Block, Left Anterior Fascicular Block, Hyperkalemia.** The rSR' pattern in V1 and wide S wave in V5 and V6 indicates the presence of a right bundle branch block (Figure 2), while the extreme left axis deviation suggests the presence of a left anterior fascicular block (Figure 3). The potassium level was 6.3 mEq/L. Hyperkalemia can, itself, cause conduction disturbances like bundle branch or fascicular blocks; however, this patient's conduction disturbances were known. Relative to prior ECGs, the QRS complex is wider and P waves are absent – both features of hyperkalemia.

8. **Ventricular Tachycardia**. The differential for regular, wide complex tachycardia includes ventricular tachycardia, supraventricular tachycardia with aberrancy, antidromic atrioventricular reentrant tachycardia, toxicologic/metabolic disturbances, and ventricular paced rhythm.[11] Although the rate is slower than typical ventricular tachycardia, features favoring ventricular tachycardia include RSr' (left R taller than the right r' in V1) and extreme right axis (Figure 5).

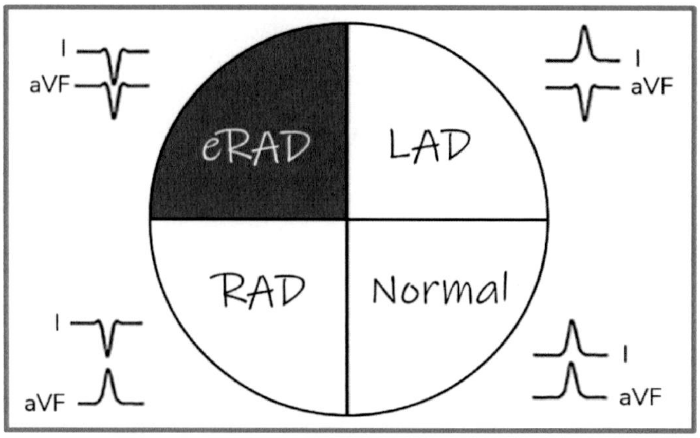

Figure 5. LAD, left axis deviation; RAD, right axis deviation; eRAD, extreme right axis deviation.

This rhythm was confirmed to be ventricular tachycardia by electrophysiology and the patient was electrically cardioverted.

While 80% of wide complex tachycardia is ventricular tachycardia, several algorithms including the Brugada algorithm,[12] the Vereckei algorithm,[13] and, more recently, the Basel algorithm[14] have been developed to differentiate ventricular tachycardia from supraventricular tachycardia with aberrancy. It is worth noting that their use in the clinical setting has shown low reproducibility, and it is safest to presume ventricular tachycardia in the absence of compelling information to suggest otherwise.[15–19]

9. **Hyperkalemia, Left Ventricular Hypertrophy**. There are signs of left ventricular hypertrophy including large QRS complexes and associated repolarization abnormalities (i.e., asymmetric T wave inversions primarily in the lateral leads).[20] Additionally, peaked T waves indicate hyperkalemia.

10. **Dextrocardia, Sinus Tachycardia.** Typically, the QRS complexes increase in amplitude across the precordium, however they decrease across the precordium in this ECG due to increased distance from the site of the cardiac impulse in this patient with dextrocardia. To obtain a more familiar appearing ECG in patients with dextrocardia, all leads (limb and precordial) should simply be reversed. The convex ST segments (especially in the inferior leads) and significantly elevated troponin prompted emergent catheterization, which revealed clean coronaries. This patient was ultimately diagnosed with myopericarditis.

11. **Hypercalcemia, Right Bundle Branch Block.** The QT interval is short with essentially zero ST segment, and there is a right bundle branch block. Shortening of

the QT interval can result in a "high-takeoff" of the ST-segment, mimicking myocardial ischemia or infarction.[21–23] The identification of ECG changes associated with hypercalcemia is critical as these are manifestations of conduction abnormalities with a rare risk of progression to potentially fatal ventricular dysrhythmias such as ventricular fibrillation.[24] The ECG findings commonly associated with hypercalcemia are QT interval shortening and Osborn J waves.[25]

12. **Inferior ST-elevation Myocardial Infarction.** There is ST-segment elevation in the inferior leads (II, III, aVF) with reciprocal changes in the anterolateral leads (I, aVL, V2 through V6). Left heart catheterization revealed an occluded right coronary artery and percutaneous coronary intervention was performed.

13. **Hypokalemia, Prolonged QT.** Hypokalemia prolongs the QT interval by way of delaying repolarization, creating a broad-based T wave, U waves, and T-U fusions (Figure 6).[26,27] This patient's potassium was 1.9 mEq/L. The repolarization changes resolved after potassium repletion.

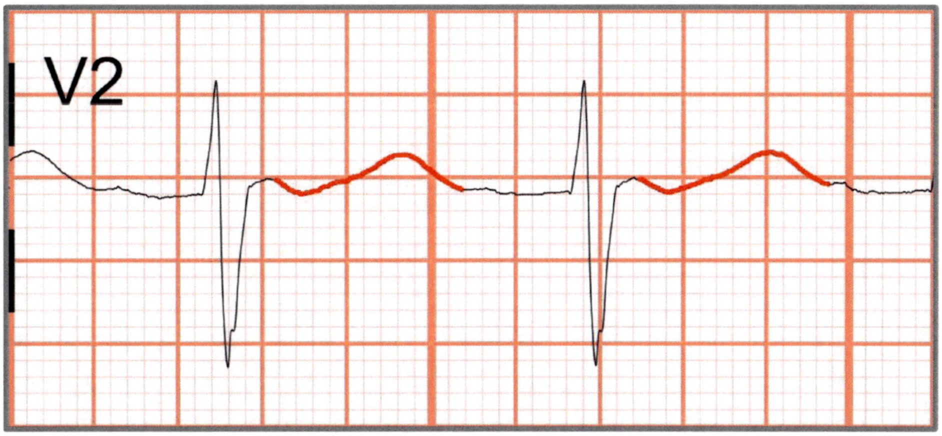

Figure 6. Wavy T-U fusion in V2 (red) characteristic of hypokalemia.

14. **Third Degree Atrioventricular Block with Ventricular Escape.** There is atrioventricular dissociation with QRS complexes occurring at regular intervals. The wide, and slow (<40 bpm) QRS complexes suggest a ventricular escape rhythm.

15. **Hyperacute T Waves, ST-elevation Myocardial Infarction.** Large amplitude T waves in the anterior precordium approach the size of the QRS complexes, making them "hyperacute." Some authors have proposed identifying hyperacute T waves using proportional T-wave "bulk," defined by the increased area under the curve (AUC) of the T-wave relative to the QRS amplitude – meaning, when the area under the T wave is relatively large compared to the QRS complex, hyperacute T waves are likely.[10,28,29] Hyperacute T waves, even in the absence of ST-segment elevation,

can be a subtle sign of vessel occlusion and an indication for emergent reperfusion.[30,31] Additional features of myocardial infarction include (reciprocal) ST-segment depressions in the inferolateral leads. Left heart catheterization revealed an acute left anterior descending artery occlusion.

16. **Orthodromic Atrioventricular Tachycardia.** This regular, narrow complex tachycardia looks like any other supraventricular tachycardia; however, the post-conversion ECG clearly shows evidence of ventricular pre-excitation including a short PR interval, a slurred QRS upstroke (i.e., delta wave), and a slightly widened QRS complex (Figure 7).

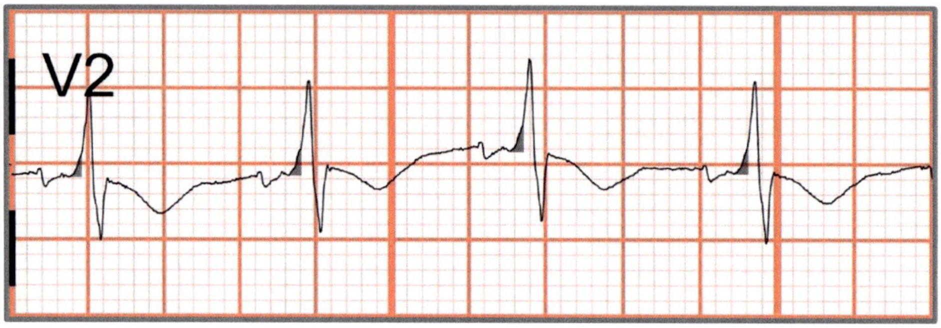

Figure 7. Delta waves seen in lead V2 represented by the shaded region.

The presence of ventricular pre-excitation suggests this rhythm was orthodromic conduction (Figure 8),[32,33] a fact later confirmed via an electrophysiology study.

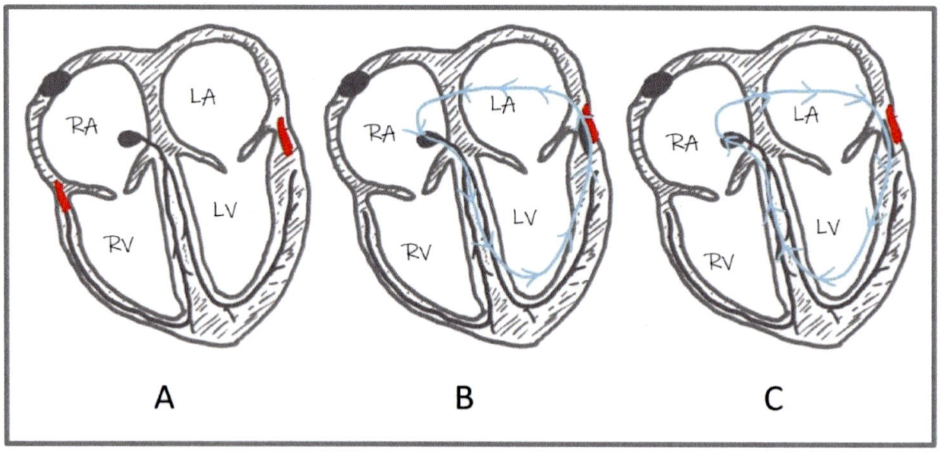

Figure 8. Orthodromic and antidromic atrioventricular reentrant tachycardia. The red bars in panel A represent possible locations of the accessory pathway (type A, between LA and LV; type B, between RA and RV). The blue line in panel B represents orthodromic conduction (narrow complex) and the blue line in panel C represents antidromic conduction (wide complex). RA, right atrium; RV, right ventricle; LA, left atrium; LV, left ventricle.

17. **Ventricular Tachycardia.** The differential for regular wide complex tachycardia includes ventricular tachycardia, supraventricular tachycardia with aberrancy, antidromic atrioventricular reentrant tachycardia, and toxicologic/metabolic disturbances.[11] The right bundle branch block pattern with the first R larger than the r' in V1 is very specific for ventricular tachycardia.

18. **Wellens Syndrome.** The presence of deep, symmetric T wave inversions in anterior precordial leads (Figure 9) is suggestive of Wellens syndrome in the appropriate clinical context.

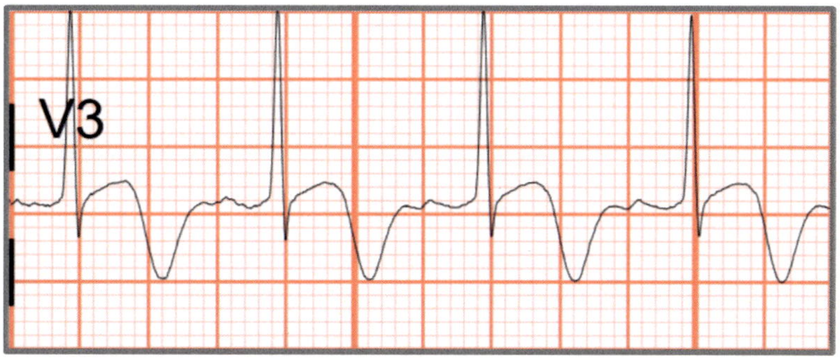

Figure 9. Deep, symmetric T wave inversions in V3.

Wellens syndrome is characterized by:

1. Biphasic T-waves with a terminal negative deflection (Type A) or deep and symmetric inverted T-waves in V2/V3 (Type B),
2. ECG findings present in pain-free state, and
3. normal or minimally elevated cardiac biomarkers.[30,34]

The syndrome is suggestive of critical left anterior descending artery stenosis. Left heart catheterization revealed a 95% proximal left anterior descending artery stenosis.

19. **Limb Lead Reversal, Sinus Bradycardia.** The extreme right axis, abnormal P wave axis (i.e., positively deflected in aVR), and concordance of complexes in aVR and V6 strongly suggest limb lead reversal (i.e., when opposing leads like aVR and V6 show QRS complexes traveling in the same direction, limb lead reversal is likely). The subsequent ECG was performed with corrected lead placement. The rhythm is sinus bradycardia and there are terminal T wave inversions that suggest ischemia; however, left heart catheterization revealed coronary ectasia without obstructive disease.

20. **Inferior ST-elevation Myocardial Infarction, Third Degree Atrioventricular Block.** The inferior ST segments are "straightened," and take-off directly from the R wave

- an early finding of evolving ST-segment elevation (Figure 10). There are reciprocal ST-segment depressions in aVL and V2. In the setting of inferior myocardial infarction, atrioventricular block is usually transient, due to ischemia or edema of the atrioventricular node, and resulting in a junctional escape rhythm.[3] Left heart catheterization revealed right coronary artery occlusion and percutaneous intervention was successful. The atrioventricular block resolved, and permanent pacing was not required.

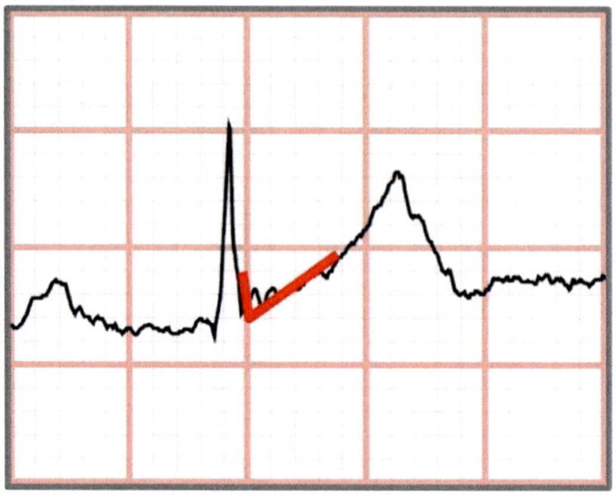

Figure 10. Lead II complex demonstrating ST "straightening," or the "checkmark sign" (red).

21. **Ventricular Tachycardia**. The differential for regular wide complex tachycardia includes ventricular tachycardia, supraventricular tachycardia with aberrancy, antidromic atrioventricular reentrant tachycardia, and toxicologic/metabolic disturbances.[11] Josephson's sign, notching near the nadir of the S wave, can be seen in V1 and V2, and suggests ventricular tachycardia (Figure 11).[5] This patient was ultimately diagnosed with ventricular tachycardia.

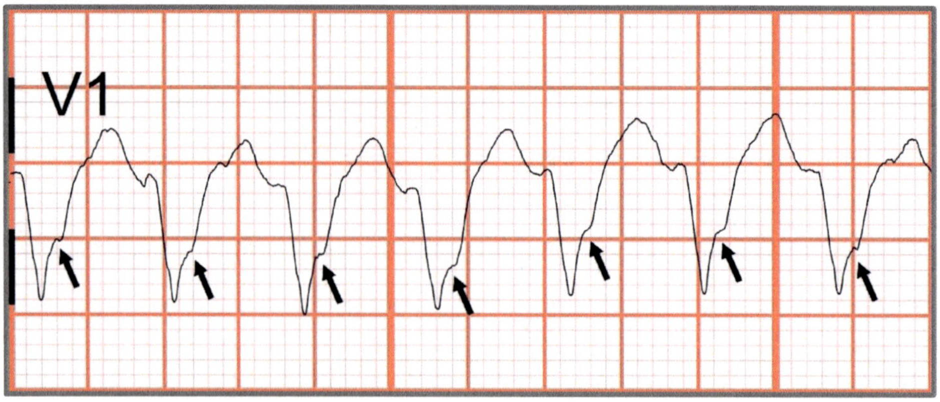

Figure 11. Notching near the nadir of the S wave in V1 (Josephson's sign, arrows).

22. **Supraventricular Tachycardia with Aberrancy.** The differential for regular wide complex tachycardia includes ventricular tachycardia, supraventricular tachycardia

with aberrancy, antidromic atrioventricular reentrant tachycardia, and toxicologic/metabolic disturbances.[11] The wide complex seen here was exactly consistent with the patient's known left bundle branch block. This is one instance when supraventricular tachycardia with aberrancy can be reliably diagnosed. This patient was successfully converted with adenosine. The prior ECG shows a left bundle branch block pattern with a wide and negatively deflected QRS complex in V1, and broad, monophasic R waves in the lateral leads (I, aVL, V5, V6). Note the expected discordant ST changes (i.e., ST deviations in the opposite direction of the QRS complexes).

23. **Inferior ST-elevation Myocardial Infarction**. The concave up ST-segment morphology along with the J wave notching might suggest early repolarization; however, the T wave inversion and slight ST-segment depression in aVL strongly suggests inferior myocardial infarction. Left heart catheterization revealed an occluded distal right coronary artery and percutaneous intervention was successful.

24. **Hypokalemia.** This bizarre rhythm was due to severe hypokalemia, which is known to increase automaticity.[35] Frequent ventricular ectopy in the setting of severe hypokalemia places this patient at risk for torsade de pointes. This patient's potassium was 1.8 mEq/L at the time of the ECG likely related to overuse of diuretics. The ectopy resolved with electrolyte repletion and a normal rhythm was restored.

25. **Anterior ST-elevation Myocardial Infarction, Hyperacute T Waves.** Hyperacute T waves, ST-segment elevation, and ST-segment straightening are present across the precordium. Note that the amplitudes of the T waves in V4 and V5 are greater than the QRS complexes. The relative size of the T waves makes them "hyperacute," an early indicator of coronary occlusion.[10,28,29] This patient had a proximal left anterior descending artery occlusion and received successful percutaneous coronary intervention.

26. **Right Bundle Branch Block, Atrial Fibrillation**. The irregularly irregular rhythm is the result of atrial fibrillation. There is a rate-dependent right bundle branch block that resolves at lower rates (see the post-conversion ECG). At higher rates, diseased fascicles can fail.[36,37]

27. **Prolonged QT**. The prolonged QT interval was likely drug-induced. This patient was on several QT-prolonging medications including amiodarone, metoclopramide, and ondansetron. Measuring the QT can be challenging, and many different methods

exist. One simple method is the "half the RR" rule – the QT interval is prolonged if it occupies more than half the R-R interval (Figure 12).[38]

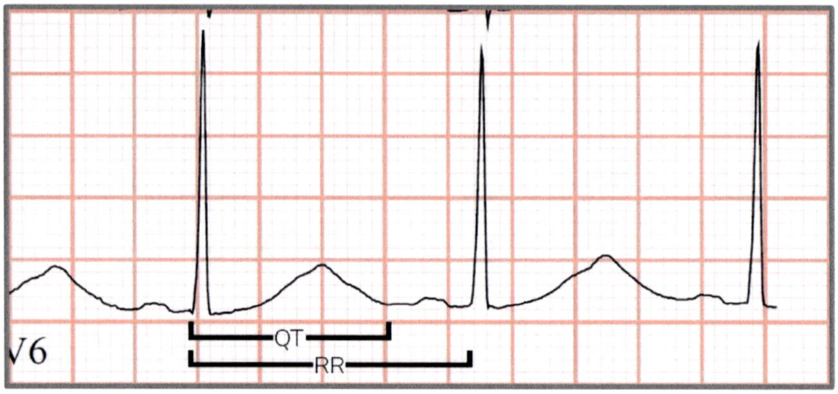

Figure 12. QT and RR intervals in lead V6. The QT interval is more than half the RR interval.

28. **Second Degree Atrioventricular Block - Mobitz I, Trifascicular Disease.** Second degree atrioventricular block, Mobitz I associated with right bundle branch block and left anterior fascicular block. This represents trifascicular disease, and the patient is at risk for progression to complete heart block.[1,32] The subsequent ECG demonstrates progression to complete heart block with junctional escape.

29. **Atrioventricular Nodal Reentrant Tachycardia.** This rhythm is regular with a narrow QRS complex, and a rate of 200 beats per minute. The differential includes sinus tachycardia, atrioventricular nodal reentrant tachycardia, atrioventricular reentrant tachycardia, atrial flutter, and atrial tachycardia. The presence of retrograde P' waves, seen immediately following the QRS complexes in lead V1 (pseudo-R waves, Figure 13) confirms the diagnosis of atrioventricular nodal reentrant tachycardia.[39] Adenosine was administered, and the rhythm converted to sinus.

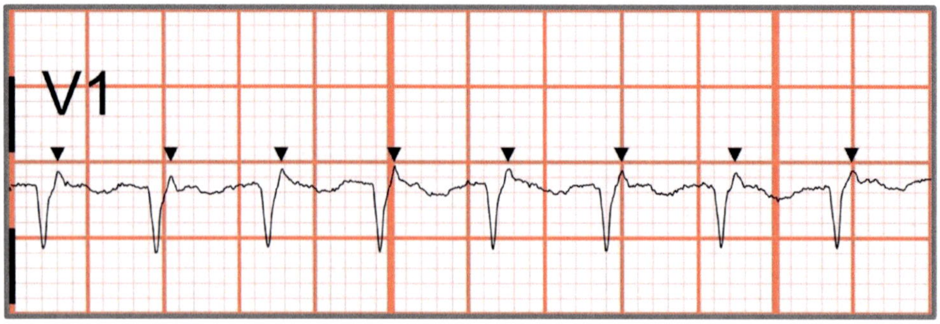

Figure 13. Pseudo-R waves in V1 represent retrograde P' waves (arrowheads).

30. **Atrial Flutter with 2:1 Conduction.** The subsequent ECG was performed with the Lewis lead and unmasked the underlying 2:1 conduction. The Lewis lead describe a different positioning of the limb leads in order to better visualize atrial activity (Figure 14).[40] Upright P waves with an atrial rate of about 280 bpm are best visualized in leads I and II (Figure 15).

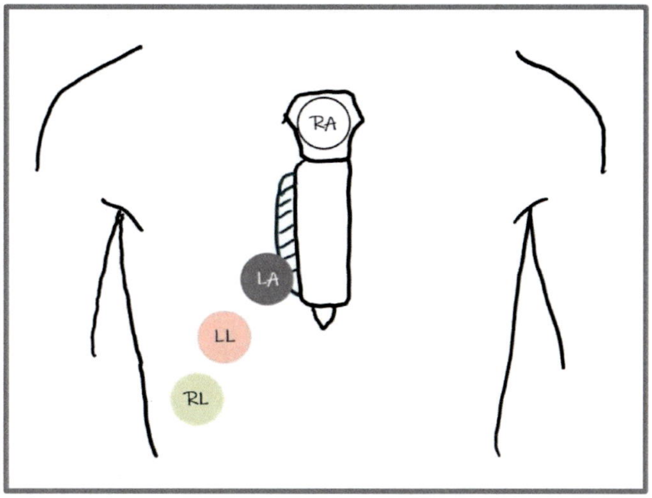

Figure 14. The Lewis lead can help better visualize atrial activity. Lead placement is demonstrated here. RA, right arm electrode; LA, left arm electrode; LL, left lower limb electrode; RL, right lower limb electrode.

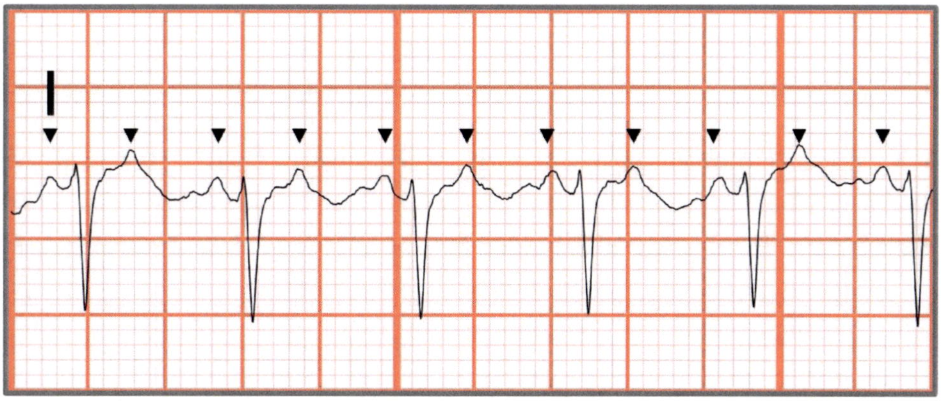

Figure 15. Atrial activity seen in lead I (arrowheads).

31. **Atypical right bundle branch block, Atrial Fibrillation with Rapid Ventricular Response.** Atypical right bundle branch block pattern in a patient with known Ebstein anomaly (i.e., downward displacement of the tricuspid valve). Right bundle branch block is present in most cases of Ebstein anomaly, but the pattern is usually atypical (i.e., the QRS complex in the right precordial leads, V1 through V3, tends to be polyphasic and Q waves are often present in V1).[5]

32. **Nonsustained Ventricular Tachycardia.** There is a run of nonsustained ventricular tachycardia in a patient with known hypertrophic cardiomyopathy. Nonsustained ventricular tachycardia is defined by at least three beats and no more than 30 seconds of consecutive complexes originating from the ventricles at a rate of greater than 100 beats per minute.[41]

33. **Acute Pericarditis.** Features of acute pericarditis include diffuse, concave up ST-segment elevations without reciprocal changes, and PR depression (with PR elevation in aVR). The diagnosis is made by meeting two of four criteria:[32,42]

    1. Typical symptoms (pleuritic, sharp chest pain relieved when leaning forward)
    2. New pericardial effusion
    3. Presence of friction rub
    4. Typical ECG findings

    This patient had worsening renal failure associated with profound uremia, typical symptoms of acute pericarditis, and a new pericardial effusion. He was diagnosed with uremic encephalopathy and uremic pericarditis, both of which improved with serial dialysis sessions.

34. **Junctional Escape, Sinus Node Dysfunction.** This junctional escape rhythm alternates with atrial fibrillation, classic for sick sinus syndrome – a collection of maladies related to sinus node dysfunction from degenerative disease.[2]

35. **Anterior ST-elevation Myocardial Infarction, Right Bundle Branch Block.** Typically, with a right bundle branch block, the ST-segments are slightly depressed in leads V1-3;[3,43] therefore, any degree of ST-segment elevation in these leads is concerning for anterior myocardial infarction. Left heart catheterization revealed a 95% culprit lesion to the left main and percutaneous coronary intervention was successful.

36. **Pseudo-Left Ventricular Hypertrophy, Pseudo-Right Atrial Enlargement, T-wave Inversions.** This ECG is a mimic of left ventricular hypertrophy and right atrial enlargement in a very young, thin individual. Just as increased soft-tissue impedance from adipose or edema can influence the surface ECG by dampening the conduction of electrical impulses, an especially slender body habitus can have the inverse effect. In this case, the various electrocardiographic abnormalities were simply amplifications of normal cardiac activity. One potentially helpful hint is the combination of left ventricular hypertrophy with right axis deviation – the former

when truly representative of ventricular hypertrophy being more commonly associated with leftward axis deviation.[5]

37. **Sodium Channel Toxicity.** This ECG represents sodium channel toxicity in a patient with tricyclic antidepressant overdose. Features of sodium channel toxicity include right axis deviation, tall terminal R wave in aVR (Figure 16), and a slightly widened QRS complex.[44]

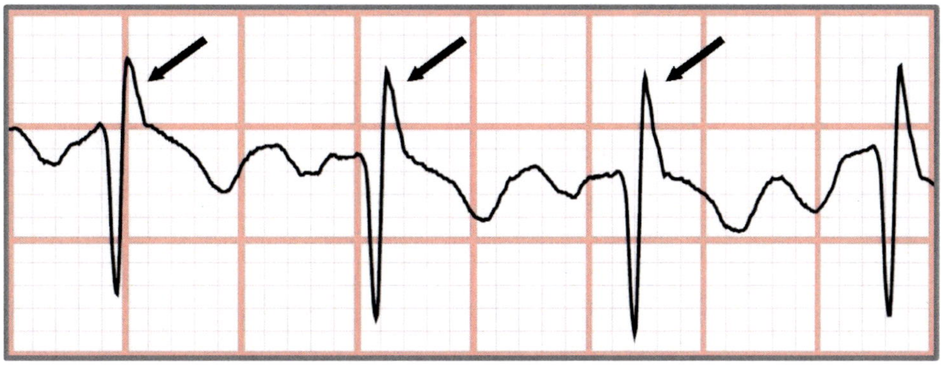

Figure 16. Tall terminal R wave in aVR (arrows).

38. **Right Heart Strain, Right Atrial Enlargement, Pulmonary Embolism.** This patient was diagnosed with a submassive pulmonary embolism. Findings of right heart strain in this ECG include early R wave progression, right axis deviation, right atrial enlargement, ST-segment depressions, and T-wave inversions in inferolateral leads.[5]

39. **Supraventricular Tachycardia with Aberrancy, Right Bundle Branch Block, Left Anterior Fascicular Block.** The differential for regular wide complex (i.e., QRS > 120 ms) tachycardia includes ventricular tachycardia, supraventricular tachycardia with aberrancy, antidromic atrioventricular reentrant tachycardia, and toxicologic/metabolic disturbances.[11] This patient had known right bundle branch and left anterior fascicular blocks with the identical morphology, at baseline, that is seen here in this ECG. The patient was successfully cardioverted with adenosine. Unless compelling evidence exists to the contrary, as with this case, ventricular tachycardia should be the presumptive diagnosis for regular wide complex tachycardia.

40. **Atrial Tachycardia.** Atrial tachycardia occurs when an ectopic atrial focus delivers impulses, typically at a rate of 150 to 250 beats per minute.[3] Normally, the P wave axis is down in lead V1 and up in lead II. The abnormal P wave axis in this ECG suggests an ectopic atrial source (Figure 17).

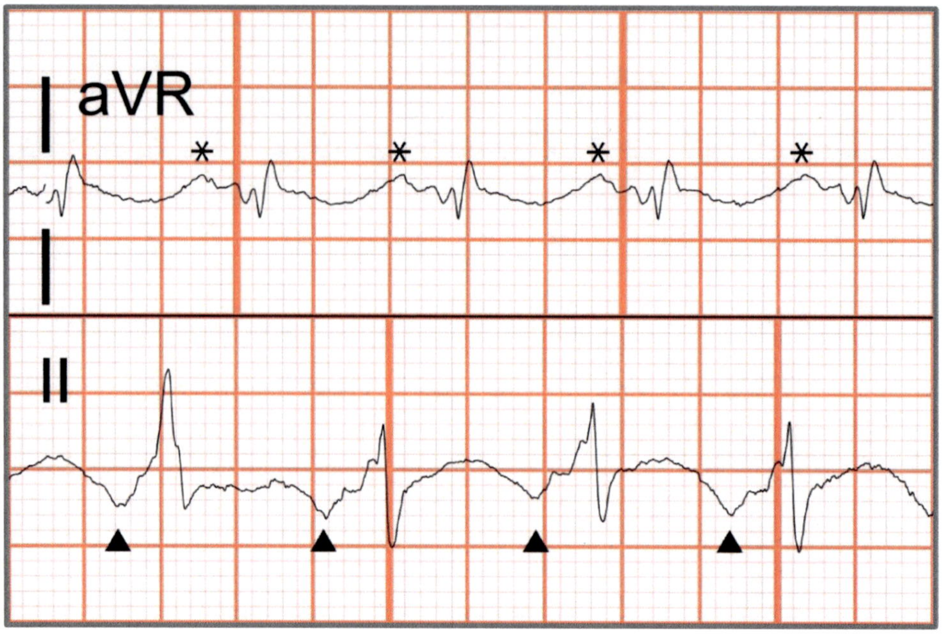

Figure 17. Abnormal P wave axis with upright P waves in aVR (asterisks) and negatively deflected P waves in lead II (arrowheads) indicating an ectopic atrial focus.

41. **Atypical Atrioventricular Nodal Reentrant Tachycardia.** Atrioventricular nodal reentrant tachycardia is a regular, narrow complex tachycardia usually between 140 and 220 beats per minute[3] (but can be slower[45] as with this case) in which a reentrant circuit is formed within the atrioventricular node. Fast and slow pathways are the necessary substrate to establish the circuit. In typical atrioventricular nodal reentrant tachycardia, the conduction travels down the slow pathway and up the fast pathway within the atrioventricular node, and retrograde P' waves can occasionally be seen immediately following the QRS complex. In atypical atrioventricular tachycardia, which conducts down the fast and up the slow pathway, retrograde atrial activity can occasionally be seen prior to or in between QRS complexes as with this case (Figure 18, Figure 19).[32,46] This patient converted with adenosine, helping to confirm the diagnosis of atypical atrioventricular nodal reentrant tachycardia.

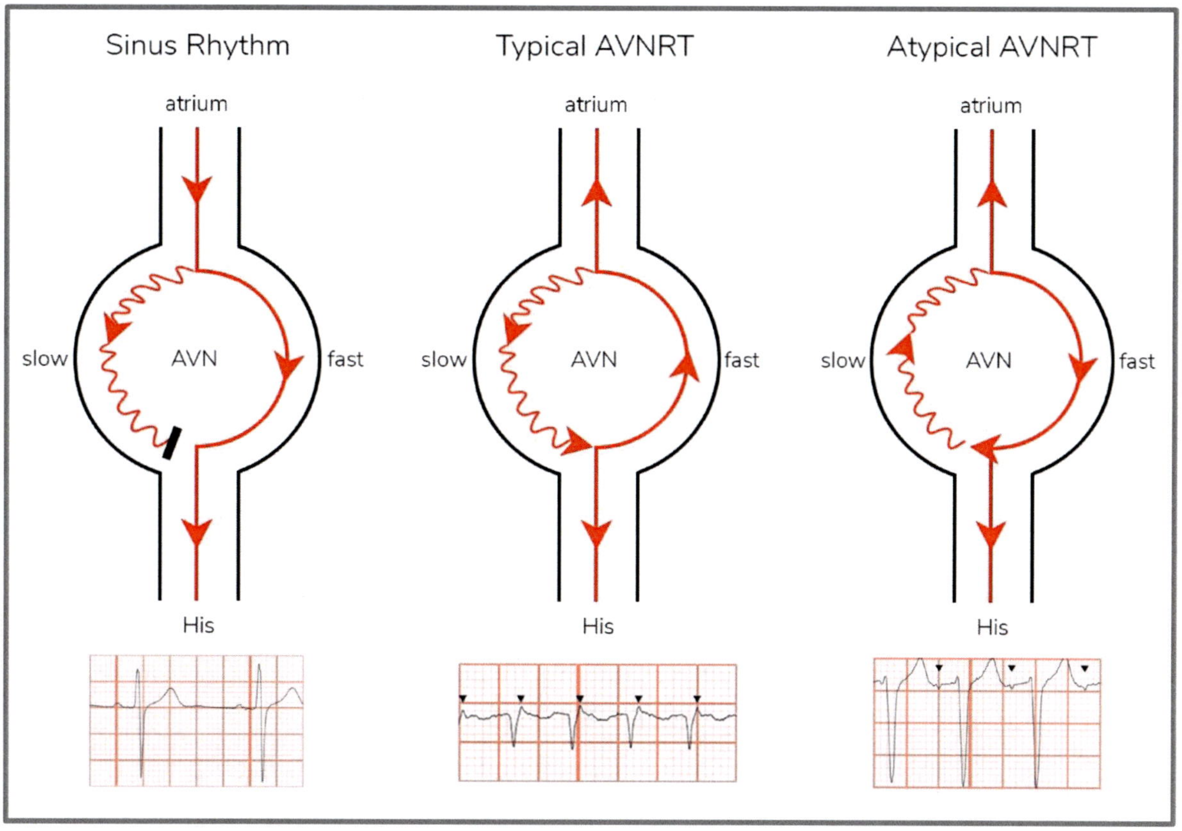

Figure 18. Slow and fast pathways providing the substrate for atrioventricular reentrant tachycardia (AVNRT). AVN, atrioventricular node.

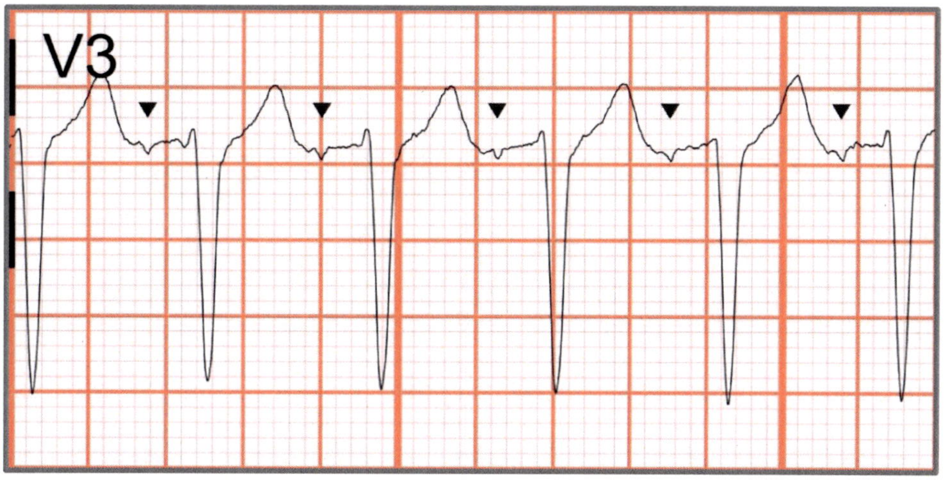

Figure 19. Retrograde atrial activity (arrowheads), forming the long RP interval of atypical AVNRT.

42. **Bidirectional Ventricular Tachycardia, Digoxin Toxicity.** Bidirectional ventricular tachycardia is near pathognomonic for digoxin toxicity.[47] The mainstay of treatment is digoxin-specific antibody fragments and is indicated with cardiac manifestations of toxicity.

43. **Limb Lead Reversal.** The presence of negative P-QRS complexes in lead I is unusual, and the P-wave axis is abnormal – with an inverted P-wave in lead I and upright in aVR (where the inverse would be expected for sinus node origin). The presence of negative P-QRS-T complexes in lead I combined with positive deflections in aVR are suspicious for LA/RA reversal. A repeat ECG was obtained, and the axis normalized. Some key electrocardiographic features of limb lead reversal are:[48–51]

    1. Opposing directions of P-QRS complexes between I and V6 (limb and precordial leads with shared axes)
    2. Positive P-QRS in aVR
    3. Extreme axis deviation (+180° and -90°)
    4. P-wave amplitude greater in lead I than II
    5. Very-low amplitude in isolated limb lead (I, II, III).

44. **Anterior ST-elevation Myocardial Infarction.** There is ST-segment elevation associated with terminal QRS distortion in lead V3, a highly specific for ST-elevation Myocardial Infarction Terminal QRS distortion is the absence of both an S and J wave in either V2 or V3 (Figure 20).[52] Left heart catheterization revealed a 100% mid left anterior descending artery occlusion.

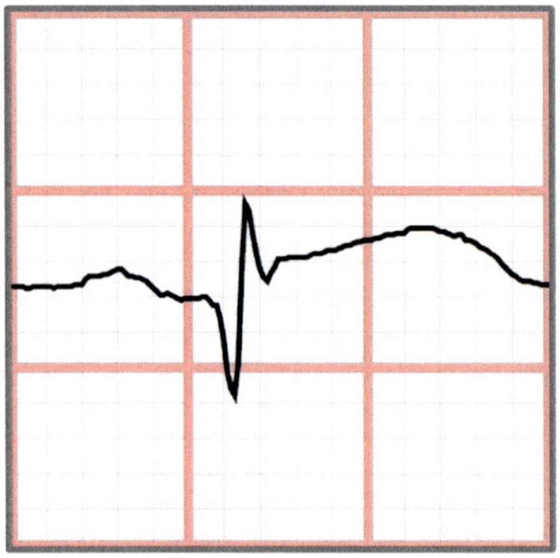

Figure 20. Terminal QRS distortion (absent S and J waves) in V3. An S wave is defined as any deflection at the end of an R wave that dips below the baseline.

45. **Right Bundle Branch Block.** Classic right bundle branch block pattern with rSR' in V1 and a wide S wave in the lateral leads (Figure 21).

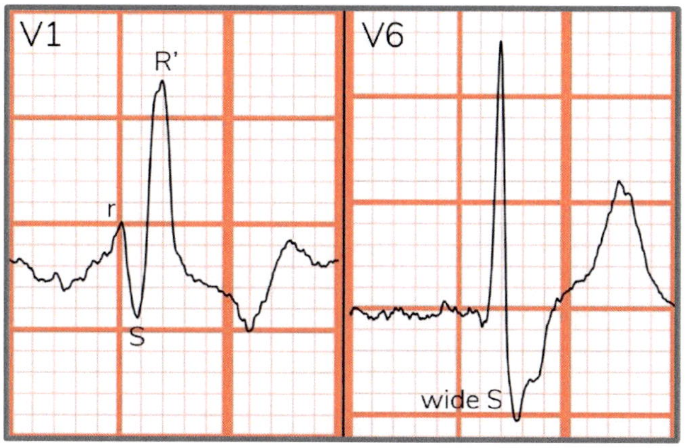

Figure 21. Classic right bundle branch block pattern with rSR' in V1 and wide S in V6.

46. **Prior Inferior Myocardial Infarction.** Causes of left axis deviation were previously reviewed in case 3. In this case, the left axis deviation is due to large Q waves from a prior infraction in the inferior leads (II, III, aVF).

47. **Accelerated Idioventricular Rhythm.** Accelerated idioventricular rhythm (AIVR) occurs under conditions of enhanced automaticity. An enhanced ectopic ventricular pacemaker outpaces superior pacemakers (e.g. sinus node) and, thus, becomes the dominant pacemaker by usurping control. AIVR occurs at rates faster than ventricular escape, but slower than ventricular tachycardia (i.e. between 50 and 110 beats/min). It can occur for many reasons including electrolyte abnormalities and drug toxicity (e.g. digoxin), however, it occurs most commonly in the setting of reperfusion – that is, after intervention for myocardial infarction or cardiac arrest. AIVR is frequently mistaken for ventricular tachycardia since both have wide, regular complexes and can have signs of atrioventricular dissociation (e.g. fusion and/or capture beats), especially when only viewed from the telemetry monitor. The feature that distinguishes the two rhythms is the rate. Rates greater than 110 beats/min are likely to be ventricular tachycardia. The distinction between AIVR and ventricular tachycardia is of paramount importance since the management differs significantly. AIVR is a self-terminating and well-tolerated rhythm that does not require intervention, unlike ventricular tachycardia.[3,5,53,54] Left heart catheterization confirmed a proximal left anterior descending artery occlusion and percutaneous coronary intervention was successful.

48. **High Lateral Ischemic T Wave Inversions.** The symmetric morphology of the T wave inversions seen in I, aVL, and V2 (biphasic with negative terminal deflection)

suggests ischemia (Figure 22). Left heart catheterization revealed 95% mid-left anterior descending artery stenosis.

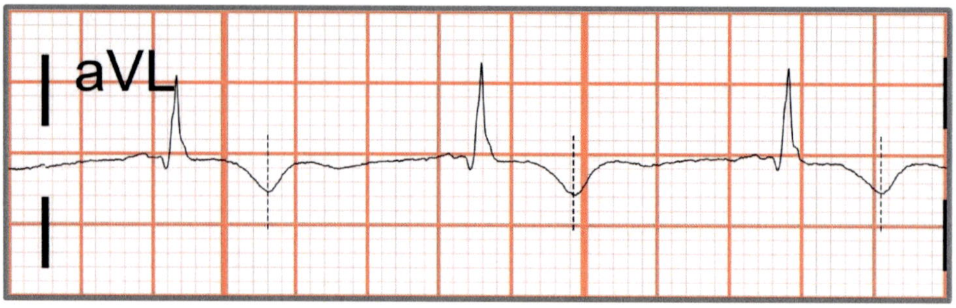

Figure 22. Symmetric T wave inversions (vertical dotted lines) are more likely to portend ischemia than asymmetric ones.

49. **ST-elevation Myocardial Infarction, Left Bundle Branch Block.** A left bundle branch block occurs when the left bundle no longer conducts, and the signal must pass to the left ventricle via myocyte-to-myocyte conduction. This pattern of conduction is slower than via the specialized conduction system, and results in a wide QRS complex (Figure 23).

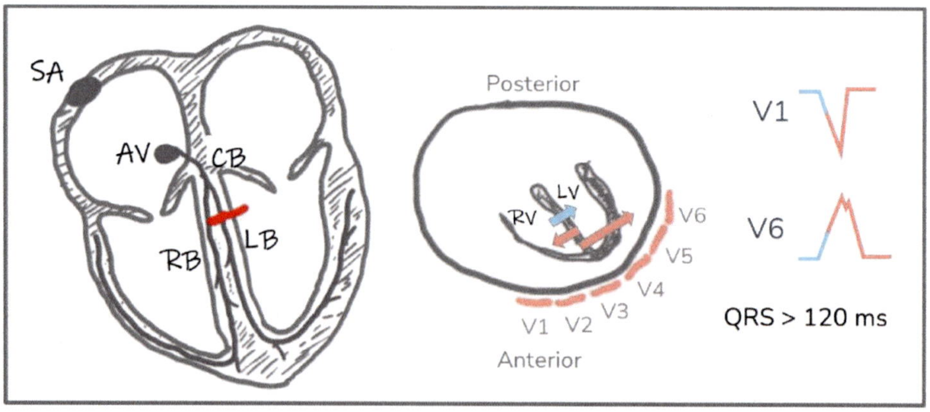

Figure 23. Direction of depolarization in left bundle branch block. The septum first depolarizes from right to left (blue arrow), followed by near simultaneous depolarization of the right and left ventricles (pink arrows). The resultant vector leads to a negative deflection in V1 and a positive deflection in V6. SA, sinoatrial node; AV, atrioventricular node; RB, right bundle; LB, left bundle; CB, common bundle; RV, right ventricle; LV, left ventricle; red dash represents a block of the left bundle.

Normally, a left bundle branch block demonstrates characteristic discordant changes – ST segments tend to deflect in the opposite direction from the QRS complex. In leads with primarily down-going QRS complexes (i.e. V1, V2, V3), ST-elevation is expected; and in leads with primarily up-going QRS complexes (i.e. I, aVL, V5, V6), ST-depression is expected. ST-segment deviation in a direction concordant with the QRS complex is specific for acute myocardial infarction and warrants emergent reperfusion.[30,31] The (modified) Sgarbossa criteria were developed to identify acute myocardial infarction in the setting of left bundle branch block, and is considered positive if any of the following criteria are met:[55–57]

1. Concordant ST elevation of ≥ 1 mm
2. Concordant ST depression of ≥ 1 mm in V1, V2, or V3, or
3. Excessively discordant ST elevation defined as the ST/S ratio greater than 0.25.

This ECG demonstrates concordant ST-segment elevation in I and aVL. Left heart catheterization revealed diffuse disease and percutaneous intervention was performed to the left anterior descending and left circumflex arteries.

50. **Pacemaker Malfunction.** Failure to capture in a patient with a dual chamber pacemaker diagnosed with Twiddler's syndrome, a rare condition in which the pacemaker malfunctions due to coiling of the device in the skin pocket with resultant lead displacement.[58,59] Pacemaker spikes (green) are seen without associated QRS complexes.

51. **Low Voltage Due to Myxedema.** The traditional definition of low voltage is QRS amplitudes less than 5 mm in all limb leads or less than 10 mm in all precordial leads.[60–62] The differential for low voltage can be broken down into two categories:

    1. Cardiac abnormalities resulting in diminished impulse generation (e.g., prior infarcts, infiltrative cardiomyopathies like amyloidosis, and hypothyroidism).
    2. Increased impedance related to attenuating substances between the heart and surface leads (fluid, air, or adipose).

    The combination of low voltage and bradycardia should raise the concern for hypothyroidism/myxedema, as was the case with this patient.[60,61,63,64]

52. **Wellens Syndrome**. Wellens syndrome (previously described in case 18) with deep, symmetric T wave inversions in the precordial leads.[30,31,34] Left heart catheterization revealed 99% proximal left anterior descending artery stenosis.

53. **Posterior Myocardial Infarction.** Features of posterior wall myocardial infarction include R wave amplitude greater than the S wave amplitude in V1-2 with "mirror" ST-segment depression (especially horizontal or down-sloping) and upright T waves (Figure 24). Posterior myocardial infarction is commonly confused with anterior subendocardial ischemia; however, the T waves are usually negatively deflected with anterior subendocardial ischemia.[30,31,65] This ECG shows ST-

segment depression and upright T waves in the precordial leads V2 through V4. In the subsequent ECG, V4-V6 represent posterior leads. At least 0.5 mm ST-segment elevation in any posterior lead is diagnostic of posterior wall infarction and can be seen in V6.

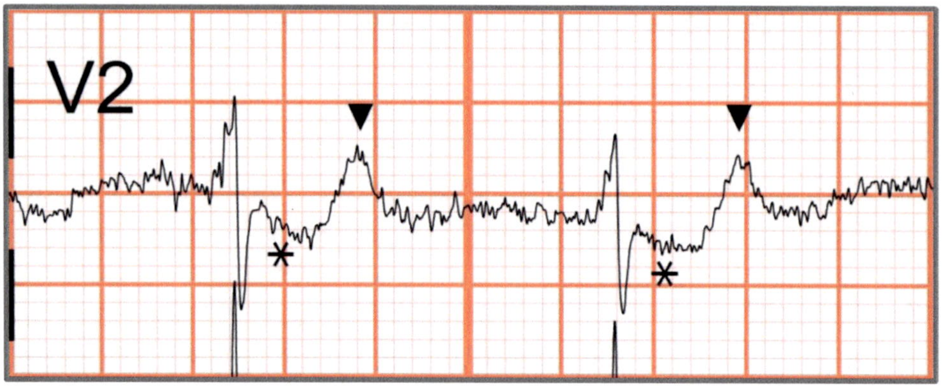

Figure 24. Lead V2 of the repeat ECG demonstrating the classic features of posterior myocardial infarction including R/S > 1, "mirror" ST-segment depression (asterisks), and upright T waves (arrowheads).

This patient received successful percutaneous coronary intervention to an occluded left circumflex artery.

54. **Atrial Fibrillation with Rapid Ventricular Response.** The differential for irregularly irregular rhythms includes at least three entities: atrial fibrillation (most common), atrial flutter with variable conduction, and multifocal atrial tachycardia. The latter two diagnoses produce coordinated atrial activity that can be visualized on the surface ECG, while the former does not.[66] Since there are no discernable P waves, the rhythm is atrial fibrillation.

55. **Left Bundle Branch Block.** Classic left bundle branch block pattern with a wide and down-going QRS complex in V1, and notched, positively deflected QRS complex in I, aVL, and V6, and left axis deviation (see Figure 23 for further explanation of left bundle branch blocks).

56. **Sinus Tachycardia, Left Bundle Branch Block.** A left bundle branch block can be misinterpreted as ventricular tachycardia, or an accelerated idioventricular rhythm, at faster rates when the P wave is buried by the preceding T wave, masking the atrial activity. This patient was in sinus tachycardia; P waves are most clearly seen in V1 (Figure 25).

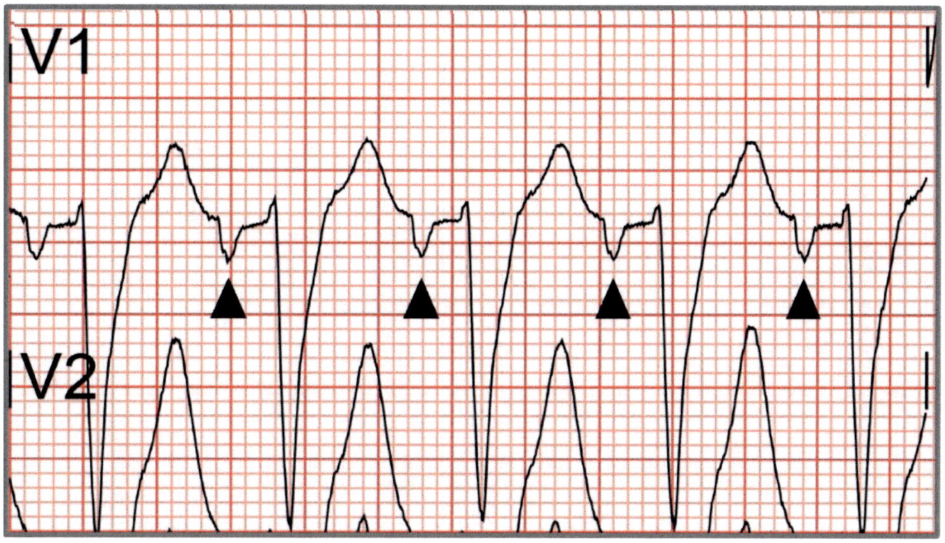

Figure 25. P waves in lead V1 (arrowheads)

57. **Atrioventricular Nodal Reentrant Tachycardia.** This is a regular, narrow complex tachycardia with a rate of 160 beats per minute. The differential includes sinus tachycardia, atrial flutter with 2:1 conduction, atrioventricular reentrant tachycardia with orthodromic conduction, and atrial tachycardia. Atrioventricular nodal reentrant tachycardia usually ranges between 140 and 220 beats per minute and occurs when a reentrant circuit is formed within the atrioventricular node (Figure 18).[3] This case converted to sinus rhythm with adenosine, confirming the diagnosis.

58. **Left Anterior Fascicular Block, Sinus Tachycardia.** This is the post-conversion ECG from the prior case. The extreme left axis deviation, qR complexes in aVL, and rS complexes in the inferior leads (II, III, aVF) are diagnostic for left anterior fascicular block (Figure 3).[2]

59. **Brugada Syndrome**. Type 1 or coved-type Brugada pattern in a patient presenting with syncope. Brugada syndrome is an inherited sodium channel mutation with a characteristic ECG pattern and increased risk of sudden cardiac death in the absence of structural disease.[67–69] The Brugada pattern has at least two variants:

    1. Type 1, coved-type: ST-segment elevation of ≥2 mm with a coved-type morphology followed by a negative T wave in ≥1 right precordial lead (Figure 26). Type 1 establishes the diagnosis.
    2. Type 2, saddleback-type: J point elevation of ≥2 mm gives rise to a gradually descending ST-segment that remains 1 mm above

the baseline followed by a positive T wave that gives a saddleback appearance in ≥1 right precordial lead (Figure 26).

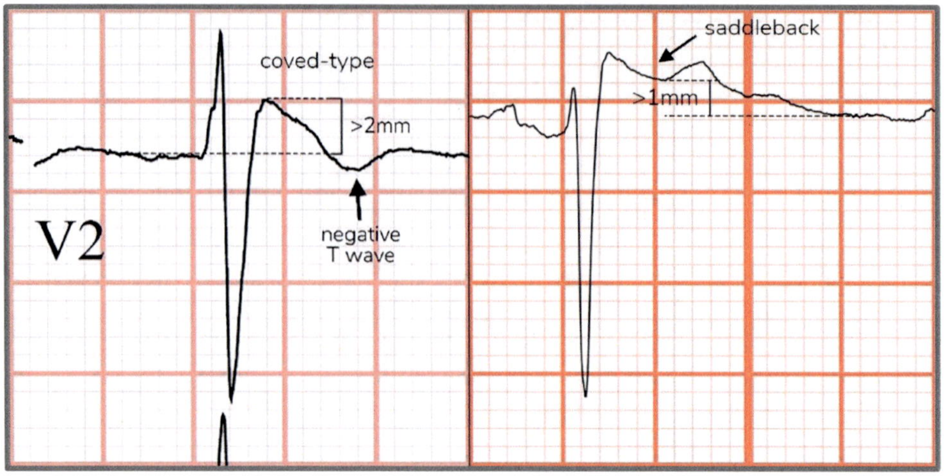

Figure 26. Coved-type Brugada pattern in V2 on the left panel, and saddleback type in V2 on the right panel.

This patient was formally diagnosed with Brugada syndrome and had an implantable defibrillator placed.

60. **Hypothermia, Junctional Bradycardia.** Electrocardiographic findings of hypothermia have been a subject of interest for over 100 years and include sino-atrial exit block, PR and QT prolongation, QRS widening, ST-segment depression, and atrial and ventricular fibrillation. Osborn waves are J point elevations immediately following the QRS complex are more specific (Figure 27).[70,71] This patient's core temperature was 26.1 °C (79 °F). Rewarming is the mainstay treatment of choice.

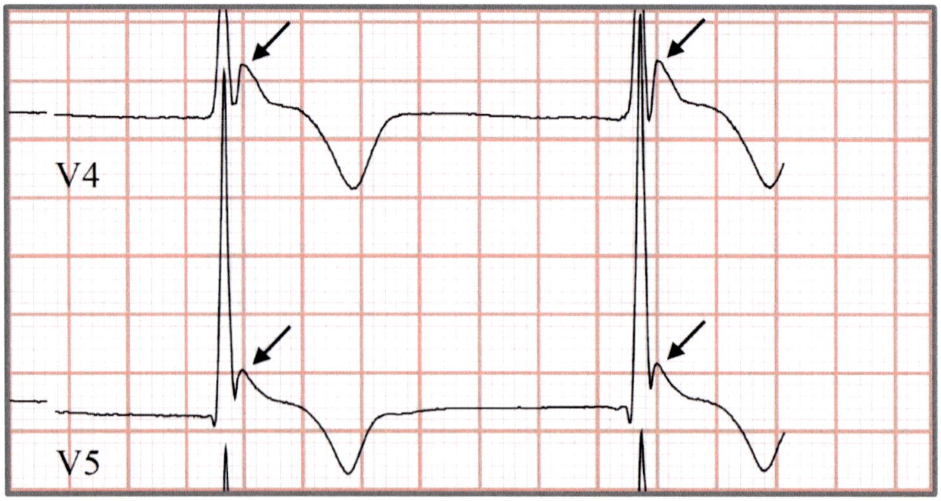

Figure 27. Osborn waves of hypothermia (arrows). Absent P waves in the setting of hypothermia suggests sino-atrial exit block.

61. **Low Voltage due to Myxedema.** The bradycardia, prolonged QT, and low voltage are all due to myxedema. This patient had a large pericardial effusion. Hypothyroidism can cause low voltage through two mechanisms: the direct effects of hormonal deficiency on the generation of cardiac action potentials and via the presence of a pericardial effusion, seen in up to one third of patients with hypothyroidism and, rarely, leading to tamponade. Patients with tamponade or large effusions due to hypothyroidism will characteristically lack a compensatory tachycardic response. [60,61,63,64] The differential diagnosis for low voltage was previously described in case 51.

62. **Inferior ST-elevation Myocardial Infarction.** Subtle inferior ST straightening with negative terminal T wave deflection in lead III suggests myocardial infarction (Figure 28). While this ECG does not meet classic ST-elevation myocardial infarction criteria,[72] it should prompt serial ECGs, early cardiology consultation, and possible emergent catheterization. Left heart catheterization revealed 90% stenosis of the left circumflex and occlusion of the second obtuse marginal branch.

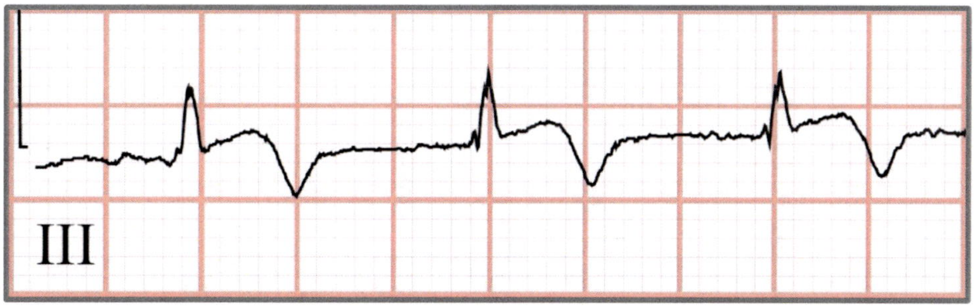

Figure 28. Subtle ST-segment straightening and elevation with negatively inverted T waves in lead III.

63. **Hyperkalemia.** Electrocardiographic findings of hyperkalemia tend to follow a progression as toxicity progresses. Often, the earliest finding is narrow-based, peaked T waves. At the extreme end of the hyperkalemia spectrum, sine wave morphology is a harbinger of impending ventricular fibrillation. [25,73,74] This ECG has a very wide QRS approaching sine wave morphology.

64. **Hypokalemia, Prolonged QT**. While there is quite a bit of baseline artifact, a prolonged QT interval with broad-based T waves is evident.[25,26,75] This patient was severely hypokalemic (2.4 mEq/L) and intermittently went into polymorphic ventricular tachycardia. Overdrive pacing via a temporary transvenous pacer was initiated to avoid further episodes of polymorphic ventricular tachycardia.

65. **Global Subendocardial Ischemia.** Any pathology that creates a supply/demand mismatch can cause this pattern of multilead ST-segment depressions and ST-segment elevation in aVR.[7–9,76] The differential diagnosis for this pattern was previously described in case 5. In the right clinical context, this pattern is recognized as a predictor of triple vessel and/or left main disease.[6] This patient had elevated troponins and left heart catheterization revealed diffuse disease not amenable to percutaneous coronary intervention; coronary bypass grafting was successful.

66. **Ventricular Tachycardia.** A fusion beat near the beginning of the rhythm strip (Figure 29) represents the fusion of a normally conducted complex with a ventricular complex and indicates the presence of atrioventricular dissociation[77] - in this case, the result of ventricular tachycardia.

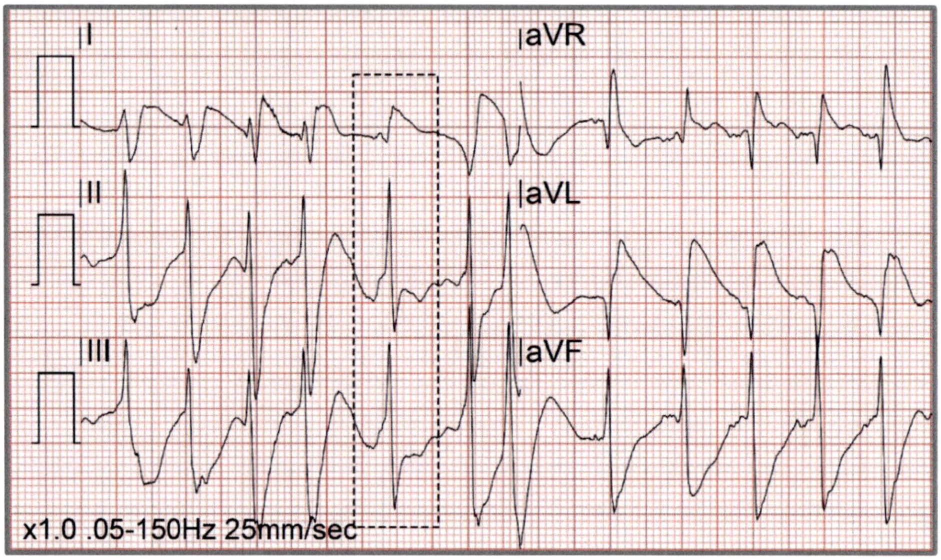

Figure 29. The fusion beat appears morphologically distinct from the other complexes (dashed rectangle).

67. **Hyperacute T Waves, ST-elevation Myocardial Infarction.** While not particularly large in amplitude, the T waves in V5 and V6 are broad-based and larger than their associated QRS complexes.[10,28,29,34,78,79] This ECG evolved into a more obvious ST-elevation myocardial infarction on the subsequent ECG. Leart heart catheterization revealed an occluded left anterior descending artery.

68. **Global Subendocardial Ischemia.** Remember to keep a broad differential with this pattern of multilead ST-segment depression and ST-segment elevation in aVR, as any pathology that creates a supply/demand mismatch can cause it (as previously described in case 5).[7–10] In this case, the pattern was the result of cardiac arrest.

69. **Left Ventricular Aneurysm.** The usual ECG findings of left ventricular aneurysm include ST elevation that persists more than two weeks after myocardial infarction, deep Q waves, and the absence of reciprocal ST depressions.[80,81] In the age of reperfusion, left ventricular aneurysms have become quite rare, but in the absence of reperfusion, it is a common structural complication of anterior myocardial infarctions.[80,82] The convex ST-elevation in V2 was consistent with prior ECGs.

70. **Third Degree Atrioventricular Block.** This is complete atrioventricular block with a junctional escape rhythm in an infant. The junction is the only part of the conduction system capable of producing a narrow escape rhythm, and rates typically range from 40 to 60 beats per minute. Infants with junctional escape tend to tolerate atrioventricular block well.

71. **Inferolateral ST-elevation Myocardial Infarction.** Inferolateral ST-segment elevation with reciprocal ST-segment depression in aVL and V2. Left heart catheterization revealed left circumflex occlusion.

72. **Global Subendocardial Ischemia.** This patient had an upper gastrointestinal bleed and was severely anemic, accounting for the multilead ST-segment depression and ST-segment elevation in aVR. The differential diagnosis for this pattern is broad and was previously described in case 5.

73. **Left Bundle Branch Block, First Degree Atrioventricular Block.** While not classically referred to as a "trifascicular block," a left bundle branch block indicates failure of two fascicles - the left anterior and posterior fascicles - and, when associated with first-degree atrioventricular block (i.e., prolonged PR interval), likely represents a diseased right bundle branch (i.e., trifascicular disease).[3] The term “trifascicular block” is a misnomer as a true block of all three fascicles (the right bundle branch, left anterior fascicle and left posterior fascicle) would result in complete heart block. Instead, the term references the presence of diseased conduction in all three fascicles with sufficient sparing of one fascicle that results in delayed conduction and manifests as a prolonged PR interval. The American Heart Association guidelines suggest that use of the term “trifascicular block” be abandoned in favor of a description of the identified blocks independently.[4] Patients with multiple fascicle disease are more likely to progress to third degree atrioventricular block.[83] This patient presented with syncope and subsequently received a permanent pacemaker after telemetry revealed intermittent high-grade atrioventricular block while inpatient.

74. **Hyperkalemia.** Electrocardiographic findings of hyperkalemia tend to follow a progression as toxicity progresses. Often, the earliest finding is narrow-based, peaked T waves.[74] Additional features of hyperkalemia seen on this ECG include a widened QRS and flat, or absent, P waves (Figure 30).

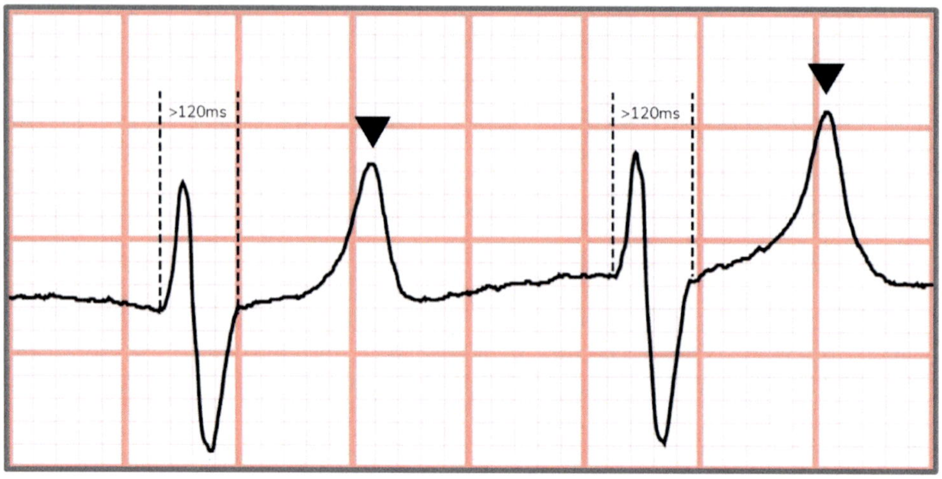

Figure 30. Wide QRS, peaked T waves (arrowheads), and absent P waves of hyperkalemia in the lead II rhythm strip.

75. **Early Repolarization.** Early repolarization is considered a normal variant in young men. It is characterized by concave ST-segment elevation, usually greatest in the precordial leads, and J wave notching.[84,85] This ECG is classic for early repolarization with J wave notching and diffuse ST-segment elevation (Figure 31). Early repolarization is generally considered benign and requires no follow up.

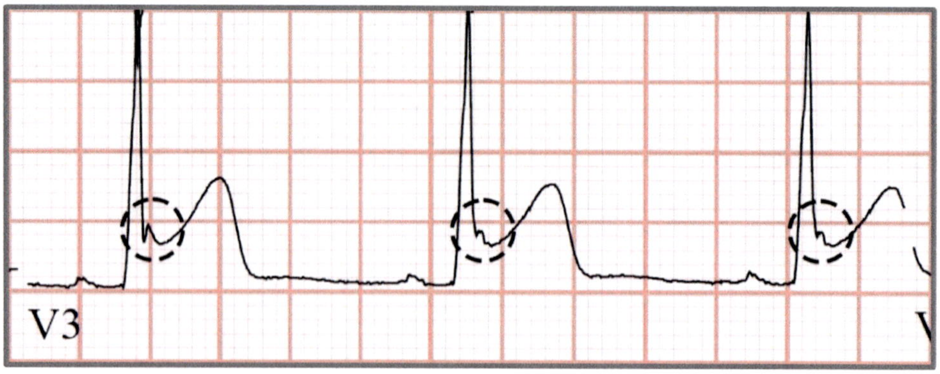

Figure 31. J wave notching (dashed circles) and concave ST-segment elevation characteristic of early repolarization.

76. **Paced Rhythm, Atrial Flutter.** Atrial flutter occurs from a reentrant circuit in the right atrium. It is an organized rhythm that is generally characterized by an atrial rate of approximately 300 beats per minute. It more commonly occurs in a counterclockwise fashion, leading to inverted flutter waves in the inferior leads (II,

III, and aVF).[5,66] This ECG demonstrates atrial flutter without native ventricular conduction and with paced ventricular activity (i.e., the vertical green bars represent pacing spikes). The pacemaker threshold was set to 40 beats per minute and was later increased to 60 beats per minute.

77. **Second Degree Atrioventricular Block with 2:1 Conduction.** P waves are conducted in a 2:1 ratio, with every other P wave "dropped", or failing to conduct through the atrioventricular (AV) node. When P waves are conducted but intermittently "dropped," it is referred to as second degree atrioventricular block, which comes in two varieties - Mobitz I (or Wenckebach) and Mobitz II. Mobitz I occurs when conduction is progressively delayed through the atrioventricular node and eventually fails. It is represented by progressively prolonging PR intervals followed by a "dropped" P wave. It does not always represent pathology, particularly when seen in younger or physically fit individuals with high vagal tone. Mobitz II occurs when the infranodal conduction system intermittently fails, resulting in intermittently "dropped" P waves but consistent PR intervals when conducted. Mobitz II usually occurs with preexisting conduction disease (e.g., combination of bundle branch and fascicular blocks), is always pathologic, and more likely to progress to complete heart block.[2,5,43] When atrioventricular block occurs in a 2:1 ratio, it is impossible to distinguish between Mobitz I and Mobitz II; therefore, 2:1 atrioventricular block is simply referred to as "second degree atrioventricular block with 2:1 conduction" (Figure 32). When the QRS is narrow, as in this case, Mobitz I is more likely; however, it is prudent to assume the worst scenario (i.e., Mobitz II).

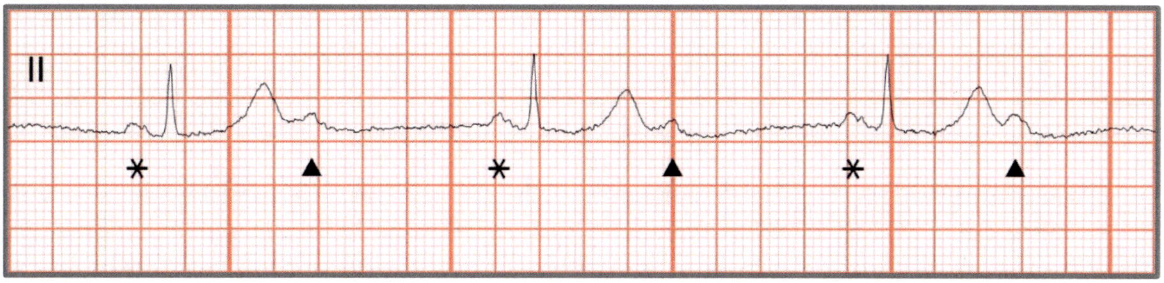

Figure 32. Second degree atrioventricular block with 2:1 conduction; conducted P waves (asterisks) and non-conducted P waves (arrowhead).

78. **Ventricular Tachycardia.** Features that suggest ventricular tachycardia include an extreme right axis, concordance of the QRS complexes across the precordium, and an initial R wave in aVR. There are established algorithms to help differentiate supraventricular tachycardia with aberrancy versus ventricular tachycardia, but

none of the established criteria perform well in the acute setting. It is safest to assume a regular wide complex tachycardia is ventricular tachycardia unless there is overwhelming evidence to the contrary.[12–16,18,19]

79. **Global Subendocardial Ischemia.** This patient with multilead ST-segment depressions and ST-segment elevation in aVR had an acute type A aortic dissection. The differential diagnosis for this pattern is broad and was previously described in case 5.

80. **Second Degree Atrioventricular Block - Mobitz I.** The initial ECG is second degree atrioventricular block with 2:1 conduction. On the repeat ECG, conduction is 2:1 at times, but there are two series (one near the beginning and the other near the end) of 3:2 conduction, confirming Mobitz I conduction (Figure 33).

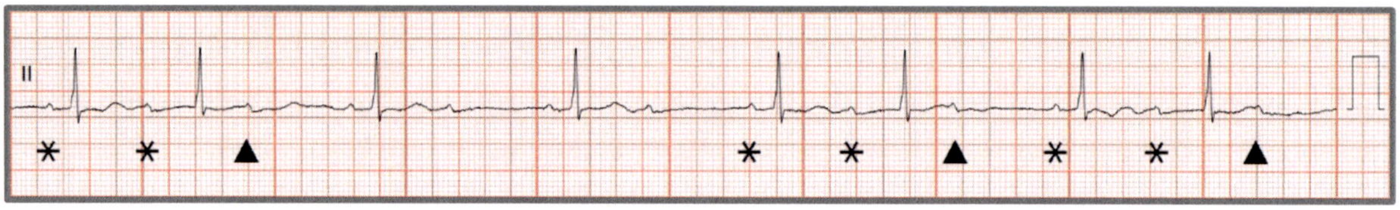

Figure 33. Lead II rhythm strip showing conducted P waves with progressively prolonging PR intervals (asterisks) followed by a dropped P wave (arrowheads).

Mobitz I conduction occurs when conduction is progressively delayed through the atrioventricular node and eventually fails. It is represented by progressively prolonging PR intervals followed by a "dropped" P wave. It does not always represent pathology, particularly when seen in younger or physically fit individuals with high vagal tone.

81. **Left Bundle Branch Block, Atrial Fibrillation.** This rhythm is irregularly irregular and the QRS is wide with left bundle branch block morphology (i.e., deep S wave in V1 and broad R wave in V6, see case 49 for further explanation of left bundle branch block morphology). The left bundle branch block was rate-dependent and resolved after rate control. In most cases, rate-related bundle branch blocks occur due to a prolonged refractory period of a diseased bundle. When a critical heart rate is exceeded, the diseased bundle fails.[36,37] Rate-related bundle branch blocks can be especially challenging to diagnose when the rate is regular and fast, creating a regular, wide complex tachycardia that appears like ventricular tachycardia.

82. **Atrioventricular Dissociation, Junctional Bradycardia.** This ECG shows atrioventricular dissociation, a condition in which the atria and ventricles act independently. The P waves appear to be sinus in origin, variable in rate, and non-

conducted. There are presumably more P waves buried within the QRST complexes, and, therefore, unable to be visualized on this surface ECG (Figure 34). There is junctional bradycardia with a ventricular rate of 48 beats per minute.

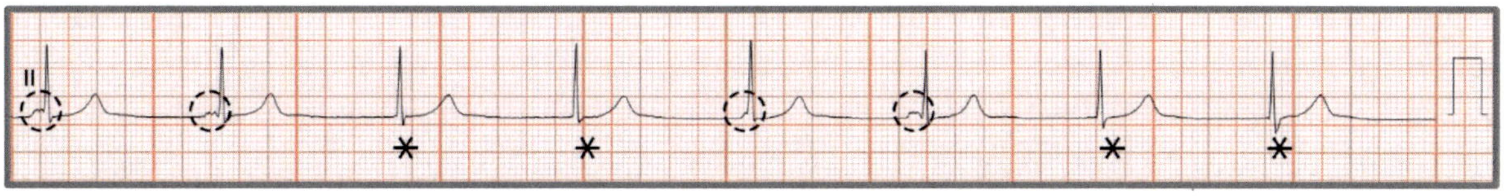

Figure 34. Lead II rhythm strip with P waves circled and presumptive location of buried P-waves designated with asterisks.

When a superior pacemaker fails to generate impulses at a rate faster than an inferior one, then the faster, more inferior, one will "escape." In this case, the sinus node failed to generate a rate that outpaced the junction, which led to a junctional escape rhythm and atrioventricular dissociation.[1,86]

83. **Sinus Bradycardia.** When the atrial wave of depolarization originates in the sinoatrial node (as is normal), the atria depolarize from superior to inferior, creating an upright P wave in the inferior leads. The sinoatrial node can depolarize more slowly than usual when the person is a well-conditioned athlete, as a normal variant, due to increased vagal tone, or from the use of beta-blocking or calcium-channel blocking agents. The rate of 48 beats per minute is unlikely to be hemodynamically significant.[3]

84. **Left Ventricular Hypertrophy, T-wave Inversions.** Classic findings of left ventricular hypertrophy include large amplitude QRS complexes and associated repolarization abnormalities (e.g., asymmetric T-wave inversion in V6). The most cited criteria for diagnosing left ventricular hypertrophy are the Sokolow-Lyon and the Cornell criteria:[20]

    1. Sokolow-Lyon Criteria: $S_{V1} + R_{V5,6} > 35$ mm *OR* $R_{aVL} > 11$ mm
    2. Cornell Criteria: $R_{aVL} + S_{V3} > 28$ mm for men *OR* > 20 mm for women

85. **Atrial Fibrillation, Digoxin Toxicity.** Differential considerations for slow atrial fibrillation include drug toxicity (e.g., atrioventricular nodal blocking agents like digoxin, beta blockers, or non-dihydropyridine calcium channel blockers), hypothermia, hypothyroidism, hyperkalemia, or conduction block. Digoxin slows conduction through the atrioventricular node and increases automaticity. Note the "scooped" ST-segments typical of the digoxin-effect (Figure 35).[3,32]

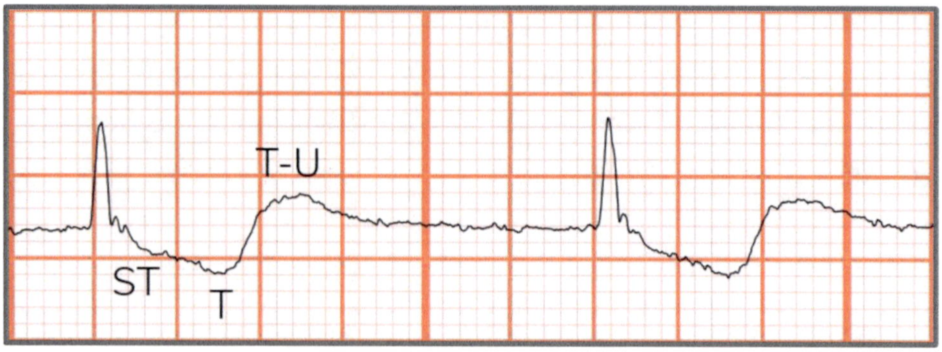

Figure 35. "Scooped" ST segment and biphasic T wave with terminal positivity (T-U fusion) in lead II typical of digoxin.

86. **Atrial Flutter with 2:1 Conduction.** There is an atypical appearance to P waves in the limb leads (specifically II, III and aVF) where the usual isoelectric baseline is replaced by identical appearing "sawtooth" waves. These atrial flutter waves occur at a rate of approximately 300 beats per minute, complemented by a ventricular rate of 150 beats per minute. In the absence of treatment or atrioventricular block, the most common atrial to ventricular response is 2:1.[5]

87. **Hyperacute T Waves, ST-elevation Myocardial Infarction.** The presence of large T waves in the inferolateral leads (II, III, aVR, V4, V5, V6), especially in proportion to their corresponding QRS complexes, suggests that they are hyperacute – an early finding of coronary occlusion.[10,28,29] Left heart catheterization revealed a mid-left anterior descending artery occlusion.

88. **Second Degree Atrioventricular Block - Mobitz II.** Second degree atrioventricular block Mobitz II is characterized by intermittently blocked P waves and constant PR intervals (Figure 36); the block is usually infranodal (as previously described in case 77).[5] The presence of a right bundle branch and left anterior fascicular blocks indicates severe infranodal conduction disease (see case 3).

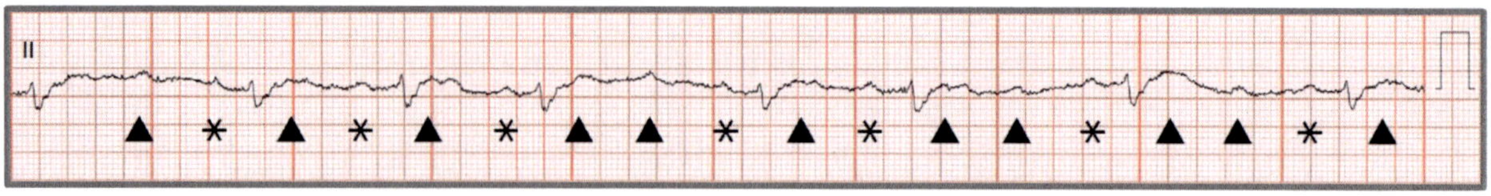

Figure 36*.* Lead II rhythm strip showing conducted (asterisks) and dropped (arrowheads) P waves. The atrial rate is 120 beats per minute. The presence of serial dropped P waves makes this a high-grade atrioventricular block.

89. **Inferior ST-elevation Myocardial Infarction.** Subtle inferior ST-segment elevation with reciprocal ST-segment depression in V1 through V3. Note the change in P wave axis indicating the presence of a competing ectopic atrial pacemaker. Left heart catheterization revealed a mid-left circumflex occlusion.

90. **Atrial Fibrillation, Ashman Phenomenon**. There are two aberrantly conducted beats with wide QRS complexes and unifocal morphology. In both instances, a long R-R interval is followed by a relatively short R-R interval, which is then terminated by an aberrant beat. Ashman phenomenon is aberrant conduction when a short cycle is preceded by a longer one (Figure 37). This occurs because the refractory period of the His-Purkinje system is proportional to the length of the preceding R-R interval, so longer R-R intervals result in longer refractory periods and vice versa. Typically, the aberrant beat will have a right bundle branch block pattern because the right bundle has a longer refractory period than the left.[32,87,88]

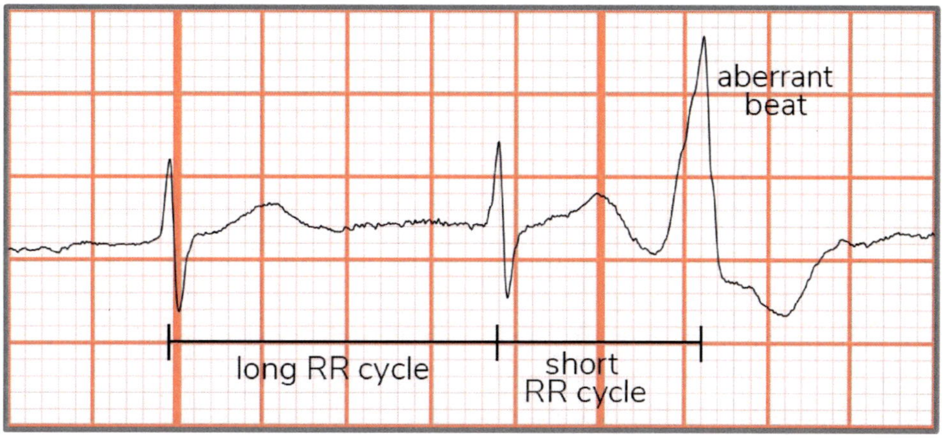

Figure 37. Ashman phenomenon is characterized by a long RR cycle followed by a short one and terminated by an aberrant beat.

91. **Ventricular Tachycardia.** The R-S time is greater than 100 ms strongly favors ventricular tachycardia (Figure 38).[12]

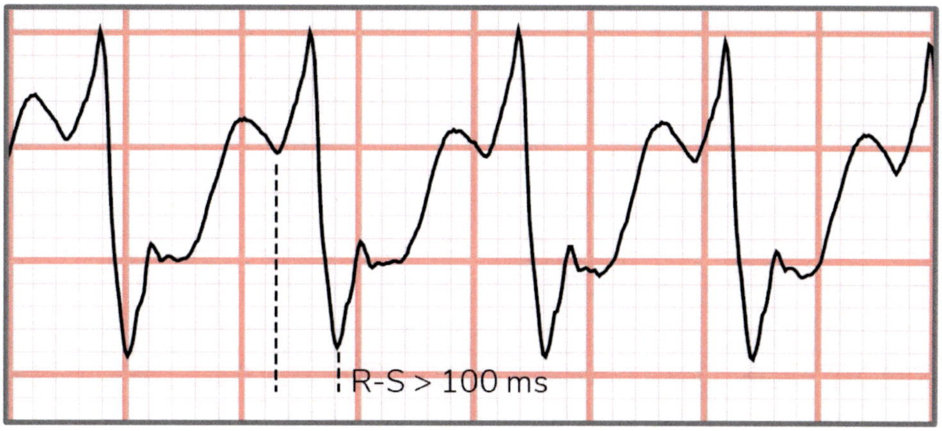

Figure 38. V6 R-S time greater than 100 ms – highly specific for ventricular tachycardia.

92. **Second Degree Atrioventricular Block – Mobitz II.** This rhythm is challenging but there are two conducted P waves and the rest are dropped. Intermittent failure of conduction is defined as second degree atrioventricular block. Mobitz II conduction

is due to infranodal conduction disease and is characterized by constant PR intervals.[5] The PR intervals for the conducted P waves are constant, therefore, this rhythm is most likely second degree atrioventricular block with Mobitz II conduction (Figure 39).

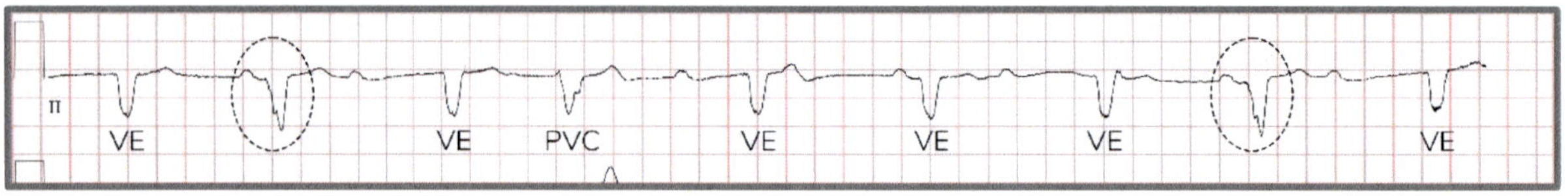

Figure 39. Lead II rhythm strip. The ventricular escape (VE) beats tend to march out at regular intervals unless interrupted by a premature ventricular contraction (PVC). The two conducted P waves and associated QRS complexes are circled.

93. **Low Voltage, Cardiac Tamponade.** Low voltage is defined as:

    1. All limb lead amplitudes less than 5 mm, or
    2. All precordial lead amplitudes less than 10 mm.[61]

This ECG meets the precordial low voltage criteria as the largest amplitude precordial QRS complex is 7 mm (in V2 and V3). The differential diagnosis for low voltage was previously described in case 51. The QRS amplitudes in the rhythm strip of lead II can be seen to alternate between larger and smaller complexes, a phenomenon known as electrical alternans. Electrical alternans often results from the pendulous-like swinging of the heart inside a fluid-filled pericardium.[89,90] The presence of electrical alternans and low voltage is specific for cardiac tamponade.

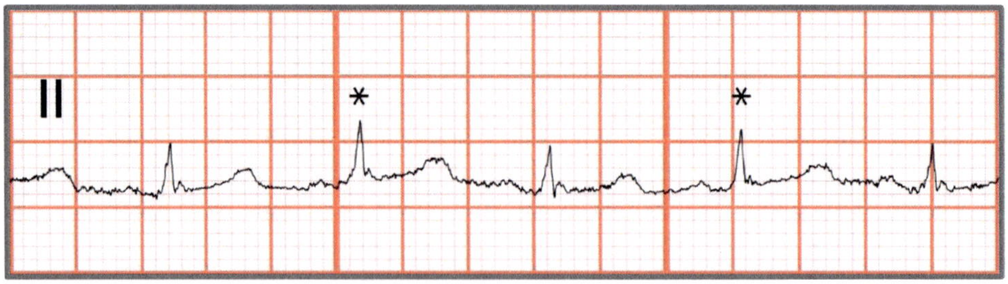

Figure 40. QRS amplitudes alternate between slightly larger (asterisks) and smaller complexes in electrical alternans.

94. **Ventricular Tachycardia.** The presence of atrioventricular dissociation confirms ventricular tachycardia. P waves can be seen marching through the rhythm strip in V1 (look for the pointed complexes preceding every third QRS complex (Figure 41). This patient was successfully treated via synchronized electrical cardioversion.

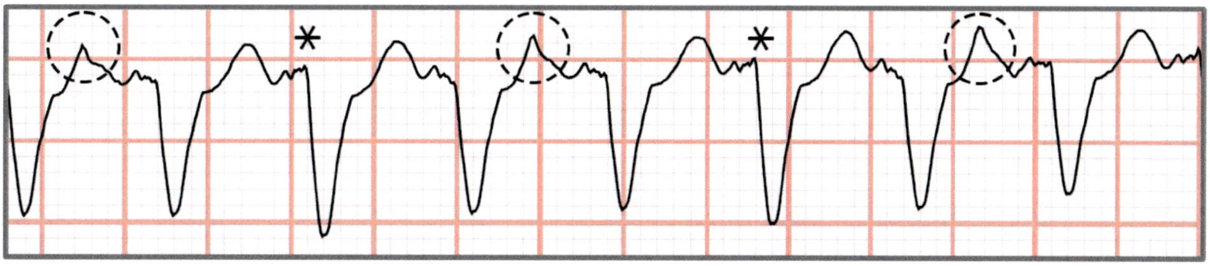

Figure 41. Pointed complexes representing P waves (dashed circles) can be seen marching throughout the V1 rhythm strip with presumptive interceding P waves buried in the QRS complex (asterisks).

95. **Accelerated Idioventricular Rhythm.** Accelerated Idioventricular Rhythm (AIVR) is a rhythm that occurs under conditions of enhanced automaticity. An enhanced ectopic ventricular pacemaker outpaces more superior pacemakers (e.g., sinus node) and, thus, becomes the dominant pacemaker by usurping control. It occurs at a rate faster than ventricular escape, but slower than ventricular tachycardia (i.e., between 50 and 110 beats/min). AIVR can occur for many reasons including electrolyte abnormalities and drug toxicity (e.g., digoxin), however, it occurs most commonly in the setting of reperfusion – that is, after myocardial infarction or cardiac arrest.[3,5,54] This patient was confirmed to have a 90% occluded obtuse marginal culprit lesion.

96. **Pacemaker Malfunction.** Pacemaker spikes occur within the QRST complexes, indicating failure-to-sense. Failure-to-sense occurs when the pacemaker fails to sense native cardiac activity which leads to asynchronous pacing; it can be caused by a lead insulation break, new intrinsic bundle branch blocks, electrolyte abnormalities, and Class IC antiarrhythmics. Failure-to-capture occurs when the delivery of a pacing stimulus does not lead to myocardial depolarization; it can be caused by mechanical lead displacement or fracture, electrolyte abnormalities, and ischemia or infarction.[91,92] This ECG exhibits both failure-to-capture and failure-to-sense due to a dislodged pacer lead (Figure 42).

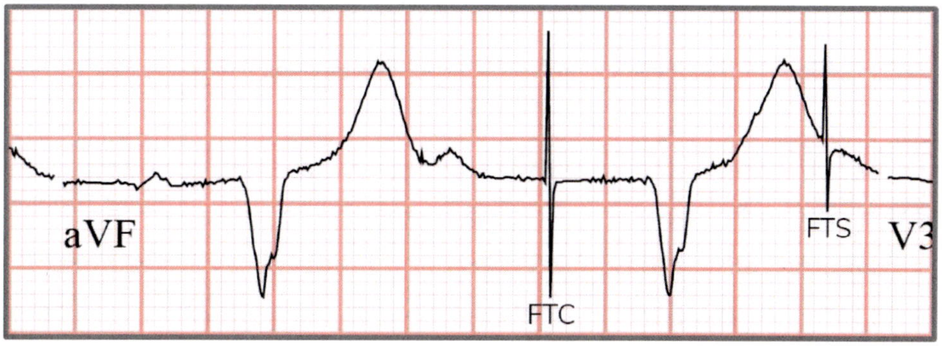

Figure 42. Two failed pacing spikes in lead aVF – failure-to-capture (FTC) and failure-to-sense (FTS).

97. **Ventricular Fibrillation.** A 12-lead of ventricular fibrillation should never be obtained on an unconscious patient. This patient had a left ventricular assist device and was awake and alert. The rhythm still warrants defibrillation because the left ventricular assist device is preload dependent and relies on right ventricular output. This patient was successfully defibrillated.

98. **Hypercalcemia.** Hypercalcemia causes shortening of the QT interval, which can result in a "high-takeoff" of the ST-segment, mimicking myocardial ischemia or infarction.[21–23] The QT interval normalized after treatment of hypercalcemia.

99. **Right Bundle Branch Block, Left Anterior Fascicular Block.** The wide QRS, rSR' in the anterior precordial leads (V1, V2), and deep S-waves in the lateral leads (I, V6) indicate the presence of a right bundle branch block. The right bundle branch block, however, does not explain the left axis deviation (recall the causes of left axis deviation from case 3). When the left anterior fascicle is disrupted, current passes along the posterior fascicle and the left ventricle is depolarized in a leftward/upward direction - producing left axis deviation and often extreme left axis deviation (Figure 3). This ECG demonstrates disruption of two fascicles – the right bundle and the left anterior fascicle – and is termed a "bifascicular" block.[2,4]

100. **Early Repolarization.** There are diffuse, mild, concave ST-segment elevations with J-point notching (Figure 43) and absence of reciprocal depressions.[32]

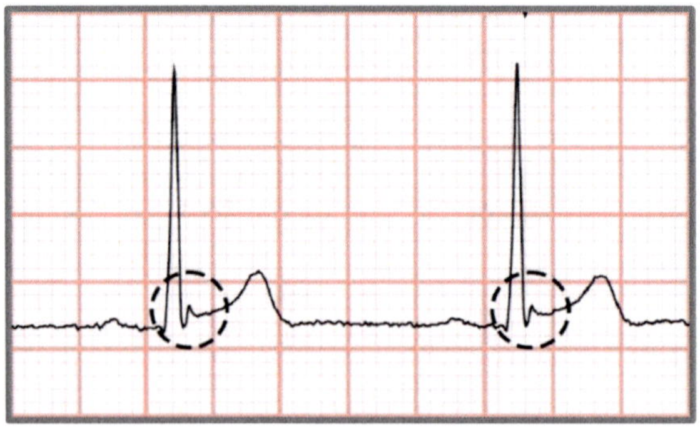

Figure 43. J wave notching (dashed circles) and concave ST-segment elevation characteristic of early repolarization.

101. **Sinus Tachycardia, Left Atrial Enlargement.** Atrial enlargement can be determined by analyzing the P waves in leads II and V1. The first half of the P wave represents right atrial depolarization, while the second half represents left atrial depolarization. There are deeply inverted P waves in V1 and wide P waves in II (Figure 44).[20] Left atrial enlargement occurs with increased pressure or volume overload and is a

precursor to atrial fibrillation. It is classically seen in mitral stenosis or conditions that lead to left ventricular hypertrophy as was the case with this patient.

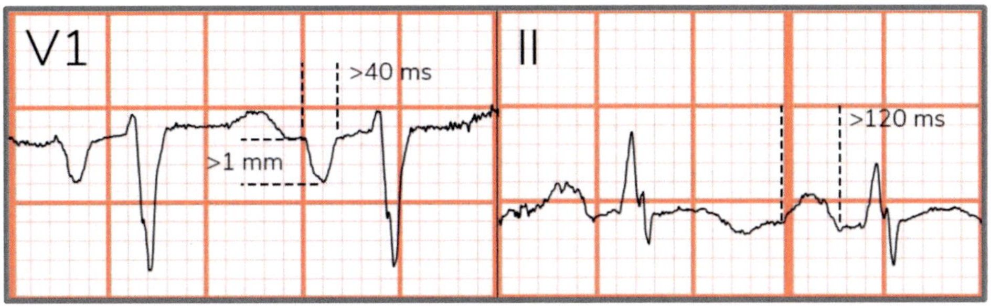

Figure 44. Left atrial enlargement is characterized by a negative P wave in V1 that's at least 1 mm deep and 40 ms wide and a wide P wave in lead II that's at least 120 ms.

102. **Pre-excited Atrial Fibrillation.** The irregularly irregular rhythm and faster-than-usual rate are the result of atrial fibrillation with pre-excitation (i.e., the Wolf-Parkinson-White syndrome). There are inconsistent QRS morphologies resulting from variable transmission of signals from the atria to the ventricles via anterograde conduction through the atrioventricular node and the accessory pathway. The rate approaches 300 beats per minute at times (Figure 45). Rates this fast are not seen with atrial fibrillation unless an accessory pathway exists.[32,33,93]

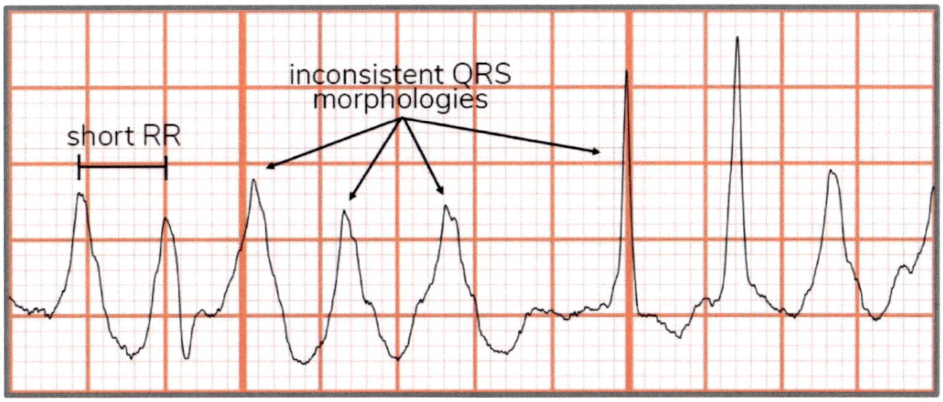

Figure 45. Lead II rhythm strip showing a shorter RR cycle than typically expected from atrial fibrillation and inconsistent QRS morphologies characteristic of pre-excited atrial fibrillation.

These patients should not receive medications that block the atrioventricular node as they can precipitate ventricular fibrillation. This patient was electrically cardioverted.

103. **Left Bundle Branch Block, First Degree Atrioventricular Block.** The wide QRS complex, dominant S wave in V1, broad notched R wave in the lateral leads (I, aVL, V6) and left axis deviation are all characteristic of a left bundle branch block (Figure

23).[4] The prolonged PR interval represents a first-degree atrioventricular block. These disturbances coupled together suggest trifascicular disease.[94]

104. **Right Bundle Branch Block.** This right bundle branch block pattern has an atypical appearance. The rsR' in V1 can have a qR appearance in some right bundle branch blocks (Figure 46). The expected wide S is present in the lateral leads (I, V5, V6).

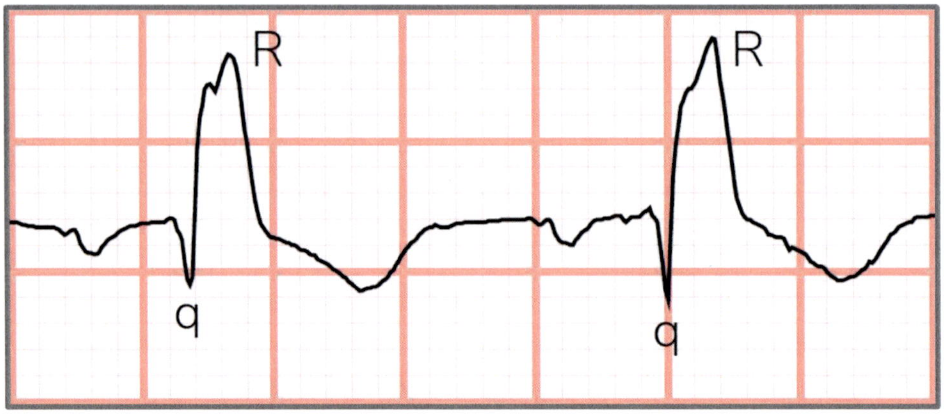

Figure 46. qR pattern of a right bundle branch block in V1.

105. **Hypertrophic Cardiomyopathy.** Hypertrophic Cardiomyopathy (HCM) is the most common cause of sudden cardiac death in individuals under 40 years of age.[95] HCM can have a variable appearance and it's not uncommon to see repolarization abnormalities like the ones seen here. Common ECG findings include large QRS complexes of left ventricular hypertrophy, T wave inversions (especially in lateral leads), and narrow, "dagger" Q waves in the lateral leads (I, aVL, V5, V6).[32,96] Symmetric T-wave inversions in the precordial leads (as seen with this ECG) is suggestive of apical HCM, although this patient had septal hypertrophy.

106. **Wellens Syndrome.** This is type B Wellens pattern with deeply inverted precordial T waves. Wellens syndrome was previously described in case 18. This patient had a 95% proximal left anterior descending stenosis.

107. **Second Degree Atrioventricular Block - Mobitz I.** There is variable decremental conduction through the atrioventricular node (i.e., progressively prolonging PR interval) that ultimately results in a dropped P wave (Figure 47).

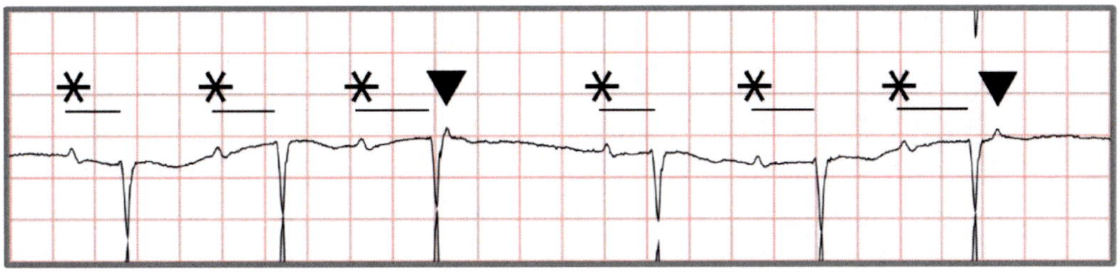

Figure 47. V1 rhythm strip showing conducted (asterisks) and non-conducted (arrowheads) P waves in Mobitz I conduction. The horizontal lines represent the progressively prolonging PR intervals preceding a non-conducted P wave.

108. **Anterior ST-elevation Myocardial Infarction.** Pay attention to the natively conducted complexes and ignore the premature ventricular complexes when looking for acute ischemic findings (Figure 48). There are anterior ST-segment elevations and hyperacute T waves in V1 through V4 and reciprocal ST-segment depressions in the inferior leads (II, III, and aVF). Left heart catheterization revealed left anterior descending artery occlusion.

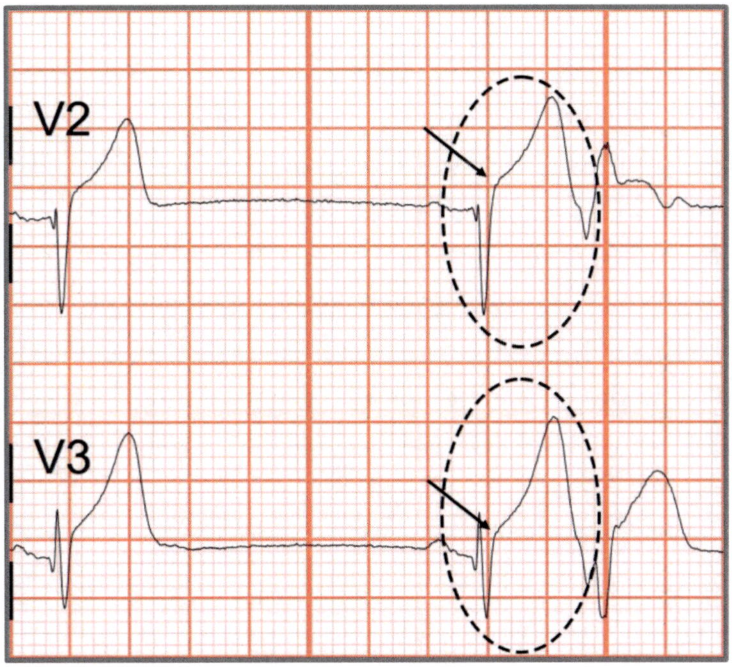

Figure 48. Natively conducted complexes (dashed ovals) and ST-segment elevation (arrows).

109. **Wellens Syndrome.** This is type A Wellens pattern – biphasic T waves with negative terminal deflections. This patient had a 90% proximal left anterior descending artery stenosis. (See case 18 for further explanation of Wellens syndrome).

110. **Anterior ST-elevation Myocardial Infarction, Sinus Tachycardia.** Notice the slight reciprocal ST depressions in the high lateral leads (i.e., I and aVL) and the presence of terminal QRS distortion in V3 (i.e., the absence of an S wave or a J notch) – a very specific finding for ST-elevation myocardial infarction (see case 44).[52] Left heart catheterization revealed a 90% mid-left anterior descending artery culprit lesion and percutaneous coronary intervention was successful.

111. **Left Bundle Branch Block.** Left bundle branch block pattern with a wide and down-going QRS complex in V1, and broad, notched R waves in the lateral leads (I, aVL, V5, V6). Expected repolarization waves (i.e., T waves in the opposite direction as the QRS complexes) and appropriate discordance (ST-segments in the opposite direction as the QRS complexes) are present.

112. **Early Repolarization.** There are diffuse, concave, (predominantly) precordial ST-segment elevations without reciprocal changes in a young patient. The precordial leads V3, V4, and V5 have the J wave notching (e.g., "fishhook" appearance) characteristic of early repolarization (see case 75).[32]

113. **Ventricular Pre-excitation.** Ventricular preexcitation with shortened PR, delta waves, and slightly prolonged QRS (Figure 49). Pre-excitation is a condition in which an accessory pathway exists between the atria and the ventricles, often referred to as the bundle of Kent.[33] When the accessory pathway conducts in an anterograde direction, the ventricles are "pre-excited," yielding the characteristic delta wave on the ECG. When dysrhythmias occur involving the accessory pathway, it is referred to as the Wolf-Parkinson-White syndrome (Figure 8).

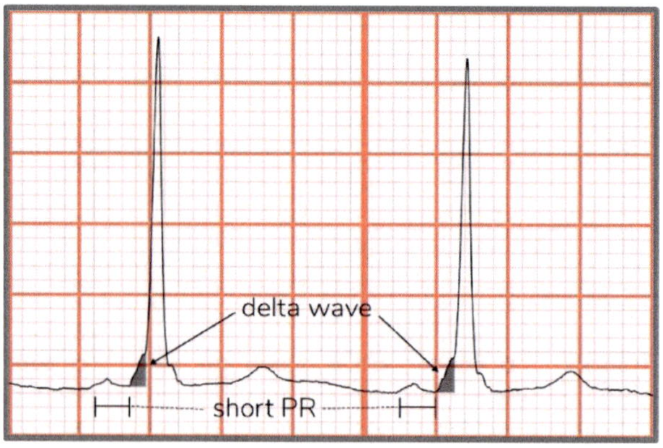

Figure 49. Short PR and delta wave (shaded region) in lead V5 characteristic of ventricular pre-excitation.

114. **Hyperacute T Waves, ST-elevation Myocardial Infarction.** Notice that the amplitude of the T waves exceeds that of the QRS complexes in some leads. Some

authors have proposed identifying hyperacute T waves using proportional T-wave "bulk," defined by the increased area under the curve (AUC) of the T-wave relative to the QRS amplitude.[10,28,29] Left heart catheterization revealed a completely occluded left anterior descending artery and percutaneous coronary intervention was successful.

115. **Left Posterior Fascicular Block.** The normal infranodal conduction divides into the right and left bundles, and the latter is further subdivided into anterior and posterior divisions or "fascicles." Disruption of both fascicles produces the familiar left bundle branch block pattern, but each fascicle can be affected independently - resulting in either left anterior fascicular block or left posterior fascicular block. Left posterior fascicular block results in depolarization in a rightward/downward direction and produces right axis deviation (Figure 50). Isolated left posterior fascicular block is rare due to its robust blood supply and is demonstrated by right axis deviation, rS complexes in the lateral leads (I, aVL) and qR complexes in the inferior leads (II, III, aVF).[2]

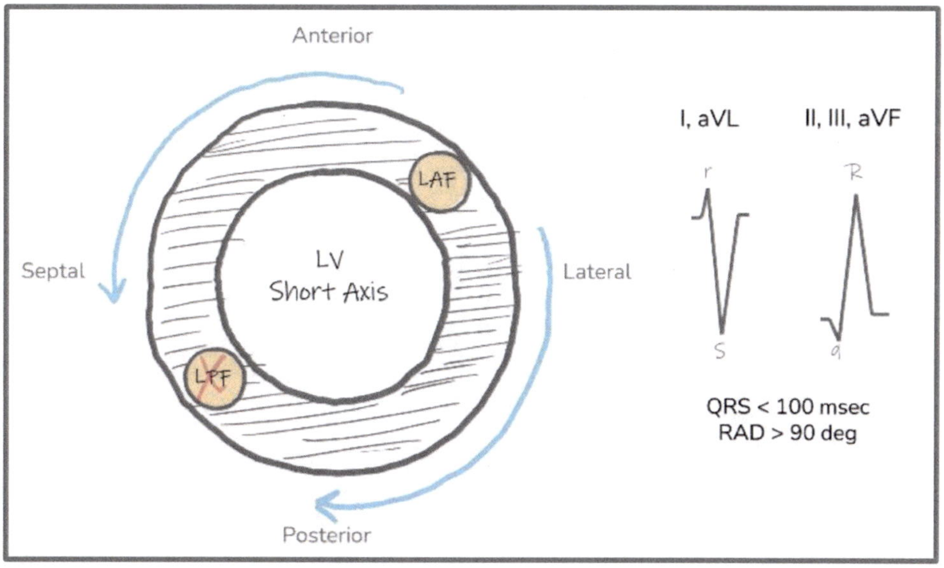

Figure 50. Relative locations of the anterior and posterior fascicles within the left ventricle. The blue arrows demonstrate the direction of depolarization with a left posterior fascicular block. LV, left ventricle; LPF, left posterior fascicle; LAF, left anterior fascicle; RAD, right axis deviation.

116. **Hypertrophic Cardiomyopathy.** Hypertrophic Cardiomyopathy is the most common cause of sudden cardiac death in individuals under 40 years of age.[95] Common ECG findings were previously described in case 105. This patient has known apical hypertrophic cardiomyopathy, a condition known to cause ischemic-

appearing repolarization abnormalities (i.e., symmetric T wave inversion) in the precordial leads.

117. **Ventricular Tachycardia.** While the baseline is difficult to establish, there is concordance across the precordium (i.e., QRS complexes in the same direction) with the QRS complexes predominately upright, strongly favoring ventricular tachycardia.[12]

118. **Acute Pericarditis.** There are diffuse concave ST-segment elevations without reciprocal ST-segment depressions. Other electrocardiographic findings of acute pericarditis include PR-segment depressions, PR-segment elevation in aVR, and down-sloping of the TP segment (Spodick's sign, Figure 51).[97] This patient had typical symptoms of pericarditis (i.e., sharp, pleuritic chest pain relieved when leaning forward), a new pericardial effusion on echocardiography, and a friction rub on exam. Diagnostic criteria were previously described in case 33.

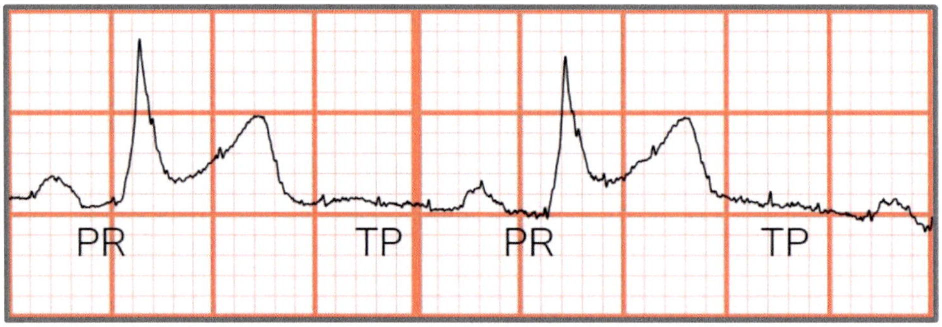

Figure 51. Serial complexes in the lead II rhythm strip showing PR-segment depression (PR), ST-segment elevation, and down-sloping of the TP segment (TP).

119. **Right Bundle Branch Block, Left Posterior Fascicular Block, Atrial Fibrillation.** The rhythm is irregularly irregular and without discernable P waves (i.e., atrial fibrillation). The wide QRS, rSR' in the anterior precordial leads (V1, V2), and deep S-waves in the lateral leads (I, V6) indicate the presence of a right bundle branch block (Figure 2). Right bundle branch blocks, in isolation, do not cause right axis deviation. The right axis deviation is most likely due to a left posterior fascicular block (Figure 50). This ECG demonstrates disruption of two fascicles, the right bundle and the left posterior fascicle, and is termed a "bifascicular" block.[2,4]

120. **Ventricular Tachycardia.** The extreme right axis (i.e., negatively deflected QRS complexes in both leads I and aVF) strongly favors ventricular tachycardia (Figure 5).

121. **Third Degree Atrioventricular Block.** There is atrioventricular dissociation and a severely bradycardic ventricular escape rhythm. The term atrioventricular dissociation refers to the independent contraction of the atria and ventricles and suggests a disturbance in the normal conduction pathway;[1] in this case, third degree (i.e., complete) atrioventricular block. The wide (>120 ms), and slow (<40 beats per minute) QRS complexes are consistent with ventricular escape.

122. **Third Degree Atrioventricular Block.** Again, there is atrioventricular dissociation and a severely bradycardic ventricular escape rhythm.

123. **Orthodromic Atrioventricular Reentrant Tachycardia.** This narrow complex tachycardia converted to sinus rhythm with adenosine. She was subsequently discovered to have a left-sided lateral accessory pathway with retrograde conduction that was successfully ablated (i.e., orthodromic atrioventricular reentrant tachycardia or orthodromic reciprocating tachycardia, Figure 8). This tachycardia is virtually indistinguishable from atrioventricular nodal reentrant tachycardia and can be safely treated with atrioventricular nodal blocking agents. It is important to keep orthodromic accessory conduction on the differential for narrow complex tachycardia and always obtain a post-conversion ECG to look for evidence of pre-excitation.

124. **Ventricular Fibrillation.** A 12-lead of ventricular fibrillation should never be obtained on an unconscious patient. This patient had a left ventricular assist device and was, therefore, awake and alert. The rhythm still warrants defibrillation because the left ventricular assist device is preload dependent and relies on right ventricular output.

125. **Ventricular Escape Complexes.** The wide complexes are ventricular escape complexes, not premature ones (Figure 52). Pacemakers "escape" from suppression when a superior one fails or is too slow. In this case, the 13-year-old female had high vagal tone, and the finding is not clinically significant.

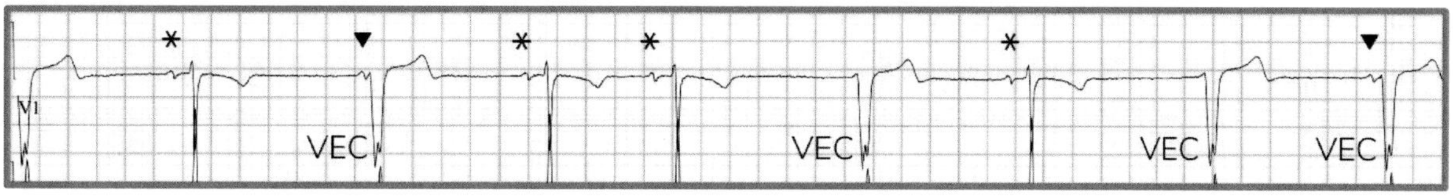

Figure 52. Conducted (asterisks) and non-conducted (arrowheads) P waves with ventricular escape complexes (VEC).

126. **Ashman Phenomenon.** There is a series of aberrantly conducted beats with wide QRS complexes and unifocal morphology near the beginning of the rhythm strip

consistent with Ashman phenomenon. Ashman phenomenon is aberrant conduction when a short cycle is preceded by a longer one.[32,87] It can be mistaken for non-sustained ventricular tachycardia when it occurs in series, as with this case; instead, these beats are not ectopic but aberrantly conducted.

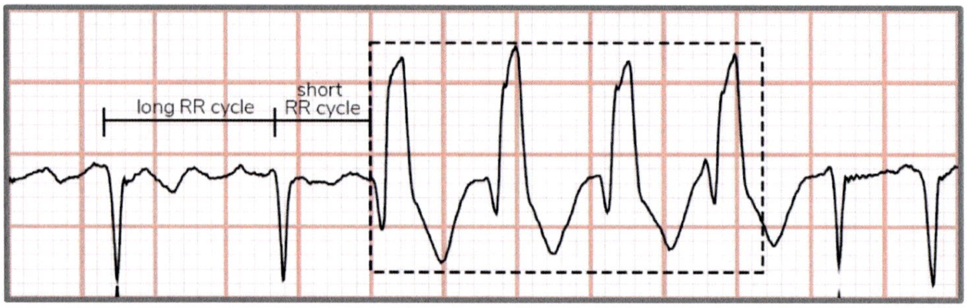

Figure 53. A long RR interval precedes a shorter one, leading to a series of aberrantly conducted beats (dashed rectangle) in the V1 rhythm strip.

127. **Second Degree Atrioventricular Block with 2:1 Conduction.** P waves are conducted to the ventricular system in a 2:1 ratio, with every other P wave being "dropped", or failing to conduct to the ventricles. When atrioventricular block occurs in a 2:1 ratio, it is impossible to distinguish between Mobitz I and Mobitz II; therefore, it is simply referred to as "2:1 atrioventricular block." Mobitz I and Mobitz II conduction was previously described in case 77. The repeat ECG confirms Mobitz II conduction (Figure 54. When consecutive P waves are non-conducted, it is referred to as "high grade" atrioventricular block and should be treated the same as complete heart block (i.e., pacemaker placement is indicated).[5]

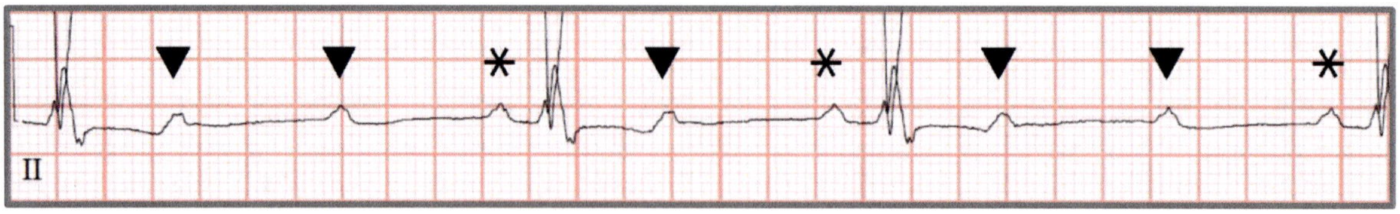

Figure 54. Conducted (asterisks) and non-conducted P waves (arrowheads). Consistent PR intervals for conducted P waves confirm Mobitz II conduction.

128. **Left Bundle Branch Block, First Degree Atrioventricular Block.** There is a left bundle branch block (Figure 23), and the PR interval is borderline prolonged (i.e., 200 ms). When a left bundle branch block accompanies first-degree atrioventricular block, it suggests trifascicular disease. First-degree blocks are usually seen it active, healthy patients without heart disease, and represent delayed conduction within the atrioventricular node itself. First-degree blocks are unlikely to progress to complete heart block. However, when accompanied by preexisting conduction disease (e.g., right bundle branch block, left bundle branch block, or bifascicular

block), it can indicate severe infranodal conduction disease.[2,4] This patient subsequently developed third-degree (i.e., complete) heart block and lost consciousness.

129. **Third Degree Atrioventricular Block.** Atrioventricular dissociation with a ventricular escape rhythm. The term atrioventricular dissociation refers to the independent contraction of the atria and ventricles and suggests a disturbance in the normal conduction pathway;[1] in this case, third degree (i.e., complete) atrioventricular block. The wide (>120 ms), and slow (<40 beats per minute) QRS complexes suggest a ventricular escape rhythm.

130. **Sodium Channel Toxicity.** Sodium channel toxicity from a tricyclic antidepressant overdose. Note the triad of right axis deviation, tall terminal R wave in aVR, and widened QRS (Figure 55).[44,98] This patient was successfully treated with sodium bicarbonate.

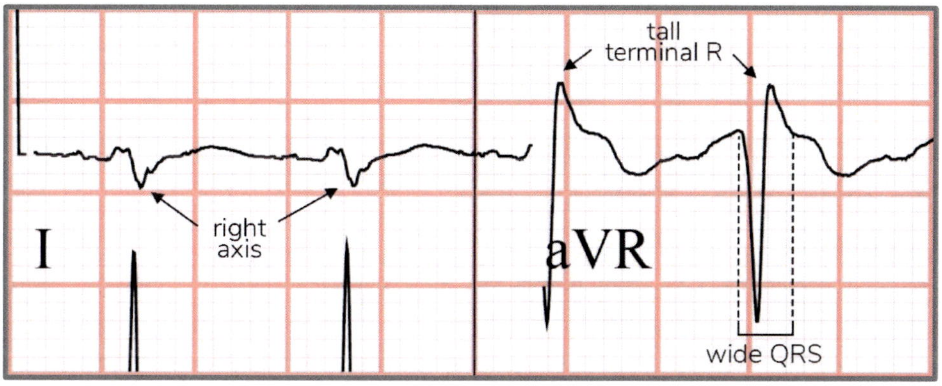

Figure 55. Right axis deviation in lead I, tall terminal R wave in aVR, and wide QRS of sodium channel toxicity.

131. **Persistent Juvenile T Wave Pattern.** The T waves in the right precordial leads (V1 through V3) are asymmetrically inverted in childhood and become upright (except for V1 and occasionally V2) by adulthood. In predominantly black women under the age of 40, this juvenile T wave pattern may persist in the absence of cardiac abnormalities.[99–101]

132. **Hyperkalemia.** Hyperkalemia can mimic STEMI, especially in leads V1 and V2, as with this case. Hyperkalemic changes include widened QRS complexes and peaked T waves.[73,102] It is not uncommon for hyperkalemia to produce findings similar to sodium channel toxicity including right axis deviation and a tall terminal R in aVR. This patient was mistaken for having an anterior myocardial infarction, and was

taken emergently for cardiac catheterization, which failed to reveal an obstructive lesion. The potassium resulted later, and was 9.1 mEq/L.

133. **Sgarbossa Criteria, ST-elevation Myocardial Infarction.** The Sgarbossa criteria are a set of rules to help identify acute myocardial infarction in the setting of a left bundle branch block and were previously described in case 49. This ECG demonstrates concordant ST-elevation in leads I and aVL, and concordant ST-depression in V3. Left heart catheterization revealed an occluded first diagonal branch of the left anterior descending artery.

134. **Hyperacute T Waves, ST-elevation Myocardial Infarction.** There are hyperacute 'de Winter T waves' that ultimately evolved into an anterior ST-elevation myocardial infarction (STEMI). Described in 2008 by de Winter, this pattern of upsloping ST depressions and hyperacute T waves in the precordial leads suggests proximal left anterior descending occlusion.[103] While this pattern does not meet classic STEMI criteria,[72] it does suggest the presence of an occlusive myocardial infarction and emergent reperfusion is recommended [30,31]. This pattern is seen in just 2% of acute left anterior descending artery occlusions and is often misdiagnosed.[104] Left heart catheterization revealed a distal left main occlusion and percutaneous coronary intervention was successful.

135. **Atrial Flutter with 2:1 Conduction.** Atrial flutter occurs when a reentrant circuit forms in the right atrium. It more commonly occurs in a counterclockwise fashion, leading to inverted flutter waves in the inferior leads (II, III, and aVF).[5,66] There is an atypical appearance to P waves in the limb leads (specifically II, III and aVF) where the usual isoelectric baseline is replaced by identical appearing "sawtooth" waves. Pediatric intervals tend to be shorter, and rates faster than in adults (e.g., > 200 beats per minute in this ECG). In the absence of treatment or atrioventricular block, the most common atrial to ventricular response is 2:1.[5]

136. **Brugada Syndrome.** Type 1 or coved-type Brugada pattern in a patient presenting with syncope.[67,69] Brugada syndrome was previously described in case 59. This patient received an implanted defibrillator.

137. **High Lateral ST-elevation Myocardial Infarction.** There is subtle ST-segment elevation in the high lateral leads (I, aVL) and V2, along with reciprocal ST-segment depressions in the inferior leads (II, III, aVF). This pattern of ST-elevation has been dubbed the "South African flag sign" because of its resemblance of the South African flag (Figure 56).[105]

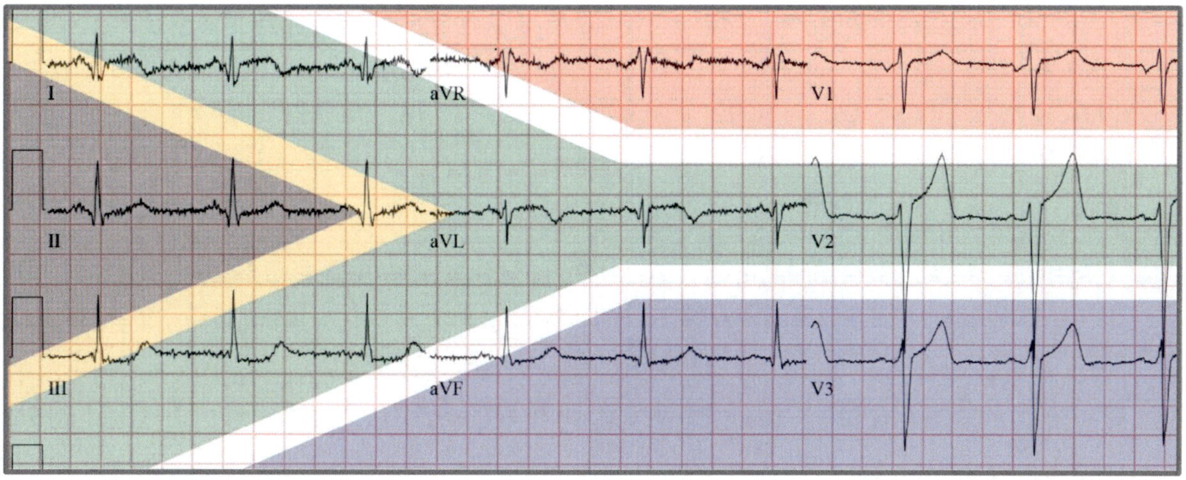

Figure 56. South African Flag Sign for recognition of high lateral myocardial infarctions. The most electrically active ST-segments follow the green pattern of distribution with leads I, aVL, and V2 showing ST-segment elevation and lead III with ST-segment depression.

The T wave in V4 is biphasic with terminal negative deflection, which is specific for ischemia. Later, in the repeat ECG, the T wave in V4 "pseudonormalized" (i.e., became upright) which suggests acute infarct. Left heart catheterization revealed 80% proximal left anterior descending artery stenosis and acute occlusion of the second diagonal branch.

138. **Right Bundle Branch Block, Left Anterior Fascicular Block.** The wide QRS, rSR' in the anterior precordial leads (V1, V2), and deep S-waves in the lateral leads (I, V6) indicate the presence of a right bundle branch block. The right bundle branch block, however, does not explain the left axis deviation. Causes of left axis deviation were previously described in case 3. This ECG demonstrates disruption of two fascicles, the right bundle and the left anterior fascicle, and is termed a "bifascicular" block.[2,4]

139. **Incomplete Right Bundle Branch Block.** This is an example of an incomplete right bundle branch block. The morphology is similar to a complete right bundle branch block, including an rSR' in V1, but the width of the QRS is less than 120 ms; therefore, it is considered incomplete.

140. **Digoxin Toxicity, Hyperkalemia.** This ECG shows the classic "dig effect" (i.e., scooped ST segment previously described in case 85) and a junctional bradycardia in a patient with acute renal failure and hyperkalemia. Digoxin is a cardiac glycoside most used in the management of systolic heart failure and atrial arrhythmias. It is a reversible inhibitor of the Na-K ATPase pump, primarily in the myocardium, leading to increased intracellular calcium and enhanced contractility. In toxic doses, digoxin can cause a multitude of arrhythmias owing to increased automaticity, shortened

refractory period, and decreased atrioventricular nodal conduction. Digoxin toxicity can cause virtually any dysrhythmia, but common dysrhythmias associated with digoxin toxicity are frequent PVCs, slow atrial fibrillation, sinus bradycardia, junctional rhythm, atrial tachycardia, atrioventricular blocks, and ventricular tachycardia (bi-directional or polymorphic).[106,107]

141. **Right Bundle Branch Block, First Degree Atrioventricular Block.** Classic right bundle branch block pattern with rSR' in V1 and a wide S wave in the lateral leads (I, aVL, V5, V6) in addition to first degree atrioventricular block (i.e., prolonged PR interval). This patient had right heart failure from obesity hypoventilation syndrome.

142. **Cerebral T waves**. The precordial T wave inversions were due to increased intracranial pressure from an acute subarachnoid hemorrhage – so called "cerebral T waves." Cerebral T waves are diffuse, symmetric, deep, and associated with a prolonged QT; they are thought to be the result of a sympathetic surge causing repolarization abnormalities. They are rare and generally resolve over time.[108,109]

143. **Hypocalcemia, Hyperkalemia.** Hypocalcemia characteristically increases the duration of the plateau phase of the cardiac action potential, manifesting as increased length of the ST-segment (Figure 57).[110,111] This form of QT prolongation is unique and distinctly different than the delayed repolarization phase experienced during hypokalemia or with QT-prolonging medications. The presence of peaked T waves also suggests hyperkalemia. The combination of electrocardiographic findings of hypocalcemia (i.e., lengthened ST-segment) and hyperkalemia (i.e., peaked T waves) is a classic manifestation of end-stage renal disease. The total calcium level was 5.2 mg/dL, and the potassium level was 6.5 mEq/L.

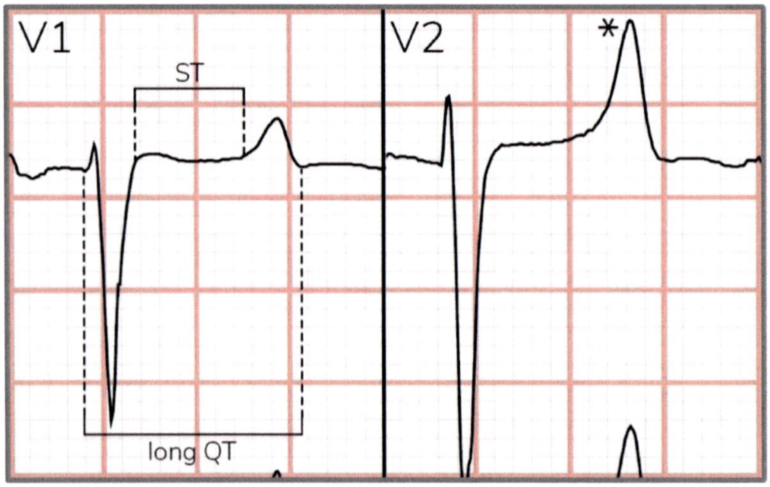

Figure 57. Lengthening of the ST-segment (ST) characteristic of hypocalcemia and peaked T wave of hyperkalemia (asterisk).

144. **First Degree Atrioventricular Block.** First degree atrioventricular block is caused by delayed conduction through the atrioventricular node. It is diagnosed when the PR interval exceeds 200 ms (Figure 58) and is considered "marked" when greater than 300 ms. It can be caused by atrioventricular nodal disease, enhanced vagal tone, ischemia (e.g., inferior myocardial infarction), infection (e.g., Lyme disease), inflammation, electrolyte abnormalities, or medications (e.g., calcium channel blockers, beta blockers, antiarrhythmics, and digoxin).[112] In isolation, it is generally benign and asymptomatic; however, it can progress to higher level blocks.

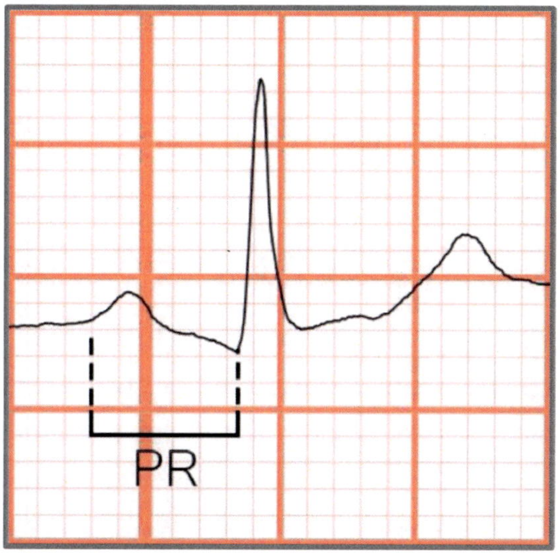

Figure 58. PR interval greater than 200 ms (or five small boxes) in lead II.

145. **Left Bundle Branch Block, Sinus Bradycardia.** Left bundle branch block pattern with a wide and down-going QRS complex in V1, and broad, notched R waves in I and aVL (Figure 23).

146. **Second Degree Atrioventricular Block with 2:1 Conduction, Right Bundle Branch Block, Left Anterior Fascicular Block.** P waves are conducted in a 2:1 ratio, with every other P wave "dropped", or failing to conduct through the atrioventricular node. When P waves are conducted but intermittently "dropped," it is referred to as second degree atrioventricular block. When atrioventricular block occurs in a 2:1 ratio, it is impossible to distinguish between Mobitz I and Mobitz II (previously described in case 77); therefore, it is simply referred to as "2:1 atrioventricular block." Given this patient's extensive conduction disease, a permanent pacemaker was placed.

147. **Multifocal Atrial Tachycardia, Low Voltage.** Multifocal atrial tachycardia is an irregularly irregular rhythm, typically between 100-150 beats per minute, that

arises from multiple ectopic foci within the atria. It is most often seen in patients with advanced lung disease, such as chronic obstructive pulmonary disease. It is defined by a rate greater than 100 beats per minute with at least three morphologically distinct atrial complexes, varying P-P intervals, and an isoelectric baseline between P waves (Figure 59).[5,113] This patient had chronic obstructive lung disease, and the low voltage (previously defined in case 51) was due to increased impedance from hyperinflated lungs.

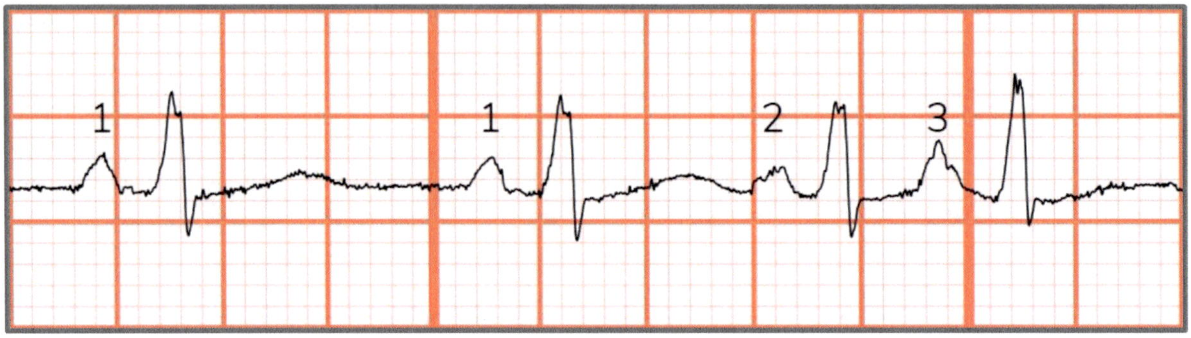

Figure 59. Three morphologically distinct P waves in a section of the lead II rhythm strip.

148. **Ventricular Tachycardia.** Concordance of the complexes across the precordium (i.e., all the QRS complexes are going in the same direction) and the presence of Josephson's sign – notching of the S wave near its nadir, best seen in the inferior leads (II, III, aVF) and previously described in case 21 – favors ventricular tachycardia. Up to 80% of cases of all wide complex tachycardia are ventricular tachycardia,[114] and none of the available algorithms for differentiating wide complex tachycardia perform well in the acute setting. When in doubt, it is safest to assume that regular wide complex tachycardia is ventricular tachycardia.[13,15,16,32]

149. **Left Ventricular Hypertrophy, T-wave Inversions.** Left ventricular hypertrophy with associated inferolateral ST-segment depressions, repolarization abnormalities, and large QRS complexes. The T-wave inversions are asymmetric consistent with a "strain" appearance (Figure 60).[20,115]

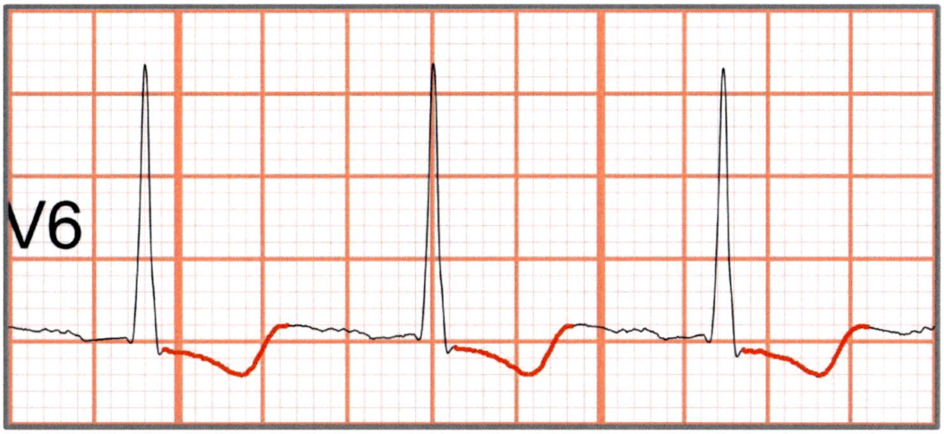

Figure 60. ST-segment depressions and asymmetric T wave inversions (red) in V6 characteristic of the "strain" pattern of left ventricular hypertrophy.

150. **Pacemaker Mediated Tachycardia, Pacemaker Malfunction.** Pacemaker-mediated tachycardia (PMT), or endless loop tachycardia, is a reentrant tachycardia in which the pacemaker forms the anterograde pathway, and the atrioventricular node forms the retrograde pathway, leading to a pacemaker-sensed retrograde P' wave. It occurs in patients with dual chamber pacemakers. The rate is usually at or near the programmed upper limit and can be terminated by slowing conduction through the atrioventricular node (e.g., adenosine) or activating asynchronous mode of the pacemaker by placing a magnet over the pacing generator.[116–118] This patient received amiodarone and the arrhythmia ceased.

151. **Junctional Bradycardia.** This is a junctional rhythm with retrograde atrial conduction. Notice the retrograde P' waves immediately following the QRS complexes. P waves conducted via sinoatrial activity are negatively deflected in V1 and upright in the inferior leads; retrograde conduction depolarizes the atria in the opposite direction, leading to upright P' waves in V1 and negatively deflected P' waves in the inferior leads (Figure 61).

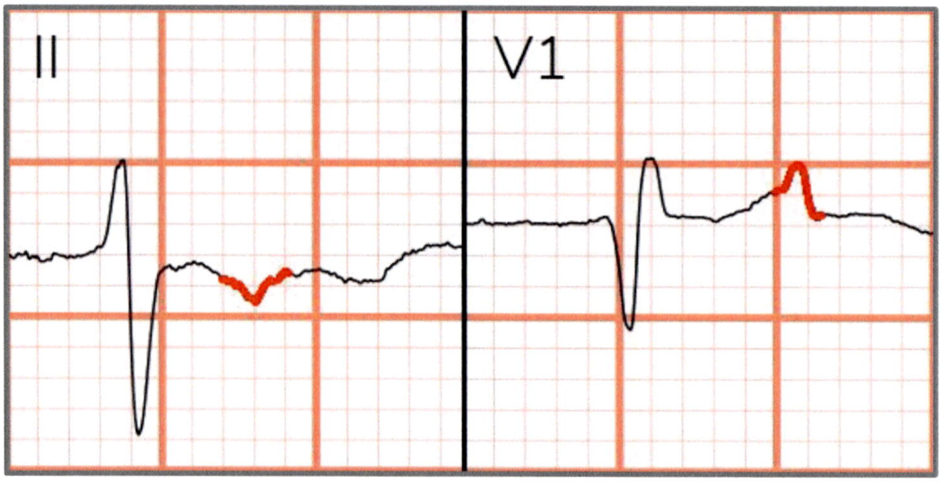

Figure 61. Retrograde atrial activity (red) is negatively deflected in lead II and upright in V1.

152. **Junctional Bradycardia.** Junctional bradycardia in a patient with beta blocker toxicity. There is no evidence of atrial activity (i.e., absent P waves). The junction refers to the part of the conduction system involving the atrioventricular node and the proximal His bundle (immediately inferior to the atrioventricular node). It is the only part of the conduction system capable of producing a narrow QRS complex, provided that the bundle branches are intact. Junctional escape rhythms generally produce a rate of 40 to 60 beats per minute, whereas more distal ventricular pacemakers are slower and less reliable.[32]

153. **Pacemaker Malfunction.** Failure to sense occurs when the pacemaker fails to sense native cardiac activity, leading to asynchronous pacing. It can be caused by a lead insulation break, new intrinsic bundle branch blocks, electrolyte abnormalities, and Class IC antiarrhythmics.[91,92] Pacing spikes (green vertical bars) can be seen within QRS complexes (Figure 62).

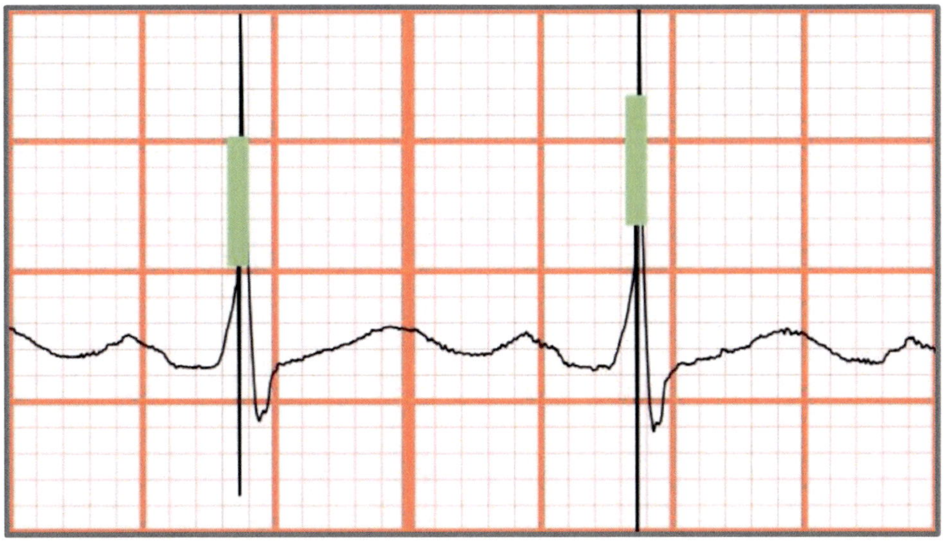

Figure 62. Failure to sense with pacer spikes (green vertical bars) within QRS complexes.

This case was caused by a temporary pacemaker that became mechanically dislodged during transport.

154. **Left Bundle Branch Block, First Degree Atrioventricular Block.** Classic left bundle branch block pattern with a wide and negatively deflected QRS complex in V1, a positively deflected and notched QRS complex in V6, and left axis deviation. There is also a first-degree atrioventricular block (i.e., prolonged PR interval), which likely represents delayed conduction through a diseased right bundle (i.e., trifascicular disease).

155. **Brugada Pattern, Type 2, or saddleback-type.** Brugada syndrome was previously described in case 59. This patient had the type 2 saddleback pattern on the resting ECG with J point elevation of greater than 2 mm that gives rise to a gradually descending ST-segment that remains 1 mm above the baseline followed by a positive T wave that gives a saddleback appearance in ≥1 right precordial lead (Figure 26). During fever, the patient developed the type 1, or coved-type pattern. Fever or drug-induced type 1 Brugada with other high-risk features might be an indication for internal defibrillator placement even in the absence of arrhythmia.[68,119]

156. **Ventricular Paced Rhythm.** Pacer spikes can be seen preceding the QRS complexes. Right ventricular pacing characteristically has a left bundle branch block appearance with negatively deflected complexes across the precordium. Biventricular pacemakers like this one often have a right bundle branch block appearance (i.e., positively deflected complex in V1) because an additional lead in

the coronary sinus paces the left ventricle (Figure 63). This is called cardiac resynchronization therapy.[3]

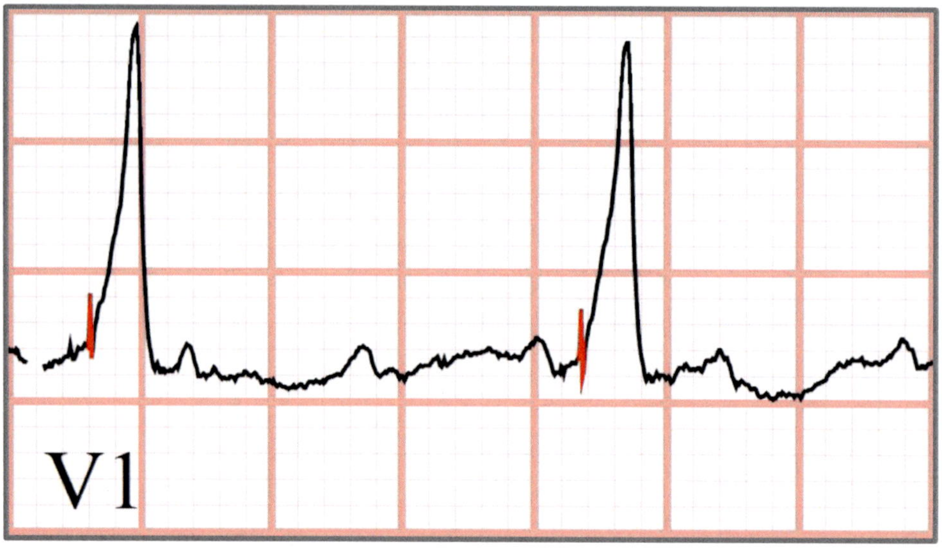

Figure 63. Pacer spikes (red) and upright QRS complexes in V1 characteristic of biventricular pacemakers.

157. **Acute Pericarditis.** There are diffuse, concave up ST-segment elevation without reciprocal changes in a cancer patient with a new pericardial effusion. PR depressions and PR elevation in aVR are typical of acute pericarditis.[42,97,120–122] Diagnostic criteria were previously described in case 33.

158. **Ventricular Tachycardia.** The presence of a narrow capture beat about a third of the way through the rhythm strip confirms atrioventricular dissociation – a specific criterion for ventricular tachycardia (Figure 64). Capture beats occur when the sinoatrial node transiently “captures” the ventricles during atrioventricular dissociation, producing a normal-appearing QRS complex.[77] (The vertical green bars can be ignored).

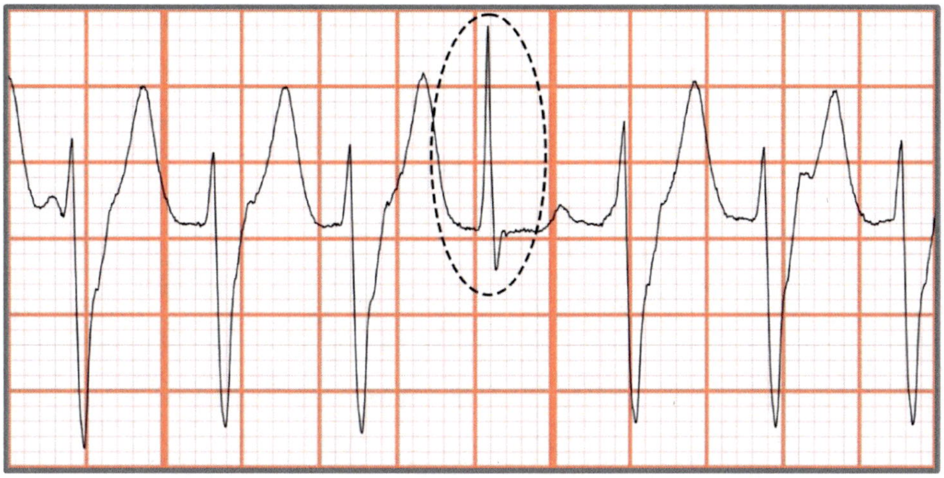

Figure 64. A capture beat (dashed oval) in the lead II rhythm strip confirming atrioventricular dissociation, and ventricular tachycardia.

159. **Pre-excited Atrial Fibrillation**. Pre-excited atrial fibrillation was previously described in case 102. Notice the more-rapid-than-usual rate for atrial fibrillation and changing QRS morphologies consistent with conduction through an accessory pathway (i.e., Wolf-Parkinson-White). Rates this fast are not seen with atrial fibrillation unless an accessory pathway exists.[32,33,93] This patient was electrically cardioverted and admitted for a successful accessory pathway ablation. On prior ECG, notice the short PR interval, delta wave, and slightly widened QRS complex.

160. **Hypothermia, Atrial Fibrillation.** Osborn waves, or J waves, are upright deflections between the end of the QRS complex and the early portion of the ST segment seen during hypothermia. They can mimic ST-segment elevation, as with this post-arrest ECG. Slow atrial fibrillation is another hallmark of hypothermia.[70] The core temperature was 76°F (24.4°C).

161. **Inferior ST-elevation Myocardial Infarction (Aslanger Pattern)**. This pattern is eponymously known as the Aslanger pattern. This pattern of isolated ST-segment elevation in lead III, ST-segment depression in V4 through V6, and ST-segment elevation in V1 greater than V2 was first introduced and published in 2020. It is a strong predictor of acute coronary occlusion in the inferior distribution (left circumflex >> right coronary artery) in patients with concomitant multi-vessel disease and is an indication for emergent reperfusion.[31,123] This patient had an occluded graft (from prior bypass) in the right coronary distribution.

162. **Hypokalemia**. This patient presented with frequent falls and had a potassium of 1.5 mEq/L. Notice the prolonged repolarization phase (i.e., QU interval). The downward

deflected T wave in the anterior precordial leads fuse with U wave and create a wavy pattern characteristic of hypokalemia (Figure 65).[25,26,124,125]

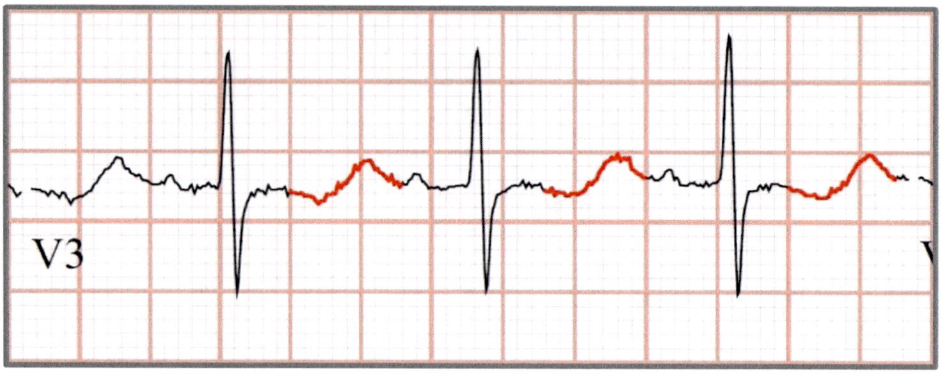

Figure 65. Wavy T-U fusion in V3 (red) characteristic of hypokalemia.

163. **High Lateral ST-elevation Myocardial Infarction**. There are subtle ST-segment elevations in the high lateral leads (I, aVL) with reciprocal ST-segment depression in the inferior leads (III, aVF).[105] While the amplitude of ST-segment elevation is sub-millimeter, it is important to consider proportionality when interpreting ST-segments (i.e., the amplitude of ST-elevation when compared to the size of the QRS complex). Lead aVL has a symmetric, terminal negative T wave deflection that is consistent with an ischemic T wave. Left heart catheterization revealed an occluded proximal left anterior descending artery.

164. **Global Subendocardial Ischemia from Submassive Pulmonary Embolism.** There are diffuse ST-segment depressions along with ST-segment elevation in aVR. As previously discussed in case 5, the differential diagnosis for the is pattern is broad, and includes any condition that creates and supply/demand mismatch.[6–10] This patient was discovered to have a saddle pulmonary embolism for which thrombectomy was performed. The ST changes and tachycardia resolved after mechanical retrieval of the embolus.

165. **Left Ventricular Hypertrophy.** Large amplitude QRS complexes, ST-segment depressions, and asymmetric T wave inversions primarily in the lateral leads (I, aVL, V5, V6) are classic for left ventricular hypertrophy.[20,115] Criteria for left ventricular hypertrophy was previously described in case 84. This patient had newly discovered heart failure with eccentric hypertrophy on echocardiography.

166. **Digoxin toxicity, Slow Atrial Fibrillation.** There is atrial fibrillation with baseline artifact and sagging or scooped ST segments best seen in the lateral precordial leads. These expected findings of digoxin, which this patient took. Digoxin toxicity

can cause virtually any dysrhythmia, but common dysrhythmias associated with digoxin toxicity are frequent premature ventricular contractions, slow atrial fibrillation, sinus bradycardia, junctional rhythm, atrial tachycardia, atrioventricular blocks, and ventricular tachycardia (bi-directional or polymorphic).[106,107]

167. **Left Ventricular Hypertrophy, Left Atrial Enlargement, Poor R Wave Progression.** The large R wave in aVL (>11 mm) is diagnostic for left ventricular hypertrophy (see case 84 for criteria).[20] The left axis deviation, slight intraventricular conduction delay, and absent R wave progression across the precordium are all explained by left ventricular hypertrophy. The large, downward deflected P wave in V1 and wide P wave in lead II (greater than 120 ms) indicates left atrial enlargement (Figure 44).[4,20]

168. **Atrial flutter with 2:1 Conduction, Sodium Channel Toxicity**. Sodium channel blockers slow phase 0 of the action potential resulting in slowing of intraventricular conduction, an effect of which the right bundle is most susceptible to. Electrocardiographically, sodium channel toxicity manifests as a widened QRS (> 100 ms) and right axis deviation.[126,127] In this ECG, note the wide and fragmented QRS, right axis deviation, and tall terminal R wave in aVR – all consistent with sodium channel toxicity. This case was due to cocaine toxicity.

169. **Poor R Wave Progression**. There is poor R wave progression and Q waves in the inferior leads. Poor R wave progression is a non-specific finding that is suggestive of prior anterior myocardial infarction. It is a poorly defined term that implies diminished amplitude of the R wave in the precordium. It has been defined as an R wave less than 3 mm in lead V3 or decreasing R wave amplitude from V2 to V3 or V3 to V4. Poor R wave progression has been implicated in left ventricular hypertrophy, right ventricular hypertrophy and can be a normal variant.[5,128] This patient had prior myocardial infarctions in both the anterior and inferior distributions.

170. **Ventricular Tachycardia**. Negative QRS concordance across the precordium (i.e. QRS complexes are all pointing downward) strongly favors ventricular tachycardia.[12] This patient was unstable and was electrically cardioverted. A post-cardioversion ECG showed anterior ST-elevation and left heart catheterization revealed a left anterior descending artery occlusion.

171. **Multifocal Atrial Tachycardia**. This ECG shows multifocal atrial tachycardia in a patient with heart failure and chronic obstructive pulmonary disease. Multifocal atrial tachycardia was previously described in case 147.

172. **Brugada Syndrome**. This is the Type 1 or coved-type Brugada pattern in a patient with a family history of sudden cardiac death. This patient was admitted for successful defibrillator placement. Brugada syndrome was previously described in case 59.

173. **Hypokalemia**. This patient presented with global weakness and was diagnosed with hypokalemic periodic paralysis. The potassium level was 1.9 mEq/L. There are T-U fusion complexes across the precordium (Figure 66).

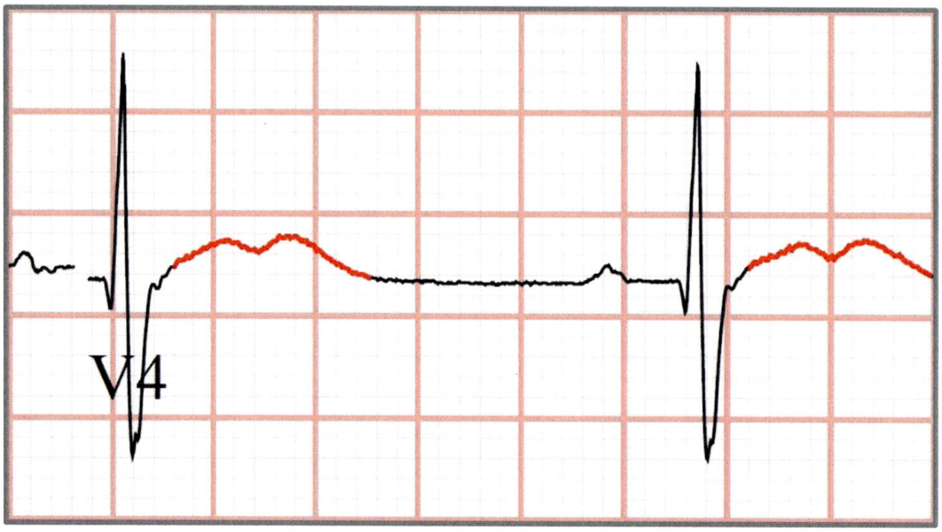

Figure 66. T-U complexes (red) in V4 are characteristic of hypokalemia.

174. **Left Ventricular Aneurysm**. In the absence of reperfusion therapy, left ventricular aneurysm is a common structural complication of anterior myocardial infarction.[80,82] Usual ECG findings include ST-segment elevation that persists more than two weeks after ST elevation myocardial infarction, deep Q waves, and the absence of reciprocal ST-segment depressions.[81] This patient presented with left sided body pain after a fall. There are large Q waves in the precordial leads V2-V4 with associated ST-segment elevation. A bedside (and then formal) echocardiogram confirmed the left ventricular aneurysm. Catheterization revealed non-obstructive coronary artery disease.

175. **Hyperkalemia**. Note the "peaked" morphology of the T waves (e.g., narrow base and pointed at the top) and slightly widened QRS. This patient's potassium was 7.5 mmol/L.

176. **Early Repolarization**. This patient received an ECG for reasons unrelated to his presentation and was incidentally noted to have diffuse, concave ST-segment elevation. The degree of ST-segment elevation is greater in the precordial leads, and

a prominent J-point notch (or "fishhook") can be visualized in V3, characteristic of early repolarization.[84,129]

177. **Ventricular Tachycardia**. The differential for regular wide complex tachycardia includes ventricular tachycardia, supraventricular tachycardia with aberrancy, antidromic atrioventricular reentrant tachycardia, and toxicologic/metabolic disturbances.[11] This ECG shows concordance across all precordial leads (i.e., the QRS complexes are going in the same direction - downwards), favoring ventricular tachycardia.[12] The patient was electrically cardioverted.

178. **Wellens Syndrome**. Wellens syndrome, previously described in case 18, represents a special category of high-risk acute coronary syndrome that should receive urgent catheterization.[30,31] This is type B Wellens pattern with deeply inverted precordial T waves obtained while the patient was pain-free. Left heart catheterization revealed a 90% proximal left anterior descending stenosis.

179. **Hyperkalemia**. This patient presented with altered mental status and was found to have ECG changes of profound hyperkalemia. The rhythm is sinus, although it is unclear whether the initial several P waves are conducted through to the ventricles because of the inconsistent PR interval. There is a right axis deviation, a right bundle branch block pattern, and a widened QRS (~240 ms, more than expected for a typical right bundle branch block).

180. **Second Degree Atrioventricular Block - Mobitz I.** Mobitz I occurs when conduction is progressively delayed through the atrioventricular node and eventually fails. The PR interval is prolonged and progressively lengthens until a P wave is "dropped," or fails to conduct to the ventricular system, resulting in the absence of an associated QRS complex. There are eight P waves for every seven QRS complexes, representing 8:7 conduction.

181. **Left Ventricular Hypertrophy, Left Atrial Enlargement.** The large QRS complexes and asymmetric repolarization abnormalities (i.e., T wave inversions) in the lateral leads are consistent with the "strain" pattern of left ventricular hypertrophy. Additionally, notice that the terminal negative deflection of the P wave in V1 is greater than 1 mm deep and 40 ms in duration, meeting criteria for left atrial enlargement (Figure 44).[20] This patient was discovered to have severe aortic stenosis.

182. **Hypokalemia.** Notice the ST-segment depressions and wavy appearance of the ST-segment and T wave, which represents T-U wave fusion.[26] The prolonged

repolarization phase is a risk for the development of dysrhythmias, specifically torsade de pointes. The potassium level was 1.6 mEq/L.

183. **Multifocal Atrial Tachycardia.** Multifocal atrial tachycardia is an irregularly irregular rhythm previously described in case 147. It is most often seen in patients with advanced lung disease, such as chronic obstructive pulmonary disease. The presence of three different P wave morphologies confirms the diagnosis in this patient with chronic obstructive lung disease.

184. **Ventricular Pre-excitation.** This ECG displays the classic features of pre-excitation: the delta wave, shortened PR interval, and slightly widened QRS. The dominant R wave in V1 is consistent with a left-sided accessory pathway, referred to as "type A."[5,32]

185. **Left Ventricular Hypertrophy.** Cornell criteria for left ventricular hypertrophy is met via the large S wave in V3 (see case 84). The discordant ST-segment elevation in leads V2 through V4 is not out of proportion given the amplitude of the R-S complex. One paper by Armtstrong, et al., defines an abnormal amount of ST-segment elevation (in leads V1 through V3 and in the setting of left ventricular hypertrophy) as greater than 25% of the R-S amplitude (Figure 67).[130]

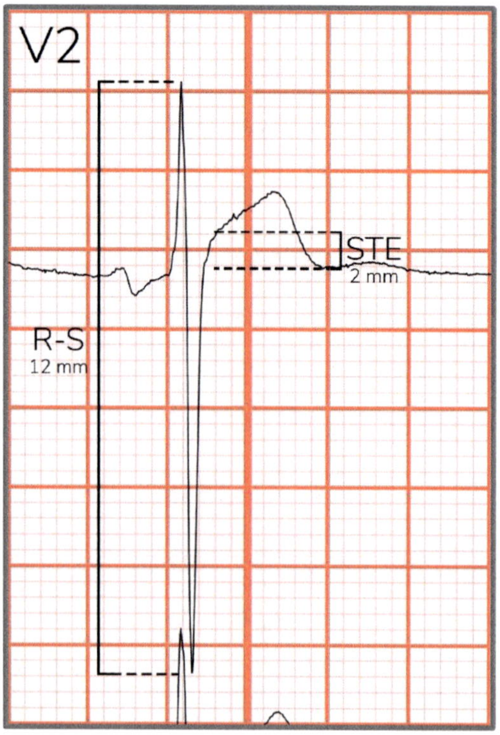

Figure 67. Appropriately discordant ST-segment elevation (STE, <25% R-S

amplitude) in the setting of left ventricular hypertrophy.

186. **Anterior ST-elevation Myocardial Infarction, Left Ventricular Hypertrophy**. Left ventricular hypertrophy is diagnosed via the Sokolow Lyon criteria (see case 84). The degree of ST-segment elevation in the anterolateral precordial leads is more than expected for appropriate discordance (Figure 68).[130] Left heart catheterization revealed complete left anterior descending occlusion and percutaneous coronary intervention was successful.

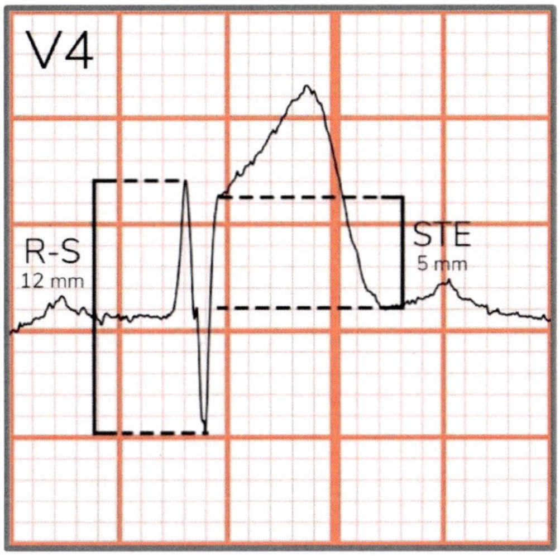

Figure 68. Inappropriately discordant ST-segment elevation (>25% R-S amplitude) in the setting of left ventricular hypertrophy.

187. **Left Ventricular Aneurysm**. In the absence of reperfusion therapy, left ventricular aneurysm is a common structural complication of anterior myocardial infarction.[80,82] Usual ECG findings include ST-segment elevation that persists more than two weeks after STEMI, deep Q waves, and the absence of reciprocal ST-segment depressions.[81] Large Q waves in the anterior precordial leads with associated ST-segment depression (consistent with prior ECGs) is consistent with anterior left ventricular aneurysm, confirmed via echocardiography.[81,131,132]

188. **Inferior ST-elevation Myocardial Infarction with Posterior Extension**. ST-segment elevation with straightening in the inferior leads suggests inferior wall myocardial infarction. The V2 ST-segment depression, large R wave, and upright T wave all suggest posterior extension. Left heart catheterization revealed an occluded distal right coronary artery.

189. **Anterior ST-elevation Myocardial Infarction, Right Bundle Branch Block, Left Posterior Fascicular Block.** The is a right bundle branch block pattern (Figure 2)

with a right axis deviation, indicating the presence of a left posterior fascicular block (Figure 50). Additionally, inferior Q waves give this ECG an unusual extreme right axis, or "northwest" axis deviation (Figure 5). Typically, a right bundle branch block has either isoelectric or slight ST-segment depressions in the anterior precordial leads (V1 through V3).[2,43] Any degree of ST-segment elevation in V1 through V3 in the setting of a right bundle branch block is worrisome for acute occlusion (Figure 69).

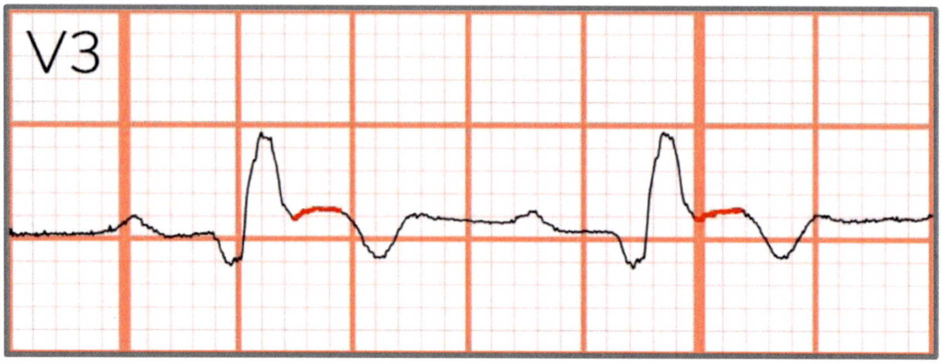

Figure 69. ST-segment straightening and slight elevation in lead V3 (red). ST-segment elevation in any V1-V3 lead in the setting of a right bundle branch block is concerning for acute occlusion.

Despite not meeting classic ST-elevation myocardial infarction criteria,[72] left heart catheterization revealed a left anterior descending artery occlusion.

190. **Acute Pericarditis.** Differentiating pericarditis from ST-elevation myocardial infarction can be challenging, but features that suggest acute pericarditis include any of the following:

   1. diffuse concave up ST elevations without reciprocal changes,
   2. PR depression,
   3. PR elevation in aVR,
   4. ST-elevation in lead II greater than lead III, and
   5. Spodick's sign – down-sloping of the TP segment.[97]

This patient developed symptoms of pericarditis during an inpatient admission and was discovered to have a new pericardial effusion. Note the diffuse concave ST-segment elevations without reciprocal changes, slight PR-segment depressions (best seen in the limb leads), and down-sloping T-P segment (best seen in the precordial leads) – so-called Spodick's sign.[42,97,120–122,133] Left heart catheterization revealed non-obstructive coronary artery disease and the patient was diagnosed with acute pericarditis. Months later, the ST-segments normalized.

191. **Right Bundle Branch Block & Left Posterior Fascicular Block.** Right bundle branch blocks do not typically cause axis deviation because the right ventricle lacks enough myocardium to cause an axis shift (in contrast to left bundle branch blocks). When a right axis deviation accompanies a right bundle branch block, there is often an associated left posterior fascicular block (Figure 50), as with this case.

192. **Atrial Flutter with 2:1 Conduction.** Atrial flutter occurs when a reentrant circuit forms in the right atrium. It is an organized rhythm that is generally characterized by an atrial rate of around 300 beats per minute. It more commonly occurs in a counterclockwise fashion, leading to inverted flutter waves in the inferior leads (II, III, and aVF).[5,66] In the absence of treatment, the most common conduction is 2:1 (atrial to ventricular conduction). Notice the sawtooth pattern in the inferior leads (II, III, and aVF), with inverted flutter waves (Figure 70).

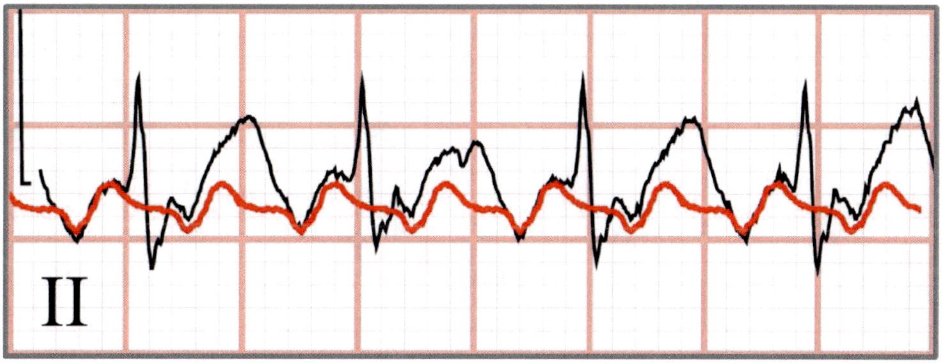

Figure 70. Atrial flutter waves (red) after rate control superimposed on the lead II rhythm strip of 2:1 conduction.

193. **Left Ventricular Hypertrophy.** There are large QRS complexes with repolarization abnormalities (i.e., T-wave inversions) in the lateral leads (I, II, aVL, V4, V5, and V6). Despite nearly 4 mm of ST-segment elevation in V2, it does not rise to the level of inappropriate discordance (Figure 71).[130] In fact, this patient had a left heart catheterization that revealed non-obstructive coronary artery disease and percutaneous intervention was not performed.

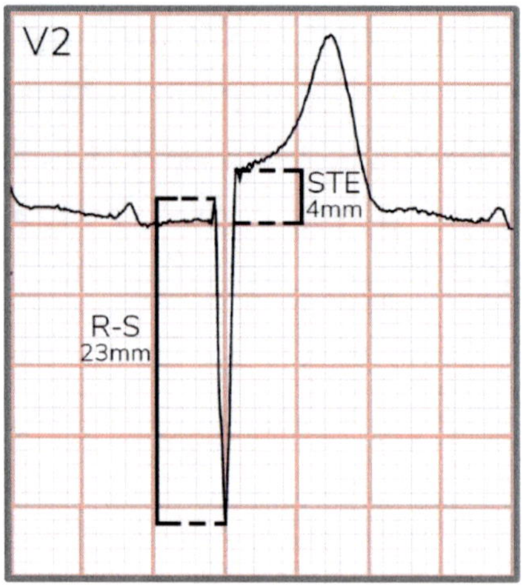

Figure 71. Appropriately discordant ST-segment elevation (<25% R-S amplitude) in the setting of left ventricular hypertrophy.

194. **Antidromic Atrioventricular Tachycardia.** The differential for regular wide complex tachycardia includes ventricular tachycardia, supraventricular tachycardia with aberrancy, antidromic atrioventricular reentrant tachycardia, and toxicologic/metabolic disturbances.[11] This wide complex tachycardia is essentially indistinguishable from ventricular tachycardia. The post conversion ECG demonstrates ventricular pre-excitation evidenced by the short PR interval and slurred upstroke (i.e., delta wave). Antidromic atrioventricular tachycardia is a macro reentrant circuit in which the signal travels anterograde through accessory pathway and retrograde through the atrioventricular node (Figure 8). The rhythm was subsequently confirmed via an electrophysiology study.

195. **Inferior ST-elevation Myocardial Infarction, Third Degree Atrioventricular Block.** There are inferior ST-segment elevations with reciprocal changes in I, aVL, and V2 along with atrioventricular dissociation. The narrow QRS (<120 ms) confirms junctional escape. In the setting of inferior myocardial infarction, atrioventricular block is usually transient, due to ischemia or edema of the atrioventricular node.[3] Left heart catheterization revealed an occluded right coronary artery.

196. **Anterior ST-elevation Myocardial Infarction, Left Ventricular Hypertrophy.** There are ST-segment elevations in V2 and V3. In the setting of Cornell criteria for left ventricular hypertrophy (see case 84).[20] Although the degree of ST-segment elevation in V2 and V3 is not out of proportion to the amplitude of the R-S complex, the convex morphology is suspicious (Figure 72). Left heart catheterization revealed mid-left anterior descending artery occlusion.

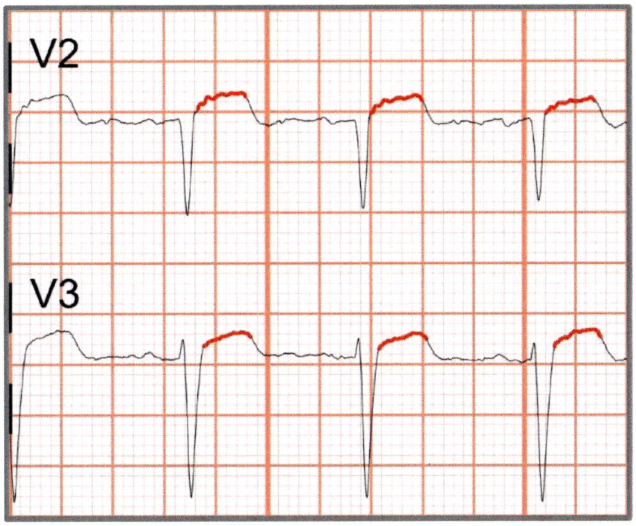

Figure 72. Convex ST-segment morphology in V2 and V3 (red).

197. **Right Ventricular Hypertrophy, Biatrial Enlargement.** Rightward forces predominate in this ECG taken from a patient with known chronic thromboembolic pulmonary hypertension. The extreme right axis deviation (Figure 5), tall P wave in lead II, anterior precordial T-wave inversions, and tall R wave in V1 are all findings of right heart strain. The qR pattern in V1 is one of the most specific signs of severe right ventricular hypertrophy.[5]

198. **Posterior Myocardial Infarction, Junctional Bradycardia**. There is a junctional bradycardia, absence of atrial activity, and ST-segment depressions in the anterior precordial leads (V2 through V4) with upright T waves, suggesting posterior myocardial infarction. Typical anterior precordial findings of posterior myocardial infarctions are R/S ratio greater than 1 (later finding), ST depressions, and upright T waves.[30,31] The appearance of tall R waves is the posterior equivalent of Q waves. 5-10% of all myocardial infarctions are isolated posterior and not associated with inferior ST-segment elevation. Isolated posterior myocardial infarctions are associated with longer door-to-balloon times and worse outcomes because they are frequently missed.[65,134] Left heart catheterization revealed an occluded left circumflex artery.

199. **Inferior ST-elevation Myocardial Infarction, Right Bundle Branch Block**. There are subtle ST-segment elevations in the inferior leads associated with reciprocal ST-segment depression in aVL. While this ECG does not meet the formal criteria for ST-elevation myocardial infarction,[72] the reciprocal changes are concerning for an occlusive process. This patient was diagnosed with an ascending aortic dissection

with retrograde dissection into the right coronary artery upon left heart catheterization.

200. **Left Ventricular Hypertrophy**. Cornell criteria for left ventricular hypertrophy is met via the large S wave in V3 (see case 84).[20] The discordant ST-segment elevation in leads V2 through V4 is appropriately discordant given the amplitude of the R-S complex.[130] The catheterization laboratory was inappropriately activated for this patient and revealed non-obstructive coronary artery disease.

References

1. Harrigan RA, Perron AD, Brady WJ. Atrioventricular dissociation. *American Journal of Emergency Medicine*. 2001;19(3):218-222. doi:10.1053/ajem.2001.22657

2. Kusumoto FM, Schoenfeld MH, Barrett C, et al. 2018 ACC/AHA/HRS Guideline on the Evaluation and Management of Patients With Bradycardia and Cardiac Conduction Delay: A Report of the American College of Cardiology/American Heart Association Task Force on Clinical Practice Guidelines and the Heart Rhyth. *Circulation*. 2019;140(8):e382-e482. doi:10.1161/CIR.0000000000000628

3. Mattu A, Tabas J, Brady W. *Electrocardiography in Emergency, Acute, and Critical Care*. 2nd ed. The American College of Emergency Physicians; 2019.

4. Surawicz B, Childers R, Deal BJ, Gettes LS. AHA/ACCF/HRS Recommendations for the Standardization and Interpretation of the Electrocardiogram. Part III: Intraventricular Conduction Disturbances A Scientific Statement From the American Heart Association Electrocardiography and Arrhythmias Committee, Council on Clinical Cardiology; the American College of Cardiology Foundation; and the Heart Rhythm Society. *J Am Coll Cardiol*. Published online 2009. doi:10.1016/j.jacc.2008.12.013

5. Surawicz B, Knilans TK. *Chou's Electrocardiography in Clinical Practice*. 6th ed. Elsevier; 2008.

6. Kosuge M, Ebina T, Hibi K, et al. An early and simple predictor of severe left main and/or three-vessel disease in patients with nonst-segment elevation acute coronary syndrome. *American Journal of Cardiology*. 2011;107(4):495-500. doi:10.1016/j.amjcard.2010.10.005

7. Kukla P, Macintyre W, Fijorek K. Electrocardiographic abnonmralities in patients with acute pulmonary emoblism complicated by cardiogenic shock. *American Journal of Emergency Medicine*2. 2014;32:507-510.

8. Brouner M, Hammock J, Doppalapudi H. Does ST Elevation in Lead aVR Require an Emergent Trip to the Catheterization Laboratory? *JAMA Intern Med*. 2023;183(3):261-262. doi:10.1001/JAMAINTERNMED.2022.5901

9. Knotts RJ, Wilson JM, Kim E, Huang HD, Birnbaum Y. Diffuse ST depression with ST elevation in aVR: Is this pattern specific for global ischemia due to left main coronary artery disease? *J Electrocardiol*. 2013;46(3):240-248. doi:10.1016/j.jelectrocard.2012.12.016

10. Miranda DF, Lobo AS, Walsh B, Sandoval Y, Smith SW. New Insights Into the Use of the 12-Lead Electrocardiogram for Diagnosing Acute Myocardial Infarction in the Emergency Department. *Can J Cardiol.* 2018;34(2):132-145. doi:10.1016/J.CJCA.2017.11.011

11. Brady WJ, Mattu A, Tabas J, Ferguson JD. The differential diagnosis of wide QRS complex tachycardia. *Am J Emerg Med.* 2017;35(10):1525-1529. doi:10.1016/J.AJEM.2017.07.056

12. Brugada P, Brugada J, Mont L, Smeets J, Andries EW. A New Approach to the Differential Diagnosis of a Regular Tachycardia With a Wide QRS Complex. *Circulation.* 1991;83:1649-1659.

13. Vereckei A. Current Algorithms for the Diagnosis of wide QRS Complex Tachycardias. *Curr Cardiol Rev.* 2014;10(3):262-276. doi:10.2174/1573403x10666140514103309

14. Moccetti F, Yadava M, Latifi Y, et al. Simplified Integrated Clinical and Electrocardiographic Algorithm for Differentiation of Wide QRS Complex Tachycardia: The Basel Algorithm. *JACC Clin Electrophysiol.* 2022;8(7):831-839. doi:10.1016/J.JACEP.2022.03.017

15. Szelényi Z, Duray G, Katona G, et al. Comparison of the "real-life" diagnostic value of two recently published electrocardiogram methods for the differential diagnosis of wide QRS complex tachycardias. *Academic Emergency Medicine.* 2013;20(11):1121-1130. doi:10.1111/acem.12247

16. Baxi RP, Hart KW, Vereckei A, et al. Vereckei criteria as a diagnostic tool amongst emergency medicine residents to distinguish between ventricular tachycardia and supra-ventricular tachycardia with aberrancy. *J Cardiol.* 2012;59(3):307-312. doi:10.1016/j.jjcc.2011.11.007

17. Kaiser E, Darrieux FCC, Barbosa SA, et al. Differential diagnosis of wide QRS tachycardias: comparison of two electrocardiographic algorithms. *Europace.* 2015;17(9):1422-1427. doi:10.1093/EUROPACE/EUU354

18. Herbert ME, Votey SR, Morgan MT, Cameron P, Dziukas L. Failure to agree on the electrocardiographic diagnosis of ventricular tachycardia. *Ann Emerg Med.* 1996;27(1):35-38. doi:10.1016/S0196-0644(96)70293-7

19. Jastrzebski M, Kukla P, Czarnecka D, Kawecka-Jaszcz K. Comparison of five electrocardiographic methods for differentiation of wide QRS-complex tachycardias. *Europace.* 2012;14(8):1165-1171. doi:10.1093/EUROPACE/EUS015

20. Wagner GS, Macfarlane P, Wellens H, et al. AHA/ACCF/HRS Recommendations for the Standardization and Interpretation of the Electrocardiogram. Part V: Electrocardiogram

Changes Associated With Cardiac Chamber Hypertrophy. *Circulation.* 2009;53(11):1003-1011. doi:10.1016/j.jacc.2008.12.016

21. Nishi SPE, Barbagelata NA, Atar S, Birnbaum Y, Tuero E. Hypercalcemia-induced ST-segment elevation mimicking acute myocardial infarction. *J Electrocardiol.* 2006;39(3):298-300. doi:10.1016/J.JELECTROCARD.2005.10.015

22. Turhan S, Kilickap M, Kilinc S. ST segment elevation mimicking acute myocardial infarction in hypercalcaemia. *Heart.* 2005;91(8):999. doi:10.1136/HRT.2003.030874

23. Ashizawa N, Arakawa S, Koide Y, Toda G, Seto S, Yano K. Hypercalcemia due to vitamin D intoxication with clinical features mimicking acute myocardial infarction. *Intern Med.* 2003;42(4):340-344. doi:10.2169/INTERNALMEDICINE.42.340

24. Kiewiet RM, Ponssen HH, Janssens ENW, Fels PW. Ventricular fibrillation in hypercalcaemic crisis due to primary hyperparathyroidism. *Neth J Med.* 2004;62(3):94-96.

25. Diercks DB, Shumaik GM, Harrigan RA, Brady WJ, Chan TC. Electrocardiographic manifestations: Electrolyte abnormalities. *Journal of Emergency Medicine.* 2004;27(2):153-160. doi:10.1016/j.jemermed.2004.04.006

26. Chua CE, Choi E, Khoo EYH. ECG changes of severe hypokalemia. *QJM.* 2018;111(8):581-582. doi:10.1093/qjmed/hcy046

27. Hoang H, Giordano JA, Cooper BL. Woman with ST Changes Following Days of Vomiting. *Ann Emerg Med.* 2021;77(4):442-444. doi:10.1016/J.ANNEMERGMED.2020.08.034

28. Emre K. A, H. Pendell M, Stephen W. S. Recognizing electrocardiographically subtle occlusion myocardial infarction and differentiating it from mimics: Ten steps to or away from cath lab. *Turk Kardiyol Dern Ars.* 2021;49(6):488-500. doi:10.5543/TKDA.2021.21026

29. Smith SW, Meyers HP. Hyperacute T-waves Can Be a Useful Sign of Occlusion Myocardial Infarction if Appropriately Defined. *Ann Emerg Med.* 2023;82(2). doi:10.1016/J.ANNEMERGMED.2023.01.011

30. Kontos MC, de Lemos JA, Deitelzweig SB, et al. 2022 ACC Expert Consensus Decision Pathway on the Evaluation and Disposition of Acute Chest Pain in the Emergency Department: A Report of the American College of Cardiology Solution Set Oversight Committee. *J Am Coll Cardiol.* 2022;80(20):1925-1960. doi:10.1016/J.JACC.2022.08.750

31. Zoni CR, Mukherjee D, Gulati M. Proposed new classification for acute coronary syndrome: Acute coronary syndrome requiring immediate reperfusion. *Catheter Cardiovasc Interv*. 2023;101(7):1177-1181. doi:10.1002/CCD.30667

32. Wagner GS, Strauss DG. *Marriott's Practical Electrocardiography*. 12th ed. Lippincott Williams & Wilkins; 2014.

33. Moore EN, Spear JF, Boineau JP. Recent Electrophysiologic Studies on the Wolff-Parkinson-White Syndrome. *New England Journal of Medicine*. 1973;289(18):956-963. doi:10.1056/nejm197311012891808

34. Zwaan D, Biir FWHM, Wellens HJJ. Characteristic electrocardiogric pattern indicating a critical stenosis high in left anteior descending coronary artery in patients admitted because of impending myocardial infarction. *Am Heart J*. 1982;103(4):730-736.

35. Helfant RH. Hypokalemia and arrhythmias. *Am J Med*. 1986;80(4A):13-22. doi:10.1016/0002-9343(86)90336-0

36. Bauer GE. Bundle-Branch Block Under Voluntary Control. *Br Heart J*. 1964;26(2):167-179. doi:10.1136/HRT.26.2.167

37. Vesell H, Friedfeld L. Critical rates in ventricular conduction. IV. Duration of unstable bundle branch block. *Am Heart J*. 1952;44(6):830-842. doi:10.1016/0002-8703(52)90129-4

38. Rischall ML, Smith SW, Friedman AB. Screening for QT Prolongation in the Emergency Department: Is There a Better "Rule of Thumb?" *Western Journal of Emergency Medicine*. 2020;226(2). doi:10.5811/westjem.2019.10.40381

39. Katritsis DG, Camm AJ. Atrioventricular nodal reentrant tachycardia. *Circulation*. 2010;122(8):831-840. doi:10.1161/CIRCULATIONAHA.110.936591

40. Bakker ALM, Nijkerk G, Groenemeijer BE, et al. The lewis lead: Making recognition of p waves easy during wide QRS complex tachycardia. *Circulation*. 2009;119(24). doi:10.1161/CIRCULATIONAHA.109.852053

41. Al-Khatib SM, Stevenson WG, Ackerman MJ, et al. 2017 AHA/ACC/HRS Guideline for Management of Patients With Ventricular Arrhythmias and the Prevention of Sudden Cardiac Death. *J Am Coll Cardiol*. 2018;72(14):e91-e220. doi:10.1161/CIR.0000000000000549

42. LeWinter MM. Acute Pericarditis. *New England Journal of Medicine*. 2017;371(25):349-359. doi:10.1016/j.pcad.2016.12.001

43. Costa D Da, Brady WJ, Edhouse J. Bradycardias and Atrioventricular conduction block. *Br Med J*. 2002;324(March):535-538. doi:10.1136/bmj.324.7336.535

44. Kerr GW, Mcguye AC, Wilkie S. Tricyclic antidepressant overdose: a review. doi:10.1136/emj.18.4.236

45. Cooper BL, Beyene JA. Atrioventricular nodal reentrant tachycardia and cannon A waves: A case report. *American Journal of Emergency Medicine*. Published online 2018. doi:10.1016/j.ajem.2018.11.016

46. Mani BC, Pavri BB. Dual atrioventricular nodal pathways physiology: A review of relevant anatomy, electrophysiology, and electrocardiographic manifestations. *Indian Pacing Electrophysiol J*. 2014;14(1):12-25. doi:10.1016/S0972-6292(16)30711-2

47. Valent S, Kelly P. Images in clinical medicine. Digoxin-induced bidirectional ventricular tachycardia. *N Engl J Med*. 1997;336(8):550-550. doi:10.1056/NEJM199702203360805

48. Harrigan RA, Chan TC, Brady WJ. Electrocardiographic electrode misplacement, misconnection, and artifact. *J Emerg Med*. 2012;43(6):1038-1044. doi:10.1016/J.JEMERMED.2012.02.024

49. Rudiger A, Hellermann JP, Mukherjee R, Follath F, Turina J. Electrocardiographic artifacts due to electrode misplacement and their frequency in different clinical settings. *Am J Emerg Med*. 2007;25(2):174-178. doi:10.1016/J.AJEM.2006.06.018

50. V. Rosen A, Koppikar S, Shaw C, Baranchuk A. Common ECG Lead Placement Errors. Part I: Limb lead Reversals. *International Journal of Medical Students*. 2014;2(3):92-98. doi:10.5195/ijms.2014.95

51. Pérez-Riera AR, Barbosa-Barros R, Daminello-Raimundo R, de Abreu LC. Main artifacts in electrocardiography. *Ann Noninvasive Electrocardiol*. 2018;23(2):e12494. doi:10.1111/anec.12494

52. Lee DH, Walsh B, Smith SW. Terminal QRS distortion is present in anterior myocardial infarction but absent in early repolarization. *American Journal of Emergency Medicine*. 2016;34(11):2182-2185. doi:10.1016/j.ajem.2016.08.053

53. Riera ARP, Barros RB, Sousa FD de, Baranchuk A. Accelerated Idioventricular Rhythm: History and Chronology of the Main Discoveries. *Indian Pacing Electrophysiol J*. 2010;10(1):40. Accessed July 28, 2021. /pmc/articles/PMC2803604/

54. Perron AD, Sweeney T. Arrhythmic Complications of Acute Coronary Syndromes. *Emerg Med Clin North Am*. 2005;23(4):1065-1082. doi:10.1016/j.emc.2005.07.002

55. Meyers HP, Limkakeng AT, Jaffa EJ, et al. Validation of the modified Sgarbossa criteria for acute coronary occlusion in the setting of left bundle branch block: A retrospective case-control study. *Am Heart J*. 2015;170(6):1255-1264. doi:10.1016/j.ahj.2015.09.005

56. Sgarbossa EB, Investigators G 1. Electrocardiographic Diagnosis of Evolving Acute Myocardial Infarction in the Presence of Left Bundle-Branch Block. *New England Journal of Medicine*. 1996;334(8):481-487. doi:10.1021/ja00009a021

57. Smith SW, Dodd KW, Henry TD, Dvorak DM, Pearce LA. Diagnosis of ST-elevation myocardial infarction in the presence of left bundle branch block with the ST-elevation to S-wave ratio in a modified sgarbossa rule. *Ann Emerg Med*. 2012;60(6):766-776. doi:10.1016/j.annemergmed.2012.07.119

58. Salahuddin M, Cader F, Nasrin S, Chowdhury M. The pacemaker-twiddler's syndrome: An infrequent cause of pacemaker failure. *BMC Res Notes*. 2016;9(1):1-5. doi:10.1186/s13104-015-1818-0

59. Lesnick J, Cooper B, Doshi P. Twiddler's Syndrome. *Clin Pract Cases Emerg Med*. 2019;3(3):299-300. doi:10.5811/cpcem.2019.4.42123

60. Madias JE. Low-Voltage Electrocardiogram in Patients with Hypothyroidism and Pericardial Effusion: Can Serial Comparative Quantitative Electrocardiography Offer More? *Cardiology*. 2010;116(1):29-31. doi:10.1159/000313463

61. Madias JE. Low QRS voltage and its causes. *J Electrocardiol*. 2008;41(6):498-500. doi:10.1016/j.jelectrocard.2008.06.021

62. Mattu A. Low Voltage on ECG. UMEM Educational Pearls. Published 2020. Accessed December 11, 2020. https://umem.org/educational_pearls/444/

63. Madias JE, Bazaz R, Agarwal H, Win M, Medepalli L. Anasarca-mediated attenuation of the amplitude of electrocardiogram complexes: A description of a heretofore unrecognized phenomenon. *J Am Coll Cardiol*. 2001;38(3):756-764. doi:10.1016/S0735-1097(01)01429-2

64. Tajiri J, Morita M, Higashi K, Sato T, Fujii H, Nakamura N. The cause of low voltage qrs complex in primary hypothyroidism pericardial effusion or thyroid hormone deficiency? *Jpn Heart J*. 1985;26(4):539-547. doi:10.1536/ihj.26.539

65. Ayer A, Terkelsen CJ. Difficult ECGs in STEMI: Lessons learned from serial sampling of pre- and in-hospital ECGs. *J Electrocardiol*. 2014;47(4):448-458. doi:10.1016/j.jelectrocard.2014.03.010

66. Link MS. Evaluation and Initial Treatment of Supraventricular Tachycardia. *New England Journal of Medicine*. 2012;367(15):1438-1448. doi:10.1056/NEJMcp1111259

67. Sieira J, Brugada P. The definition of the Brugada syndrome. *Eur Heart J*. 2017;38(40):3029-3034. doi:10.1093/eurheartj/ehx490

68. Marsman EMJ, Postema PG, Remme CA. Brugada syndrome: update and future perspectives. *Heart*. 2022;108(9):668-675. doi:10.1136/HEARTJNL-2020-318258

69. de Luna A, Garcia-Niebla J, Baranchuk A. New Electrocardiographic Features in Brugada Syndrome. *Curr Cardiol Rev*. 2014;10(3):175-180. doi:10.2174/1573403x10666140514101546

70. Doshi HH, Giudici MC. The EKG in hypothermia and hyperthermia. *J Electrocardiol*. 2015;48(2):203-209. doi:10.1016/j.jelectrocard.2014.12.001

71. Vassallo SU, Delaney KA, Hoffman RS, Slater W, Goldfrank LR. A prospective evaluation of the electrocardiographic manifestations of hypothermia. *Acad Emerg Med*. 1999;6(11):1121-1126. doi:10.1111/J.1553-2712.1999.TB00114.X

72. Thygesen K, Alpert JS, Jaffe AS, et al. *Fourth Universal Definition of Myocardial Infarction (2018)*.; 2018. doi:10.1016/j.gheart.2018.08.004

73. Durfey N, Lehnhof B, Bergeson A, et al. Severe Hyperkalemia: Can the Electrocardiogram Risk Stratify for Short-term Adverse Events? *Western Journal of Emergency Medicine*. 2017;18(5):963-971. doi:10.5811/westjem.2017.6.33033

74. Mattu A, Brady WJ, Robinson DA. Electrocardiographic manifestations of hyperkalemia. *Am J Emerg Med*. 2000;18(6):721-729. doi:10.1053/AJEM.2000.7344

75. DeFilippis EM, Yeh J. Electrocardiographic changes in a woman with anorexia nervosa. *JAMA Intern Med*. 2018;178(6):849-851. doi:10.1001/jamainternmed.2018.0981

76. Miranda D, Lobo A, Walsh B. New insights into the use of the 12-lead electrocardiogram for diagnosing acute myocardial infarction in the emergency department. *Canadian Journal of Cardiology*. 2018;34:132-145.

77. Akhtar M, Shenasa M, Jazayeri M, Caceres J, Tchou PJ. Wide QRS complex tachycardia. Reappraisal of a common clinical problem. *Ann Intern Med*. 1988;109(11):905-912. doi:10.7326/0003-4819-109-11-905

78. Goldberger AL. Hyperacute T waves revisited. *Am Heart J*. 1982;104(4):888-890. doi:10.1016/0002-8703(82)90038-2

79. Graham GK, Laforet EG. An electrocardiographic and morphologic study of changes following ligation of the left coronary artery in human beings: a report of two cases. *Am Heart J*. 1952;43(1):42-52. doi:10.1016/0002-8703(52)90023-9

80. Meizlish JL, Berger HJ, Plankey M, Errico D, Levy W, Zaret BL. Functional Left Ventricular Aneurysm Formation after Acute Anterior Transmural Myocardial Infarction. *New England Journal of Medicine*. 1984;311(16):1001-1006. doi:10.1056/nejm198410183111601

81. Engel J, Brady WJ, Mattu A, Perron AD. Electrocardiographic ST segment elevation: Left ventricular aneurysm. *American Journal of Emergency Medicine*. 2002;20(3):238-242. doi:10.1053/ajem.2002.32634

82. Mills RM, Young E, Gorlin R, Lesch M. Natural history of S-T segment elevation after acute myocardial infarction. *Am J Cardiol*. 1975;35(5):609-614. doi:10.1016/0002-9149(75)90045-4

83. McAnulty JH, Rahimtoola SH, Murphy E, et al. Natural history of "high-risk" bundle-branch block: final report of a prospective study. *N Engl J Med*. 1982;307(3):137-143. doi:10.1056/NEJM198207153070301

84. Mehta MC, Jain AC, Mehta A. Early repolarization. *Clin Cardiol*. 1999;22(2):59-65. doi:10.1002/CLC.4960220203

85. de Bliek EC. ST elevation: Differential diagnosis and caveats. A comprehensive review to help distinguish ST elevation myocardial infarction from nonischemic etiologies of ST elevation. *Turk J Emerg Med*. 2018;18(1):1-10. doi:10.1016/J.TJEM.2018.01.008

86. Cooper BL, Waller-Delarosa JC. Electrocardiographic Slow Dancing: Who Takes the Lead? *J Emerg Med*. 2022;63(1):106-108. doi:10.1016/J.JEMERMED.2022.04.002

87. Gouaux JL, Ashman R. Auricular fibrillation with aberration simulating ventricular paroxysmal tachycardia. *Am Heart J*. 1947;34(3):366-373. doi:10.1016/0002-8703(47)90487-0

88. Singla V, Singh B, Singh Y, Manjunath CN. Ashman phenomenon: a physiological aberration. *BMJ Case Rep*. 2013;2013. doi:10.1136/BCR-2013-009660

89. Ingram D, Strecker-McGraw MK. Electrical Alternans. *StatPearls*. Published online August 11, 2021. Accessed January 3, 2022. https://www.ncbi.nlm.nih.gov/books/NBK534229/

90. Goyal M, Woods KM, Atwood JE. Electrical alternans: a sign, not a diagnosis. *South Med J*. 2013;106(8):485-489. doi:10.1097/SMJ.0B013E3182A1456C

91. Mulpuru SK, Madhavan M, McLeod CJ, Cha YM, Friedman PA. Cardiac Pacemakers: Function, Troubleshooting, and Management: Part 1 of a 2-Part Series. *J Am Coll Cardiol*. 2017;69(2):189-210. doi:10.1016/j.jacc.2016.10.061

92. Berberian JG, Levine BJ, Brady WJ. *EMRA EKG Guide*. 1st ed. Emergency Medicine Residents' Association; 2017.

93. Benson DW, Cohen MI. Wolff-Parkinson-White syndrome: Lessons learnt and lessons remaining. *Cardiol Young*. 2017;27(S1):S62-S67. doi:10.1017/S1047951116002250

94. Rosenbaum MB, Elizari M V., Lazzari JO, Nau GJ, Levi RJ, Halpern MS. Intraventricular trifascicular blocks. Review of the literature and classification. *Am Heart J.* 1969;78(4):450-459. doi:10.1016/0002-8703(69)90478-5

95. Semsarian C, Ingles J, Maron MS, Maron BJ. New perspectives on the prevalence of hypertrophic cardiomyopathy. *J Am Coll Cardiol.* 2015;65(12):1249-1254. doi:10.1016/J.JACC.2015.01.019

96. Ommen SR, Mital S, Burke MA, et al. 2020 AHA/ACC Guideline for the Diagnosis and Treatment of Patients With Hypertrophic Cardiomyopathy: A Report of the American College of Cardiology/American Heart Association Joint Committee on Clinical Practice Guidelines. *J Am Coll Cardiol.* 2020;76(25):e159-e240. doi:10.1016/J.JACC.2020.08.045

97. Witting MD, Hu KM, Westreich AA, Tewelde S, Farzad A, Mattu A. Evaluation of Spodick's Sign and Other Electrocardiographic Findings as Indicators of STEMI and Pericarditis. *J Emerg Med.* Published online March 2020. doi:10.1016/j.jemermed.2020.01.017

98. Boehnert MT, Lovejoy FH. Value of the QRS duration versus the serum drug level in predicting seizures and ventricular arrhythmias after an acute overdose of tricyclic antidepressants. *New England Journal of Medicine.* 1985;313(8):474-479. doi:10.1056/NEJM198508223130804

99. Kaid KA, Maqsood A, Cohen M, Rothfeld E. Further characterization of the "persistent juvenile T-wave pattern" in adults. *J Electrocardiol.* 2008;41(6):644-645. doi:10.1016/J.JELECTROCARD.2008.08.028

100. Walsh BM, Smith SW. "Persistent Juvenile" T-Wave Pattern May Not Be Persistent: Case Series and Literature Review. *J Emerg Med.* 2015;49(6):e165-e172. doi:10.1016/J.JEMERMED.2015.06.064

101. Kligfield P, Gettes LS, Bailey JJ, et al. Recommendations for the Standardization and Interpretation of the Electrocardiogram. Part I: The Electrocardiogram and Its Technology A Scientific Statement From the American Heart Association Electrocardiography and Arrhythmias Committee, Council on Clinical Cardiology; the American College of Cardiology Foundation; and the Heart Rhythm Society Endorsed by... *J Am Coll Cardiol.* 2007;49(10):1109-1127. doi:10.1016/J.JACC.2007.01.024

102. Long B, Warix JR, Koyfman A. Controversies in Management of Hyperkalemia. *Journal of Emergency Medicine.* 2018;55(2):192-205. doi:10.1016/j.jemermed.2018.04.004

103. de Winter RJ, Verouden NJW, Wellens HJJ, Wilde AAM. A New ECG Sign of Proximal LAD Occlusion. *New England Journal of Medicine.* 2008;359(19):2071-2073. doi:10.1056/NEJMc0804737

104. Verouden NJ, Koch KT, Peters RJ, et al. Persistent precordial “hyperacute” T-waves signify proximal left anterior descending artery occlusion. *Heart*. 2009;95(20):1701-1706. doi:10.1136/HRT.2009.174557

105. Littmann L. South African flag sign: a teaching tool for easier ECG recognition of high lateral infarct. *Am J Emerg Med*. 2016;34(1):107-109. doi:10.1016/J.AJEM.2015.10.022

106. Gheorghiade M, Adams KF, Colucci WS. Digoxin in the management of cardiovascular disorders. *Circulation*. 2004;109(24):2959-2964. doi:10.1161/01.CIR.0000132482.95686.87

107. Ehle M, Patel C, Giugliano RP. Digoxin: clinical highlights: a review of digoxin and its use in contemporary medicine. *Crit Pathw Cardiol*. 2011;10(2):93-98. doi:10.1097/HPC.0B013E318221E7DD

108. Burch GE, Meyes R, Abildskov JA. A new electrocardiographic pattern observed in cerebrovascular accidents. *Circulation*. 1954;9(5):719-723. doi:10.1161/01.CIR.9.5.719

109. Stone J, Mor-Avi V, Ardelt A, Lang RM. Frequency of Inverted Electrocardiographic T Waves (Cerebral T Waves) in Patients With Acute Strokes and Their Relation to Left Ventricular Wall Motion Abnormalities. *American Journal of Cardiology*. 2018;121(1):120-124. doi:10.1016/j.amjcard.2017.09.025

110. Nijjer S, Ghosh AK, Dubrey SW. Hypocalcaemia, long QT interval and atrial arrhythmias. *BMJ Case Rep*. 2010;2010:bcr0820092216. doi:10.1136/bcr.08.2009.2216

111. Bradley TJ, Metzger DL, Sanatani S. Long on QT and low on calcium. *Cardiol Young*. 2004;14(6):667-670. doi:10.1017/S1047951104006134

112. SH O, BS QR, AN M. First-Degree Heart Block. *StatPearls*. Published online 2023. Accessed October 22, 2023. https://pubmed.ncbi.nlm.nih.gov/28846254/

113. Kastor JA. Multifocal atrial tachycardia. *N Engl J Med*. 1990;322(24):1713-1717. doi:10.1056/NEJM199006143222405

114. Steinman RT, Herrera C, Schuger CD, Lehmann MH. Wide QRS Tachycardia in the Conscious Adult: Ventricular Tachycardia Is the Most Frequent Cause. *JAMA*. 1989;261(7):1013-1016. doi:10.1001/JAMA.1989.03420070063031

115. Devereux RB, Reichek N. Repolarization abnormalities of left ventricular hypertrophy. Clinical, echocardiographic and hemodynamic correlates. *J Electrocardiol*. 1982;15(1):47-53. doi:10.1016/S0022-0736(82)80044-7

116. Abu-haniyeh A, Hajouli S. *Pacemaker Mediated Tachycardia*. StatPearls Publishing; 2020.

117. Batehnb J, Gunderson T, Forfang K. Tachycardias Related to Atrial Synchronous Ventricular Pacing. *Pacing and Clinical Electrophysiology*. 1982;5(4):471-475. doi:10.1111/j.1540-8159.1982.tb02263.x

118. Den Dulk K, Lindemans FW, Bar FW, Wellens HJJ. Pacemaker Related Tachycardias. *Pacing and Clinical Electrophysiology*. 1982;5(4):476-485. doi:10.1111/j.1540-8159.1982.tb02264.x

119. Antzelevitch C, Yan GX, Ackerman MJ, et al. J-Wave syndromes expert consensus conference report: Emerging concepts and gaps in knowledge. *Europace*. 2017;19(4):665-694. doi:10.1093/EUROPACE/EUW235

120. Spodick DH. Electrocardiogram in acute pericarditis. Distributions of morphologic and axial changes by stages. *Am J Cardiol*. 1974;33(4):470-474. doi:10.1016/0002-9149(74)90603-1

121. Spodick DH. Diagnostic electrocardiographic sequences in acute pericarditis. Significance of PR segment and PR vector changes. *Circulation*. 1973;48(3):575-580. doi:10.1161/01.CIR.48.3.575

122. Ginzton LE, Laks MM. The differential diagnosis of acute pericarditis from the normal variant: New electrocardiographic criteria. *Circulation*. 1982;65(5):1004-1009. doi:10.1161/01.CIR.65.5.1004

123. Aslanger E, Yıldırımtürk Ö, Şimşek B, et al. A new electrocardiographic pattern indicating inferior myocardial infarction. *J Electrocardiol*. 2020;61:41-46. doi:10.1016/J.JELECTROCARD.2020.04.008

124. Marti G, Schwarz C, Leichtle AB, et al. Etiology and symptoms of severe hypokalemia in emergency department patients. *European Journal of Emergency Medicine*. 2014;21(1):46-51. doi:10.1097/MEJ.0b013e3283643801

125. Hoang H, Giordano JA, Cooper BL. Woman with ST Changes Following Days of Vomiting. *Ann Emerg Med*. 2021;77(4):442-444. doi:10.1016/j.annemergmed.2020.08.034

126. Nattel S, Keable H, Sasyniuk BI. Experimental amitriptyline intoxication: electrophysiologic manifestations and management. *J Cardiovasc Pharmacol*. 1984;6(1):83-89.

127. Niemann JT, Bessen HA, Rothstein RJ, Laks MM. Electrocardiographic criteria for tricyclic antidepressant cardiotoxicity. *Am J Cardiol*. 1986;57(13):1154-1159. doi:10.1016/0002-9149(86)90691-0

128. Zema MJ, Kligfield P. ECG Poor R-Wave Progression: Review and Synthesis. *Arch Intern Med*. 1982;142(6):1145-1148. doi:10.1001/ARCHINTE.1982.00340190101018

129. Brady WJ. *Benign Early Repolarization: Electrocardiographic Manifestations and Differentiation from Other ST Segment Elevation Syndromes*. Vol 16. W.B. Saunders; 1998:592-597. doi:10.1016/S0735-6757(98)90226-1

130. Armstrong EJ, Kulkarni AR, Bhave PD, et al. Electrocardiographic criteria for ST-elevation myocardial infarction in patients with left ventricular hypertrophy. *American Journal of Cardiology*. 2012;110(7):977-983. doi:10.1016/j.amjcard.2012.05.032

131. Klein LR, Shroff GR, Beeman W, Smith SW. Electrocardiographic criteria to differentiate acute anterior ST-elevation myocardial infarction from left ventricular aneurysm. *American Journal of Emergency Medicine*. 2015;33(6):786-790. doi:10.1016/j.ajem.2015.03.044

132. Cooper BL, Fisher KM, Chathampally Y. Man With Left-Sided Chest Pain. *Ann Emerg Med*. 2018;72(5):558-561. doi:10.1016/j.annemergmed.2017.09.006

133. Imazio M, Squarotti GB, Andreis A, et al. Diagnostic and prognostic role of the electrocardiogram in patients with pericarditis. *Heart*. 2022;108(18):1474-1478. doi:10.1136/HEARTJNL-2021-320443

134. Waldo SW, Brenner DA, Li S, Alexander K, Ganz P. Reperfusion times and in-hospital outcomes among patients with an isolated posterior myocardial infarction: Insights from the National Cardiovascular Data Registry (NCDR). *Am Heart J*. 2014;167(3):350-354. doi:10.1016/j.ahj.2013.11.011

Index

Made in United States
Orlando, FL
04 November 2026

90200395R00121